15.95

Endorsements

"*Sunfood Traveler* is a comprehensive guide to the why's and how's of changing your diet for the better. Beautifully written and practical, it lays out exactly what you need to know, and may even save your life."

– **Neal D. Barnard**, MD; President, Physicians Committee for Responsible Medicine

"Filled with great information."

– **Cherie Soria**, Chief co-author *Raw Food Revolution Diet*; Founder and Director Living Light Culinary Institute. RawFoodChef.com

"There are endless books on the market but *Sunfood Traveler* by John McCabe is a must-have. Not only is it a valuable guide to raw resources around the globe, it is packed with impressive information and inspiration. A real gem. I love all of John McCabe's books, and I highly recommend them."

– **Natasha Kyssa**, author of *SimplyRaw Living Foods Detox Manual*; SimplyRaw.ca

"*Sunfood Traveler* is an excellent resource to carry with you whenever you are traveling. I highly recommend this book!"

– **Jesse Jacoby**, The Raw Cure

"Packed with educational information and of course, where to find everything raw. It is the most comprehensive guide to raw living available."

– **Anand Wells**, of Australia's LiveFoodEducation.com

"I have been involved with the raw food movement for over 12 years and I've seen and heard a lot of things. My experiences with raw foods have been amazing over the years, and just keep getting better. I am thankful for John McCabe and his extraordinary work. He has gone above and beyond in his research, some of the best I've seen actually - especially since there are so many books on the subject. John is a great writer who passionately exposes truths. He is a breath of fresh air!"

– **Angela Elliott**, Author of *Alive in Five*; she-zencuisine.com

"I think *Sunfood Traveler* is a great book. Best raw food/ecological book ever written."

– **Harley "DurianRider" Johnstone**, co-founder of 30BananasADay.com

"*Sunfood Traveler* and all the others written by John McCabe should be a staple on everyone's shelf – if you don't have it yet, now is a great time to buy it as a gift for yourself or for someone else."

– **Cindy Williams**, Tucson Natural Awakenings Magazine

"Thank you for creating such a resource."

– **Karin Dina** of Living Light Culinary Instutute

"I am absolutely loving it. I don't think I'll ever visit another city without it… I have a feeling I'll have quite a few new goals on how to live more sustainably after reading more of this book."

– **Lenette Nakauchi** of Chicago's GoRawHaveFun.com

"John McCabe's books are the best source of information for health and nutrition."

– **Masood Ali Khan**, MasoodAliKhan.com

"With such a vast knowledge of raw vegan food, John McCabe has a voice to be heard. No one I have met in the raw food movement has written books like John has. Modest as he is, as a ghost-writer he is even responsible for the content of some of the most well-known raw food books by other authors. I am so grateful for John as such an amazing being and source of information."

– **Brian James Lucas** aka Chef BeLive, ChefBeLive.com

"*Sunfood Traveler* is the most used book of all my raw food books. Amazing how much info you share in this book. When I saw the title, I almost didn't purchase it because I thought it would be only for someone who travels a lot. It is so much more."

– **Eileen Allen**, Half Moon Bay, California

"I have read this book and it is fantastic."

– **Ronnie Skurow**, UBRaw.com

SUNFOOD TRAVELER

GLOBAL GUIDE TO RAW FOOD CULTURE

BY JOHN McCABE

AUTHOR OF

SUNFOOD DIET INFUSION
Transforming Health
And Preventing Disease Through Raw Veganism

IGNITING YOUR LIFE
Pathways to the Zenith of Health and Success

MARIJUANA & HEMP
History, Laws, Uses, and Controversy

EXTINCTION
The Death of Waterlife on Planet Earth

SURGERY ELECTIVES:
What to Know Before the Doctor Operates

Carmania Books
FOOD • BODY • MIND • SPIRIT • WILDLIFE • AIR • WATER • SOIL • WORLD

Sunfood Traveler, by John McCabe **$15.95 US**

Disclaimer: This book is sold for information purposes only. How you interpret and utilize the information in this book is your decision. Neither the author nor the publisher and/or distributor will be held accountable for the use or misuse of the information contained in this book. This book is not intended as medical advice because the author and publisher of this work are not recommending the use of chemical drugs or surgery to alleviate health challenges. It also does not stand as legal advice, or suggest that you break any laws. Because of the way people interpret what they read, and take actions based on their intellect and life situations, which are not in the author's, publisher's, and/or distributor's control, there is always some risk involved; therefore, the author, publisher, and/or distributor of this book are not responsible for any adverse effects or consequences from the use of any suggestions, foods, substances, products, services, procedures, or lifestyles described hereafter.

ISBN: 978-1-884702-09-9
Library of Congress Control Number: 2010920340
Dewey CIP: 641.563. **OCLC:** 213839254
Edition: First edition: Jan. 2010; Revised 2011, 2012
Cover photo: California sunset, John McCabe
Cover graphis: Steve Minard, minardsteve@yahoo.com

Copyright © 2010, 2011, 2012 by John McCabe
All intellectual rights owned by John McCabe and reserved in perpetuity throughout the universe. No part of the author's words in this book may be reproduced in any form or by any electronic, mechanical, or other means, including on the Internet, through cell phone and/or personal, educational, public, and/or business communication and technology systems, or through any and all information storage and retrieval systems, including book sample and publicity Web sites, without permission in writing from the author, and only the author, except by a reviewer, who may quote brief, attributed passages of the final published book in a review; and as fair use by authors wishing to use short, credited quotations of the author's words.

Carmania Books POB 1272, Santa Monica, CA 90406-1272, USA
Wholesale: Nelson's Books, NelsonsBooks.com, 800-877-1267; and Ingram
Retail: Amazon.com, BarnesAndNoble.com, natural food stores, bookstores, raw restaurants.

Books by John McCabe

Sunfood Diet Infusion: Transforming Health Through Raw Veganism
Igniting Your Life: Pathways to the Zenith of Health and Success
Sunfood Traveler: Guide to Raw Food Culture
Marijuana & Hemp: History, Uses, Laws, and Controversy
Sunfood Living: Resource Guide for Global Health
Extinction: The Death of Waterlife on Planet Earth
Surgery Electives: What to Know Before the Doctor Operates

TABLE OF CONTENTS

“How often I found where I should be going only by setting out for somewhere else.”
– R. Buckminster Fuller

“If there is to be an ecologically sound society, it will have to come the grass roots up, not from the top down.”
– Paul Hawken

THE HUMAN BODY

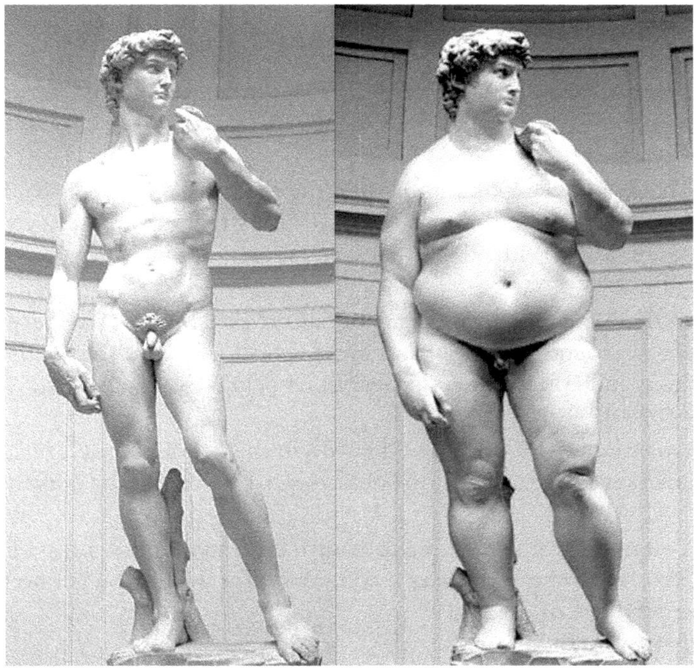

The human body is an amazing mechanism that responds to what the person thinks, eats, says, and does. The physical appearance of the body reflects what is going on with the person. This is often most evident in the shape of the body. Because of this, it can be very easy to tell certain things about how a person lives simply by observing their body shape.

Because of low-quality dietary choices and lack of movement, more and more people are suffering from obesity, heart disease, diabetes, arthritis, kidney disease, cancers, back strains, knee injuries, hernias, learning disorders, and a slew of other problems.

You are making a choice with the quality of foods you consume and the physical activities you do or don't engage in.

A person who remains physically active while following a diet consisting chiefly of raw fruits and vegetables is more likely to resemble the person on the left. A person lacking physical activity while following the modern junk diet is more likely to resemble the body on the right.

Which diet would you rather follow?

For more on food and health, read my other book, *Sunfood Diet Infusion: Transforming Health Through Raw Veganism.*

"In today's environment, hoarding knowledge ultimately erodes your power. If you know something very important, the way to get power is by actually sharing it."
– Joseph Badaracco

"The boundary between ourselves and other people and between ourselves and nature, is illusion. Oneness is reality."
– Charlene Spretnak

"The deeper we look into nature, the more we recognize that it is full of life, and the more profoundly we know that all life is a secret and that we are united with all life that is in nature."
– Albert Schweitzer

"In the Native way we are encouraged to recognize that every moment is a sacred moment, and every action, when imbued with dedication and commitment to benefit all beings, is a sacred act."
– Dhyani Ywahoo

"Our true wealth is the good we do in this world. None of us has faith unless we desire for our neighbors what we desire for ourselves."
– Muhammad

"You must give some time to your fellow men. Even if it's a little thing, do something for others – something for which you get no pay but the privilege of doing it."
– Albert Schweitzer

"It is one thing just to use the earth: it is quite another thing to receive the blessing of the earth and to become at home in the law of this reception, in order to shepherd the mystery of being and to pay attention to the inviolability of the possible."
– Martin Heidegger

"There is a way that nature speaks, that land speaks. Most of the time we are simply not patient enough, quiet enough, to pay attention to the story."
– Linda Hogan

"We are earth people on a spiritual journey to the stars. Our quest, our earth walk, is to look within, to know who we are, to see that we are connected to all things."
– Lakota Seer

"The universe is the primary revelation of the divine, the primary scripture, the primary focus of divine-human communion."
– Thomas Berry

"Something will have gone out of us as a people if we ever let the remaining wilderness be destroyed."
– Wallace Stegner

• INTRODUCTION

> "We shall require a substantially new manner of thinking if mankind is to survive."
>
> – Albert Einstein

WELCOME to *Sunfood Traveler.* This book contains the most complete listing of raw food restaurants and businesses. It is also a compilation of material I have gathered while working on various books and researching ways people can live more sustainabley.

If anything, the book is a reference book for Earth-friendly living – especially through food. It isn't meant to provide the complete picture of the raw food world, or of sustainable living, but is meant to present basic information and reference material for people to find out more – such as by reading other books, watching documentaries, and doing personal research into the various topics associated with raw food nutrition and the full spectrum of healthful living.

While the book is a guide to raw food culture, it also includes information commonly of interest to people who are into following a plant-based diet. These very same people are often aware, or are becoming aware, of issues relating to sustainable living, organic foods, home gardening, composting, natural products, protecting wildlife, and restoring and preserving wildlands, rivers, lakes, and other natural features of Earth.

> "I think the environment should be put in the category of our national security. Defense of our resources is just as important as defense abroad. Otherwise what is there to defend?"
>
> – Robert Redford, Yosemite National Park dedication, 1985

When people hear about sustainable living, many still do not know what the term means. To me, it largely means following a plant-based diet, because a plant-based diet is the least environmentally invasive diet, and following one can be the most important thing a person can do to both reduce their carbon footprint, including by using fewer fossil fuels, and improve the condition of the environment.

> "Beauty and vitality are gifts from nature for those who live by her laws."
>
> – Leonardo da Vinci

As many scientific studies have concluded, it is clear that a plant-based diet improves health, and is key to reducing the chances of experiencing degenerative diseases, including obesity, diabetes, arthritis, osteoporosis, macular degeneration, Alzheimer's, kidney disease, liver disorders, cardiovascular disease, and cancers of the breasts, colon, prostate, and reproductive organs, and also strokes, and heart attacks.

To me, sustainable living not only includes following a plant-based diet, it means growing some of your own food, and localizing most or all of your other food choices, such as by shopping at farmers' markets and natural food co-ops, and perhaps bartering with or helping friends or neighbors who have abundant gardens. It means learning about the local wild edible plants, nurturing them, and including some of these in your diet. In other areas of your life, sustainable living means reducing the use of fossil fuels, including petroleum plastics, soaps, waxes, and the chemicals derived from petroleum, coal, and natural gas.

To many people, sustainable living means transitioning human culture to live closer to nature, to use natural products, to reduce use, to reuse, to recycle, to compost, to look at daily choices, and to factor better choices that not only do less harm to the planet, but that also nurture the local land back to health.

Many people are constantly blaming others for the state of the planet and the conditions of their local environment. How much better could their environment be if they would stop placing blame, consider how they could change, become more involved in changing things, and take steps to live more sustainbly?

> "The world is a dangerous place to live; not because of the people who are evil, but because of the people who don't do anything about it."
>
> – Albert Einstein

Sustainable living means so many things that it can involve everything we think, do, purchase, and use. Transitioning to a more sustainable lifestyle can mean changing everything about our lives – from the food we eat to the soaps and clothing we use, to the types of entertainment and exercise we enjoy, to what we consider purchasing, and what we do with our kitchen scraps and used goods.

> "The care of the Earth is our most ancient and most worthy, and after all our most pleasing responsibility. To cherish what remains of the Earth and to foster its renewal is our only legitimate hope of survival."
>
> – Wendell Berry

Since I was a small boy and spent a lot of time in the woods and natural surroundings I have been aware of the harm humanity has been doing to Earth, which also harms wildlife – and humans. When I saw snow turn black from pollution, saw rivers and shorelines cluttered with trash, saw factory smoke stacks spewing pollution into the air, saw forests cut down to clear land for urban sprawl, and saw landfills packed with disposable products, I knew that something had to be done. And now the observations continue, with the world watching as more petroleum disasters take place, mountaintops are being removed to get to coal, Canadian forests are being decimated to get to tar sand, land is being violated by natural gas fracking, wetlands and rainforests are being obliterated for the spread of the monocropping and cattle industries, plastic pollution is spreading throughout the oceans and land, ice caps are melting, and species are being threatened, becoming endangered, or extinct.

I am glad that a growing number of people are becoming involved with improving the conditions of wildlife, forests, streams, rivers, lakes, oceans, and the air and environment. Having a whole lot more people involved would be much better – and that is what is needed ASAP.

> "Great things are done by a series of small things brought together."
>
> – Vincent Van Gogh

While I am far from a perfect example of what one could do to live a green life, I continue to make changes and adjustments in my daily life that bring me closer to sustainable living, including by maintaining an organic garden, by composting my food scraps, by purchasing second hand (or by avoiding the treadmill of working to gain money to purchase things), by often using a bike to get around, and by eating a more localized diet (My diet has been vegan for 20 years).

Putting this book together so others may learn and live closer to nature is one of my ways of creating the change I wish to see.

Thank you for using it.

If you know of any additions you feel should be included in future editions, please email them to information@sunfoodliving.com, or snail them to:

John McCabe
C/O Carmania Books
POB 1272
Santa Monica, CA 90406-1272, USA

Please, plant some trees.
Peace your path.

John

> "There isn't a problem in this world that cannot be solved. The hard part is convincing people that we are all part of the solution – that each of us has something to give which cannot otherwise be given."
>
> – Jon Kabat-Zinn

"There is an entire history behind the relationship of man towards nature. Our indigenous ancestors like the Incas, Aucas, and other native tribes used to acknowledge the power and crucial relationship between nature and man. Therefore, they respected, cherished and took care of Mother Nature. Man lives because nature is the mother who takes care of her children. Man feels that he is the dictator when in fact he would die if the mother ceased to exist."
– Alex Leonidas Pusternak

"The relationship you have with the world is the same as the relationship you have with yourself."
– Dorothy Rowe

"In the long term, the economy and the environment are the same thing. If it's unenvironmental it is uneconomical. That is the rule of nature."
– Mollie Beattie

"Every morning I awaken torn between the desire to save the world and the inclination to savor it."
– E.B. White

"Man is at his highest when nature is his teacher."
– Mervyn Brady

"The have-nots can be out of sight and even out of mind, but they breathe the same air, drink from the same scant supply of fresh water, and birth children who will grow up to work with our children to finish the job we've barely started; they will have to find a way for all of us to live well within the Earth's means."
– Vicki Robin

"If we sell you the land, you must remember that it is sacred, and you must teach your children that it is sacred and that each ghostly reflection in the clear water of the lakes tells of events and memories in the life of my people. The water's murmur is the voice of my father's father."
– Chief Seattle

"In the hopes of reaching the moon men fail to see the flowers that blossom at their feet."
– Albert Schweitzer

"Every flower is a soul blossoming in nature."
– Gerard De Nerval

"Human subtlety will never devise an invention more beautiful, more simple or more direct than does nature, because in her inventions, nothing is lacking and nothing is superfluous."
– Leonardo da Vinci

• The Restoration of Nature

> "Good health is about being able to fully enjoy the time we do have. It is about being as functional as possible throughout our entire lives and avoiding crippling, painful, and lengthy battles with disease. The enjoyment of life is greatly compromised if we cannot see, if we cannot think, if our kidneys do not work, and if our bones are fragile or broken."
>
> – T. Colin Campbell, author of *The China Study;* TColinCampbell.org

THE biology of the human naturally works to be in sync with that which is most healthful. It is also the design of your cells to be in tune with nature. Evidence of this is displayed by how the forces within each cell work toward cleaning out that which does not belong, bringing in that which is healthful, and building cellular structures in a fixed pattern.

The intricate activities taking place inside and among your cells are part of a system continually striving to create what is best with what is provided. The level of your health is in direct correlation with what you are supplying to your system. If you desire to experience vibrant health, it is up to you to provide the quality materials necessary for creating that level of health.

The sunfood diet is in tune with nature. It transforms health by supplying your ever-restorative cellular structures with the nutrients necessary to form healthy tissue, using the substances your body should have been ingesting all along: raw edible plants.

A sunfood diet also allows for the transfer of the subtle and powerful resonating energy of living plants into your system. Your cells will then function with vibrancy in tune with the energy of nature. This will trigger your system to release damaging residues left over from low-quality foods. As your cells become cleaner, the energy previously spent dealing with the junk you were eating finally becomes an energy used to generate health. The tissues of your brain, including the pineal gland, begin to function at a higher level. Your thinking becomes clearer and your intuition awakens. You have a stronger desire to use your talents and intellect to succeed, and to experience satisfaction.

A diet relying purely on plants benefits the planet in many different ways. Most significantly, it eliminates the dependence on the wasteful meat, dairy, egg, processed, and corporate food industries. Instead, the sunfood diet consists of edible plant substances, requiring more fruiting trees and culinary plants to be grown. More plants clean the air, provide oxygen, filter water, create homes for wildlife, and manifest a more healthful environment for all forms of life on the planet. Additionally, with fewer people consuming meat, land previously used to raise farm animals – and used to grow tremendous amounts of food for those animals – is turned over to the wilds of nature.

In addition to healthful food choices, the sunfood diet advocates daily exercise, intentional living, intellectual stimulation, nurturing relationships, a sustainable lifestyle, the protection of wildlife, and the restoration of nature.

On a sunfood diet your power will awaken from a dormant state induced by unhealthful foods, low-quality life choices, and slothful thinking patterns. Your perceptions will enlighten. What you are capable of accomplishing will become clear to you as you transform into a happier, more healthful and satisfied being in tune with your instinct, intellect, talent, and essence.

The sunfood diet provides for the restoration of your inner nature, which benefits outer nature.

Begin it now.

> "A younger generation is growing up with greater awareness of the need for a mutually enhancing mode of human presence to the Earth. We see quite clearly that what happens to the nonhuman happens to the human. What happens to the outer world happens to the inner world. If the outer world is diminished in its grandeur, then the emotional, imaginative, intellectual, and spiritual life of the human is diminished or extinguished. Without the soaring birds, the great forests, the sounds and coloration of the insects, the free-flowing streams, the flowing fields, the sight of the clouds by day and the stars by night, we become impoverished in all that makes us human."
>
> – Thomas Berry

• Colors in Plants

> "Beauty and vitality are gifts from nature, for those who live by her laws."
>
> – Leonardo da Vinci

I like to visit and support animal sanctuaries where animals that were once sickly from being caged or mistreated are able to live in natural surroundings and reclaim their health by eating a natural diet. Many of the animals that I have visited on these sanctuaries were once on the brink of death and have truly been transformed into healthy beings with a zest for life.

Just as the animals that have been rescued from the horrible living and diet conditions of factory farms can become healthier through improved nutrition and more healthful surroundings, the human body that has been mistreated and/or neglected can also regain much of its luster and vigor. This is obvious in those who have gone from obesity to a healthy weight simply by changing their food choices, increasing their physical activity, improving their atmosphere, and restructuring their thought processes to become more positive and successful.

> "That which we persist in doing becomes easier for us to do; not that the nature of the thing itself is changed, but that our power to do is increased."
>
> – Ralph Waldo Emerson

The body works to generate health. The microscopic activities deep in the cells work toward health in the best way possible using whatever nutrients provided.

> "Food is that material which can be incorporated into and become a part of the cells and fluids of the body. Non-useful materials, such as chemical additives and drugs, are all poisons. To be a true food, the substance must not contain useless or harmful ingredients."
>
> – Dr. Herbert Shelton, author of *Food Combining Made Easy*

Health comes from within. To assist this activity, it is wise to supply the body with the best form of nutrients available. Doing less than that is limiting the ability of the body to produce vibrant health.

> "Bring the power of plants into your body. There's nothing like freshly made juices to nurture your 100 trillion cells."
>
> – Jay Kordich, the juiceman

According to the U.S. Centers for Disease Control and Prevention, in 2009 only 26.3% of Americans were eating vegetables three or more times per day, and only 32.5% of Americans were eating fruit two or more times per day. Through its Healthy People 2010 program, the CDC set a goal of getting 50% of people aged two and older to consume three or more servings of vegetables per day, and 75% of people aged two and over to consume two or more servings of fruit per day. While increasing the consumption of fruits and vegetables is a good thing, for the best of health, the goals set by the CDC didn't go far enough.

> "A diet high in fruits and vegetables can reduce the risk for many leading causes of death."
>
> – U.S. Centers for Disease Control and Prevention, 2010

Raw plant substances are what the body needs if a person desires to experience the best health.

Consider the colors on fruits and vegetables that capture our attention when selecting them. Would you consider the unadulterated, vibrant botanical colors to be nutrients? There is more than meets the eyes to the colors within the plants that we eat.

The spectrum of botanical pigments existing inside plant cells contain molecules that absorb specific wavelengths of sunlight energy. In turn the cells of the plant store and carry different levels of vibrational energy fields, including tiny specs of light called biophotons. These frequencies contained in the unheated substances of plants have a function when a person consumes them. There are photoreceptor proteins in the brain that are similar to those in the eyes, and they also exist throughout the body. The biophotons that exist within all living cells are part of the cellular communication system. Some people refer to biophotons as our *life force energy*. As you may expect, those following a diet largely consisting of a variety of raw plant matter have been found to contain richer banks of biophotons in their body tissues than those following a diet that is cooked and otherwise highly processed.

> "Nothing will benefit human health or increase the chances for survival of life on earth as the evolution to a vegetarian diet."
> – Albert Einstein

A diet rich in raw plant matter is also rich in antioxidants.

Your body wants and desires to be around certain colors of nature. You automatically are attracted to the piece of fruit that has reached its peak level of ripeness, be it the radiant peach, the passionately red strawberry, the gleaming plumpness of melon, the practically glowing colors of fresh bananas, tomatoes, cherries, grapes, persimmons, citrus, and apples, or the richness of green vegetables. Once fruits and vegetables have passed their prime and their colors have begun to fade, they don't elicit the same response from us.

The pigments synthesized within plants often work as defense mechanisms for the plants much in the same way the immune system of the human body works to protect health. The plant chemicals have been described as "plant antibiotics." They work to protect plants from the elements, such as fungi, bacteria, tissue damage, extreme temperatures, and ultraviolet light. It is understood that there is some interaction between the plant and a pathogen that will trigger the manufacture of certain chemicals within the plant to defend it against the pathogen. Plants will also manufacture certain chemicals when the plant is exposed to certain stresses, such as wind, temperatures, moisture, and dryness.

Plants that are not provided with sufficient nutrients and conditions through soil, light, water, and temperature become weak and do not produce the chemicals they need to protect themselves from pathogens and environmental stresses.

Amazingly, when humans consume plants, the very same natural chemicals that protect the plants have been found to protect human health. They lower cholesterol, prevent heart disease, regulate blood sugar, and function as antioxidants. A diet rich in raw plant matter is also rich in antioxidants.

Similar to plants, a human body that is not provided with the right combination of nutrients and atmosphere will also fail to defend itself from pathogens and stresses.

There are thousands of plant chemicals that benefit human health. Probably the most commonly known beneficial plant color is the beta-carotene that is found in apricots, cantaloupe, carrots, peaches, pumpkin, and spinach. There is also alpha-carotene that is found in carrots, red and yellow peppers, and in pumpkins. Lutein, a carotenoid that is found in avocado, corn, kale, and spinach, has been found to prevent cataracts. Zeaxanthin is a carotenoid that helps give color to corn and saffron, and has been found to protect vision. Then there is lycopene in pink grapefruit, guava, tomatoes, and watermelon, and many other plant colors. These are only a few of over 600 identified plant chemicals that give plants their colors. Many more are being identified and studied. But, because there are at least thousands in each plant, the identifying and study process can go on for many, many years. With each new discovery comes research that looks into the health benefits of the phytochemical, how the chemical works with others, and how the enzymatic systems of the human organs metabolize them.

By the process of photosynthesis, antioxidants form in plants, not in animals. To experience the best of health, we need to consume a diet rich in antioxidants, and there are more of them in raw plant matter than in heated plant matter. As mentioned in the previous chapter, there are only slight amounts of antioxidants in meat, milk, and eggs, and they are only there because the animal consumed plants. What meat, milk, and eggs do contain much more abundantly are free radicals, and you don't want be putting foods rich in free radicals in your body, especially when they are accompanied by the saturated fat and cholesterol found in meat, milk, and eggs.

While all areas of the body are reliant on antioxidants, one area that relies on antioxidants in a very specific way is the macula of the eyes. The continual chemical changes in and around the macula are what brings us site. It is in the macula that light waves are turned into energy recognized by our nerves. The light waves also continually react with the fatty acids of the macula, which is a process that creates low levels of free radicals. To counteract this free radical activity, we need antioxidants, which we obtain from eating fresh plant matter. Raw fruits and vegetables like mangoes, apricots, melon, citrus fruits, berries, red and yellow peppers, carrots, broccoli, broccoli leaves, squash, spinach, and collard greens contain the carotenoids that are particularly beneficial to eye function. Green leafy vegetables contain an antioxidant called lutein, which is specifically beneficial to the lenses of the eyes. As mentioned earlier, lutein helps to prevent cataracts – another condition associated with long term diets lacking in antioxidants. Raw edible plant matter also happens to contain the essential fatty acids we need to obtain from food, and some of these fatty acids are utilized by the macula and the nerves servicing the eyes. These are more reasons why it is good to consume raw fruits and raw vegetables, sprouts and germinates, and raw seaweeds, as they all contain essential fatty acids. Those who consume a diet rich in raw fruits and vegetables have been found to experience better vision later in life.

Animal protein, including eggs, dairy, and meat of all varieties, contain free radicals, saturated fats, and foreign cholesterol, all of which are not good for the eyes. Meat, dairy, and eggs also lack antioxidants, making them a quadruple threat to long-term eye health. The condition labeled "age-related blindness" is largely the degeneration of the macula, is the leading cause of blindness, and you do not need to experience it. Kick out meat, dairy, and eggs, and foods that contain them, from your diet, and follow a diet rich in raw fruits, vegetables, sprouts, and germinates, and you are more likely to avoid macular degeneration and cataracts.

While some people believe they are protecting their vision by taking vitamins specifically identified as being beneficial to sight, such as vitamins C and E, they would be much better off consuming raw fruits and vegetables that naturally contain the vitamins, essential fatty acids, amino acids, antioxidants, and likely an unknown number of substances beneficial to eye health, brain health, heart health, muscle and bone health, skin health, and whole body health. Pills containing one vitamin and not the whole host of substances it would be accompanied with in edible plant matter may not provide the benefits the marketing material may claim. In other words, for true nutrition, eat raw fruits and vegetables.

One plant chemical that has received a lot of attention as an antioxidant is one given the tongue-twisting name pterostilbene (pronounced tero-still-bean). This chemical is present in colorful fruits like blueberries. It is sensitive to light and air, which means it is more present in fruits that have not been processed or heated.

Another plant chemical that is rightly touted as a health-enhancer is resveratrol. This chemical is present in the skin of grapes, cranberries, and in some berries. It has been shown to improve liver and neuron tissue health, and may contribute to a longer life among those who consume an abundance of plants that contain it.

Resveratrol survives the winemaking process, and is present in red wine, which is a raw food. (If you purchase wine, make sure it is organic and that the company does not use any animal by-products in their processing. Some wines will indicate on the label that they are "vegan." If you have any problems with alcohol, please stay away from it.)

Each edible plant consists of a different variety of healthful, natural chemicals that work as nutrients when consumed by humans. To gain the benefits of these chemicals, eat a variety of unheated, raw, organically grown vegetables, fruits, nuts, seeds, sea vegetables, and edible flowers. Allow your diet to consist of a kaleidoscope of colors. The biological functions the colors play within the plants will also play a part in maintaining your health.

Many nutrients are transported into the system by way of dietary fats. Carotenoids are fat-soluble. With a belief that including oil in the diet helps to assimilate nutrients, many raw foodists add olive oil, hemp oil, grapeseed oil, flax oil, or coconut oil to their foods. However, oil is present in all plant substances because each cell naturally contains some oil. You may notice that when you squeeze lemon into water, there will be natural oil from the lemon floating on top of the water. It is true that the oils in olives, avocado, nuts, and all plant substances work to help the body absorb the nutrients of the foods accompanying those plant substances. But, there is no need to be concerned with getting enough oil, because all of the raw plant substances you eat naturally contain some oil. Even lettuce contains oils within its cells. Raw seeds, such as hemp, flax, and sesame seeds are oil-rich and can be ground first in a coffee grinder to increase the availability of the nutrients.

We know that humans respond both emotionally and physically to colors. Being around certain colors can trigger emotional responses, such as alarm or calm that illicit changes among the molecules within body tissues. The molecules within living plants carry specific color ratios and these are resonations of energy. There is an interaction going on between the frequencies of the molecules within the plants and the molecules within your body.

The energy frequency of the foods you eat is reflected in your body tissues, from your skin to your bones. It becomes obvious who is eating a deadening diet consisting of hightly cooked matter and heated oils and meats and little to no fresh plant matter as much as it is obvious who is eating an abundantly nutritious diet that is rich in fresh, raw, edible plant matter.

When you cook plants, the colors throughout the plant tissues change, the order of the molecules changes, and the energy fields fade. When you are putting deadened plants inside a body that relies on living plants to bring in nutrients, you are not getting the full benefit of the plants.

In other words, plants collect substances from the soil, air, atmosphere, and light and turn these into their structures, which nourish us when we eat them – especially if we eat them when they are unheated and fresh. The raw plant matter carries a resonating energy that is in tune with the quality of nourishment they received as they grew.

> "The answer to the American health crisis is the food that each of us chooses to put in our mouths each day. It's as simple as that."
> – T. Colin Campbell, author of *The China Study;* TColinCampbell.org

To experience vibrant health, partake of foods containing their full spectrum of colors and living frequencies of energy. Eat vibrant, radiant, raw, living, edible plant matter that has been organically grown in healthy soil.

> "There is more to us than we know. If we can be made to see it, perhaps for the rest of our lives we will be unwilling to settle for less."
> – Kurt Hahn

To make this process of consuming fresh fruits and vegetables more easily available to you, get involved in growing food, and in composting your food scraps to make rich soil for growing your garden. By doing so, I believe you will be participating in one of the most basic human experiences, and that is: growing and harvesting your own food.

• Your Life is Happening Now

> "For a long time it had seemed to me that life was about to begin – real life. But there was always some obstacle in the way, something to be gotten through first, some unfinished business, time still to be served, a debt to be paid. Then life would begin. At last it dawned on me that these obstacles were my life."
> – Alfred D. Souza

ARE you someone who is always getting ready and preparing for something to happen, and it never does, and you never arrive at the event you were setting yourself for?

Consider that maybe the reason your life isn't happening the way you want it to happen is because you are not working to make it happen, are not setting goals, do not have a game plan, are not visualizing what you want your life to be, are not spending your time wisely, and are not taking the actions to formulate the life you want.

> "What I am learning is that if you want to be more, do more, and have more in your life, you have to have more integrity. Look at the results of your life and check where you are not in your integrity."
> – Nwenna Kai

Don't be one who is caught in the neverending whirlpool of thinking that your life is going to begin when and if something is going to be done, happen, be purchased, or pass. Your life is happening now. Live in a way that uses your talents and intellect to bring about a better society and a better you right where you are, continually. Love yourself. Love others. Be your potential.

"The ones who are hardest to love are usually the ones who need it the most."

– Dan Millman

"No one saves us but ourselves. No one can and no one may. We ourselves must walk the path."

– Buddha

"Very often I watch a lot of young people sort of meander around without any idea about why they are doing what they are doing. I mean, to want and to be ambitious, and to want to be successful is not enough. That's just desire. To know what you want, to understand why you are doing it – to dedicate every breath in your body to achieve. If you feel you have something to give, if you feel that your particular talent is worth developing. is worth caring for, then there is nothing you can't achieve. You're going to grow up with your colleagues, you're going to watch them have success and watch them have failure and you're going to watch how they deal with it. And they can be as much a teacher for you as anyone."

– Kevin Spacey

"Develop yourself according to your own tradition and the call of your heart. But remember to respect differences, and strive for unity. Eat wisely. A lot of food is corrupt in either subtle or gross ways. Pay attention to what you are taking into your body. Learn to preserve food, and to conserve energy. Learn some good breathing techniques, so you have mastery of your breath."

– Sherif Kamal, NaturesFitnessModel.com

"I prefer to be true to myself, even at the hazard of incurring the ridicule of others, rather than to be false, and to incur my own abhorrence."

– Fredrick Douglas

"A man's errors are his portals of discovery."

– James Joyce

"Aim at the sun, and you may not reach it; but your arrow will fly far higher than if aimed at an object on a level with yourself."

– J. Hawes

"The great aim of education is not knowledge, but action."

– Herbert Spencer

• Dream Another Dream

"A dream you dream alone is only a dream. A dream you dream together is reality."

– John Lennon

"Consider that you are living in a dream. You say that may be a silly thought. But, similar to a dream, many people lead their daily lives making decisions based on perceptions they believe to be true, but that actually are not. Some perceptions are formed in their minds, and some are taught to them by others who may have created them, or who have passed along myths formed over the years by their culture, or by those with an agenda.

Perhaps it is time to dream another dream.

You know that there were things you believed that you eventually realized were untrue. Now think back and realize that you made decisions, and may have lived your days, based on those falsehoods. Consider that some of these falsehoods may have limited your joy and satisfaction in life."

– John McCabe, Igniting Your Life, IgnitingYourLife.com

• Piloting Your Energy Toward Health

"It is more important to know what sort of person has a disease than to know what sort of disease a person has."

– Hippocrates

SOME people think disease is the result of one thing. They may think that disease is simply because of bad eating habits, because of cleanliness, because of stress, because of environmental toxins, because of lack of exercise, or because of genetic expression. But disease is almost always a combination of these, and more – including the way the person conducts the theatre of their mind.

You can do many things that work in symphony to bring you into an excellent state of health. You can also do things that work in the opposite manner, such as engaging in damaging emotions; false and limiting beliefs; denial; procrastination; risky activities (including laziness and anonymous sex); stifled expression of intellect, talent, and love; the general unhealthful atmosphere in which you live; and in how you communicate.

The toxic combination of unhealthful living, low quality foods, lack of exercise, and dysfunctional relationships are a most common damaging combo leading to tension and disease. This is especially true if alcohol and other addictive substances are included in the combination.

When the body becomes diseased, it is not something that happens at an instant. It is the result of weeks, months, or years of some combination of unhealthful living, neglect, exposure to hazardous substances, low quality food, unhealthful thinking, or absorbing damaging forms of energy from ruinous, abusive, and/or dysfunctional relationships and situations.

A growing number of people not only eat unhealthful foods saturated with what cause disease, they also eat way too many calories, don't get enough exercise, do little to stimulate their talents and intellect, and lead a life that is far below their potential.

Obesity is an increasing problem, and it has been for decades. There are more people who are suffering from being overweight on the planet than there are people suffering from a lack of food. This is an indication of how many people are living unhealthful lives, not experiencing true health, and who are also using more than their share of resources – which damages Earth.

People began to get fatter with the mass production of automobiles and refrigerators. They stopped walking and riding bikes or horses to get places, and they began driving everywhere. They stopped the physical labor that was involved in growing and harvesting their food, and began instead to rely on stores and restaurants to supply them with their food. Then the mass production of the television and its meaningless drivel together with the introduction of processed foods and invasive television commercials brought people to become more stagnant. Then came mega-superstores where people can do all of their shopping in one stop – buying more stuff they don't need, and more stuff to make their lives cozier and lazier. This resulted in more dependency on international companies to make and sell everything people want for creating home settings reflective of those they see in advertising. It resulted in even fewer calories being used to finish chores, and mixed it with candy and junk food. Along with the mass use of the Internet and palm-based electronic entertainment people have become even heavier. Not only do they not grow their food, not build the things in their homes, and not go out to do chores that require some physical activity, they are increasingly dependant on the Internet to do their shopping. Instead of going to the store, they can now sit in a chair and, with a few strokes of the computer keys, do their shopping – purchasing more stuff that they don't need – and often going into debt to do so. Children used to be outside playing games, climbing trees, and even helping to grow family food gardens and maintain household structures and landscapes, but now a large number of children sit in chairs playing with their computer games and chat with each other on the Internet and cell phones. They often do this while consuming processed foods containing corn syrup, trans fats, fried substances, processed salts, MSG, and chemical preservatives, dyes, scents, and flavors. So now, as the population settles into being obese, and hating it, the fad diet book authors and diet product manufacturers are stuffing money into their bank accounts, and on the TV news there are liposuctioned, Botoxed, and surgically adjusted "journalists" reading stories about how fat everyone is getting – news stories told between advertisements for fast foods, desserts, candy, sodas, high tech gadgets, stomach surgery for the morbidly obese, and over-the-counter and pharmaceutical drugs.

Numerous studies have concluded that the obesity problem in America is going to cancel out all of the advances in preventative health and medicine experienced in the last few decades. It will cause more problems in society than the combined effects of cigarette smoking, alcoholism, and automobile accidents. This still holds true even though, according to 2008 studies, the number of overweight children in the U.S. seems to be leveling off, and it is doing so at a high weight. The average weight of children on the planet still continues to rise. In 2009 the Centers for Disease Control and Prevention reported that the average U.S. citizen was 23 pounds overweight. It also said that the average American was consuming 250 calories more per day than the average American did in the 1970s, and much of those calories were the result of sodas, corn syrup, junk snacks, and fried and high-fat foods. As this trend continues, other countries will be experiencing a dramatic increase in healthcare spending.

A study conducted by a number of researchers and institutions and that was published in the July 27, 2009 edition of the journal *Health Affairs* concluded that U.S. spending on healthcare doubled in ten years. The study concluded that obesity in the U.S. increased 37 percent in ten years and that the healthcare of obese people is 10 percent more than for people of a healthful weight. The cost includes the expense of treating ailments that are much more common in those who are obese, including diabetes, knee damage, heart disease, breathing difficulties, skin ulcers, foot amputations, and depression.

> "We have been brought up in a culture in which relies heavily on experts and authorities to show us the way. If we want to deal with sickness we go to a doctor or a health professional, if we want to know about God we go to a priest, if we want to educate our children we send them to a school, if we want our children entertained we put them in front of a TV or a computer game.
>
> By giving up responsibility for our own lives in so many ways we are much more vulnerable to being manipulated and molded by external forces such as BIG business and the powers that be."
>
> – Anand Wells and Runi Burton of Australia's LiveFoodEducation.com

If you want to get healthful: Turn off your TV. Stop paying attention to TV characters that are simply a figment of the imaginations of scriptwriters, producers, and marketing wizards in Hollywood and Manhattan. Spend time talking with people rather than spending time staring at a TV with them. Walk, jog, run, ride a bike, or even rollerskate to get places. Unplug from your wires and engage in craft and talent. Stop buying things that you don't need that often sit next to other stuff you bought that you don't need. Realize that health does not come in a bottle or can of diet liquid, nor is true health achieved through slimming pills, liposuction, or stomach stapling surgery. Stop eating candy, smoking cigarettes, and drinking soda pop and/or brewed and distilled alcohol. Don't eat processed foods, and foods that contain animal products, corn syrup, trans fats, clarified oils, MSG, processed salts and sugars, bleached grains, gluten grains, or synthetic dyes, scents, sweeteners, flavors, and preservatives. Do not eat fried or sautéed food of any sort – and know that foods sautéed in oil are similarly unhealthy.

> "Miracles are fantastic events which utilize hidden laws of nature that most people are not aware of. Miracles do not break the laws of nature, they are actually based on them."
>
> – Master Choa Kok Sui

> "For many years, researchers have been studying how foods affect arthritis. Some of the early studies were not of the best quality, but by 1991, the issue was settled beyond any reasonable doubt. In *The Lancet*, a prominent British medical journal, researchers reported that a specially designed vegetarian diet can greatly reduce the signs and symptoms of arthritis. In the study, researchers found that a vegetarian diet lessened joint stiffness, swelling, and tenderness, and improved grip strength. The benefits lasted long after the study was over.
>
> Here is why it works: Certain foods act as an arthritis trigger, stimulating the inflammatory process that attacks the tender synovial lining that is inside joints. The most common trigger foods are dairy products. Because it appears that a dairy protein is the culprit, even fat-free versions can trigger the inflammation that causes pain. A switch to soymilk or rice milk can help. Eggs and meat can contribute to joint pain for some people, which is why researchers are especially fond of vegan diets."
>
> – Dr. Neal Barnard, author of *Foods that Fight Pain*

A study conducted at McMaster and McGill universities in Canada, and published on the October 11, 2011 by *PLoS Medicine* journal (published by Public Library of Science) reported that a diet rich in raw fruits and vegetables favorably modified the chromosome 9p21 region genetic variant, which had been identified as a marker for heart disease. The study, titled, The Effect of Chromosome 9p21 Variants on Cardiovascular Disease May Be Modified by Dietary Intake: Evidence from a Case/Control and a Prospective Study, included data of over 27,000 people from a variety of ethnic ancestries, including Chinese, European, Latin American, and Arabian. The study authors concluded that the people with the genetic variant could, if they followed a diet rich in raw fruits and vegetables, reduce their risk of heart disease to the level experienced by those who do not have the genetic variant. The authors of the study concluded that, "The risk of myocardial infarction and cardiovascular disease conferred by chromosome 9p21 SNPs appears to be modified by a prudent diet high in raw vegetables and fruits."

Scientists have known that certain chemicals that form in cooked food, including acrylamides, glycotoxins, polycyclic aromatic hydrocarbons, d-Nitrosodiethanolamine, and heterocyclic amines, can damage DNA and trigger the growth of cancer cells. But, the McMaster and McGill study identified how a diet rich in raw plant matter favorably alters human genes to prevent disease. This was no surprise to me. I have read many studies concluding that dietary choices certainly can trigger genes to express favorable or unfavorable health events.

That being said, I should also mention that the vast variety of degenerative diseases are not initialized by genes, but are triggered by bad diet, lack of exercise, toxic environment, and substance abuse, including cigarettes and drugs. In his book, *The China Study*, T. Colin Campbell reinforces the fact that genes are a lesser part of the puzzle when it comes to common diseases, and as little as 3% of common diseases can really be blamed on genes. Even among those diseases that are triggered by genes, there is something that sets the genetic expression in motion, such as an environmental toxin, horrible dietary choices, cigarettes, and otherwise, unhealthful lifestyle. As Campbell states, "The genes that you inherit from your parents are not the most important factors in determining whether you fall prey to any of the ten leading causes of death." What matters most for disease prevention and reversal? A clean diet, and especially one that is low fat and free of synthetic chemicals and of animal protein – as in, vegan.

If you want to experience the miracle of vibrant health: Eat foods as they are presented to us from nature – living, raw fruits, berries, vegetables, herbs, nuts, seeds, sprouts, mushrooms, edible flowers, and water vegetables. Get involved in growing some of your own food by creating an organic culinary garden that will benefit you, your family, and your community. Nurture wild edible plants. Support local organic farmers. Read books that will exercise your brain and improve your intellect, talents, and life. Unclutter your brain by uncluttering and organizing your life. Take out the garbage in all areas of your life. Stop being lazy. Don't waste any more of the precious moments of your life. Stop living a life of nonsense involved with replicating corporate imagery and celebrity culture in your life. Don't listen to negativity or to those who undermine your intellect, belittle you, and otherwise keep you down. Be around people who love you and respect your drive to improve. Volunteer for organizations that help protect the environment and wildlife. Practice self-discipline and live intentionally with a list of priorities and a goal-oriented mindset. Realize that you are an amazing being capable of creating the life you want. Get inspired. Respect yourself. Access your intellect. Develop your talents. Begin living up to your potential. Know that you are worthy of love.

> "We are indeed much more than what we eat, but what we eat can nevertheless help us to be much more than what we are."
> – Daisie Adelle Davis

As you simplify, purify, and make your life more vibrant through high quality plant-based nutrition and intentional success-oriented principles and actions, you will start to understand how much nonsense you put yourself through by living a toxic life. You will let go of things you don't need. You will have more energy, will feel better, and will experience clarity of thought. Your intuition will start to make itself known to you and will be displayed in your reasoning, words, and actions. Solutions to your problems will randomly enter your mind and life. You will feel a radiance in your being that you may have never known. You will be more in alignment with and able to access infinite intelligence. The longer you live healthfully the stronger the frequency will become. You will feel an amplification of all of your senses. You will begin to understand what it is like to be radiantly alive.

> "Health is a blessing that money cannot buy."
> – Izaak Walton

Allow health to be your energy. Choose it, work for it, and make it yours.

> "You are held within the web of life, within flows of energy, and intelligence far exceeding your own."
> – Joanna Macy

> "Make sure that the things you do keep us alive."
> – Graham Nash

• Brain and Heart Nutrition

BRAIN nutrition begins before birth as billions of brain cells are forming. Because of this, women who are planning on becoming pregnant, and those who are pregnant, would benefit their babies by striving for the most excellent nutritional foods available to them.

Excellent prenatal nutrition is beneficial in many ways. Women who consume a variety of fresh fruits and vegetables during pregnancy are found to have babies with more healthful lung function, less susceptibility to asthma, and fewer complications. It should be obvious that the mother benefits in many ways be following a healthy diet prior to and during pregnancy, and during the breast-feeding stage.

> "Either it is appropriable material for tissue building – a food, or it is not. If not, then it is a foreign substance – a poison – and as such can only damage and cannot possibly ever benefit the organism."
>
> – Dr. Hereward Carrington

Substances in fresh fruits and vegetables are particularly beneficial to brain function. It is known that the neurotransmitter acetylcholine is key to cell communication and a healthful memory. That brain chemical tends to decline with age. Antioxidants in raw, dark-colored fruits and vegetables, and especially in apples, apricots, broccoli, cantaloupe, chard, kale, mangos, blueberries, goji berries, spinach, and watermelon, help to preserve a healthful level of acetylcholine.

Blueberries are often mentioned as a brain-friendly food because they contain anthocyanins, which stimulate neural regeneration and improve neural connections. Because they are rich in antioxidants, blueberries have been mentioned in various studies as being particularly beneficial for maintaining long-term memory, and also for reducing the chances of Parkinson's and Alzheimer's disease. If you are able, plant and maintain some blueberry bushes so that you will have access to the freshest blueberries at the lowest cost.

Goji berries are especially brain-friendly. Gojies contain even higher levels of antioxidants than blueberries, and more of the antioxidant beta-carotene than in carrots. Gojies contain sesquiterpenoids, which stimulate the pineal and pituitary glands. The amino acids l-glutamine and l-arginine in gojies increase the production of human growth hormone, which protects against aging. Gojies contain polysaccharides, which are long-chain sugars that help to feed the brain. The berries also stimulate the production of choline, which combats free-radicals attributed to neurological degeneration. The zeaxanthin in gojies is beneficial to the eyes. Zeaxanthin is also found in the highly nutritious fresh water algae, spirulina. Goji berries grow in a variety of terrains. Perhaps you can grow some in your garden or on nearby wildland.

Among other nutrients, bananas contain vitamin B6, potassium, and tryptophan. B6 helps to maintain blood sugar, which is the brain's food. Potassium regulates blood pressure, protecting the fine blood system in the brain. The tryptophan in bananas is used to create serotonin in the body, including in the intestines and brain cells. Serotonin is a neurotransmitter that stabilizes the mood and improves attention. Serotonin also helps a person to sleep better, which helps the brain to function at a higher level.

Flax seeds are known for containing essential fatty acids, but they are a particularly excellent source of alphalinolenic acid (ALA). This omega-3 fatty acid has been shown to aid in the function of the cerebral cortex, the area of the brain involved in processing sensory information, such as pleasure. Many people purchase flax seed oil and use this in their foods. Instead of using clarified flax oil, I purchase whole flax seeds, soak them in water, and then grind them in a coffee grinder. It is good to grind the seeds after soaking them in water for several hours or overnight, and letting them dry at room temperature for a day (spread a quarter cup of them on a ceramic tray), as this will ignite the enzymes and other nutrients in the seeds. This powder, which is also rich in fiber, can be used in salads, added to juices and smoothies, mixed in with hummus, pesto, and dips, used as an ingredient in vegetable pate, and included in dehydrated vegetable crackers made with the antioxidant-rich pulp left over from juicing vegetables. By consuming the freshly ground flax seeds, you will be consuming not only the oil, but also the other nutrients in the seeds.

Some people mix together raw flax oil, hempseed oil, and pumpkin seed or grapeseed oil for a particularly nutrient-rich oil combo they use in salad dressings and other raw foods. However, there is no sense in going overboard with consuming oils. No added oils are necessary when consuming a diet rich in raw fruits and raw vegetables. The heart-health expert, Dr. Caldwell Esselstyn, advises against adding any oils to the diet, and instead to eat the whole plant foods. Many people have found they do much better by not using bottled oils, and only eating the whole foods that contain the oils, such as raw flax, pumpkin seeds, hemp seeds or hemp seed powder, raw walnuts, germinated buckwheat and germinated chia, and raw greens, such chard, kale, spinach, and cilantro, and wild purslane. As I mention elsewhere, all raw fruits, vegetables, nuts, seeds, and seaweeds naturally contain some essential fatty acids in every cell, and getting enough calories in a raw food diet rich in fruits and vegetables easily provides a sufficient amount of both essential fatty acids and amino acids.

Raw sesame seeds are rich in the brain, neuron, heart, and bone nutrients methionine, tryptophan, other amino acids, vitamin E, B6, folic acid, riboflavin, thiamine, niacin, zinc, potassium, magnesium, manganese, copper, phosphorous, calcium, iron, and essential fatty acids, and contain more omega-6 than omega-3 (best to get sesame seeds raw, unheated, and organic). Sesame seeds are rich in fiber, and the phytosterols contained in the seeds lower blood cholesterol. The sesamin lignan in sesame seeds is an antioxidant phytoestrogen that has been identified as having anti-cancer properties. The delicate polyunsaturated fats in sesame seeds are particularly easy to damage by heating.

When raw, unheated sesame seeds are rinsed in a fine mesh strainer and kept wet for a few hours, it allows for the nutrients in the seeds to multiply. These soaked seeds can be used in various raw recipes, tossed into salads, and also used to make raw tahini, which is commonly used in raw hummus, dips, dressings, and desserts. Raw sesame seeds are also used in raw piecrust, dessert truffles, gomashio, halvah, baba ghanoush, and dehydrated sesame cracker recipes found in many of the popular raw food recipe books. One way of making raw vegan ice cream is to blend two frozen bananas with a tablespoon each of raw tahini and vanilla, and then spoon mixing in one or more of the following: berries, sliced soft fruit, raw walnuts, cinnamon, or raw carob powder.

Sesame seeds have been a common food throughout history, including for oil, and especially in the Middle East, parts of Africa, and India. The sesame plant is probably native to the sub-Saharan Africa or the East Indies. The Romans ground sesame seeds with herbs to make a spread. Buddhist monasteries in Japan commonly use sesame oil in many of their foods. Raw sesame oil has been used as a skin moisturizer for thousands of years. Ancient Chinese used sesame seed oil as an ingredient in ink. According to Assyrian legend, the gods drank sesame wine the night before they created Earth. African slaves are said to have brought sesame seeds to the Caribbean and the Americas. Sesame grows easily in many parts of the world.

Raw sesame seeds can be purchased in the bulk sections of many natural foods stores. I don't use sesame oil, but if you choose to do so, look for oil that is cold-pressed (raw), organically grown, and that does not contain other oils. It is good to keep sesame seeds stored in glass bottles in a cool, dry, dark place. Because the hull protects and preserves the seed, dehulled sesame seeds tend to go rancid within months, so it is good to purchase only what will be used within three or fewer months. They can also be frozen.

Another source of essential fatty acids are germinated buckwheat seeds, which are about 10% oil, including omega-3 essential fatty acids. Buckwheat seeds are also known as buckwheat groats. The raw seeds can be purchased at most natural foods stores. Similar to sunflower seeds, buckwheat has a thick outer hull. Before they are sent to markets, the hull of the seeds is removed. The seeds should be kept in a cool, dry, dark place, and in an airtight container to preserve the delicate polyunsaturated fatty acids. Glass bottles work best. Because the oils naturally contained in buckwheat are subject to degradation, buckwheat isn't good for long-term storage, but can be frozen.

Buckwheat seeds contain the minerals calcium, copper, iron, magnesium, manganese, phosphorus, potassium, and zinc. Like all fruits, vegetables, nuts, seeds, and seaweeds, they also contain the eight amino acids essential for human health. Buckwheat seeds are especially rich in lysine and arginine. Lysine and cystine are two of the amino acids that are easily damaged or destroyed by heat.

It is easy to germinate buckwheat seeds by soaking them in water for a few hours, then draining the water, transferring them to a clean bowl and keeping them slightly wet by using a screen strainer to rinse them two- to three-times per day for two or three days. Germinating buckwheat for two or three days greatly increases the presence of linoleic acid, and also triggers the production of enzymes. As with other seeds, germinating buckwheat more than quadruples the amino acid content, which means that buckwheat is an excellent source of protein. Germinated buckwheat is also a source for vitamins B1, B6, and C.

Because buckwheat is free of gluten, it is safe for those who have been diagnosed with celiac disease, and for those with a history of anxiety, depression, bi-polar disorders, and autism.

Buckwheat is also rich in fiber, and has been shown to absorb cholesterol from the digestive tract, which means it is excellent for cardiovascular health. Buckwheat is also beneficial to coronary health because the seeds contain alpha tocopherol, delta tocopherol, and gamma tocopherol, which protect against cardiovascular disease.

Trace nutrients in buckwheat include the polyphenols rutin and quericitrin, which are beneficial in lowering blood plasma cholesterol (and are also heart-friendly nutrients present in red wine). Rutin helps to strengthen capillary walls while improving circulation. The cholesterol-lowering substances in buckwheat also reduce the incidence of gallstones.

The chlorogenic acid in buckwheat protects health because it is antibacterial, antifungal, and antiviral. Chlorogenic acid also helps to slow the release of glucose into the blood stream.

The D-chior-inositol in buckwheat helps to maintain the balance of insulin, which means that germinated buckwheat is an excellent food for those with blood-sugar issues, which can also affect brain function.

In very rare cases, some people are allergic to buckwheat. In rare cases, buckwheat can trigger asthma-like symptoms. I know one person who has experienced a mild reaction to eating germinated buckwheat, including itching mouth and slight and temporary problems swallowing.

Boiled porridge made of buckwheat and/or hemp seeds has been a common breakfast food in Asia and Eastern Europe. In the raw food diet, freshly germinated buckwheat is a common breakfast food. Freshly germinated buckwheat can be used in fruit salad as a breakfast food, which is more healthful than common packaged cereals. However, although buckwheat resembles a grain, it is not a cereal, a grain, or a grass, but has been defined as a fruit. Typically this salad includes germinated buckwheat mixed with a chopped apple, bananas, and/or berries, a squeeze of lemon, and a dash of cinnamon.

Germinated buckwheat seeds can also be dried, which is used as kasha. Traditionally, kasha is roasted buckwheat. In the raw food diet, kasha consists of buckwheat that has been germinated and then dried, either at room temperature by spreading it out on a clean, dry cloth, or in a dehydrator. This kasha can be used in raw granola, and for adding crunch to raw piecrust, raw carob treats, and dehydrated vegetable crackers, and mixing in banana or mango whip (frozen bananas and/or mangos put into a high-speed blender or in a food processor until whipped [peel the ripe bananas and mangos before freezing!]).

Chia seeds also contain brain and heart nutrients. Chia seeds were cultivated along with beans and corn by the Nahuatl culture (Aztecs). Chia seeds are more than 25% oil, and raw chia seeds are another excellent source of essential fatty acids. Similar to hemp seeds, chia seeds are particularly rich in omega-3 fatty acids. Chia oil contains about 64% omega-3 fatty acid, which is more than what is in flax seeds. Chia seeds are rich in amino acids, quickly absorb water, and form an enzyme-rich gel coating. Germinating chia seeds greatly increases their amino acid content, which means that they are an excellent source of protein. Chia seeds are rich in the antioxidants caffeic acid, chlorogenic acid, kaempferol, myricetin, and quercetin, which make chia seeds excellent protectors of cellular and neural health. They are also rich in soluble fiber, making them a heart-healthy food. Similar to buckwheat, chia seeds are free of gluten, making them safe for those who are sensitive to that protein, including those with celiac disease, and for those with bi-polar disorders, anxiety, a history of depression, and autism.

When consumed, germinated chia seeds are a slowly digested form of carbohydrate, which prevents the sugar rush that can be experienced after eating other forms of carbohydrates, such as wheat and rice. Many raw foodists include chia seeds in their smoothies and non-dairy mylks, such as hemp milk (blend water, hemp seed powder, dates, banana, vanilla, chia. Optional: lucuma powder and/or berries.).

> "Chia seed is a superfood that resembles black sesame seed and is nutty to the taste. It is an excellent source of minerals and antioxidants. According to the U.S. Department of Agriculture, 2 tablespoons of chia seeds provide approximately 100 milligrams of

calcium, 7.5 grams of dietary fiber, and 3 grams of protein. Chia seeds are also high in alpha-linolenic acid, an omega-3 fatty acid, with 3.5 grams of alpha-linolenic acid in 2 tablespoons."

– Julia Driggers, RD, *Vegetarian Journal*; VRG.org

Similar to buckwheat, germinated Chia seeds can be used in a breakfast salad with chopped fruit; tossed into salads; used as an ingredient in vegetable burgers and dehydrated vegetable pulp crackers; and dried for use in raw granola and raw pie crust. A pudding that is similar to tapioca can be made from Chia seeds, and this is also popular among raw foodists. In Latin America, Chia fresca is made of Chia seeds soaked in water and fruit juice. Some raw foodists stir chia seeds into kombucha juice. Because Chia seeds absorb water, fruit juice, or coconut water so quickly, it only takes less than a half hour to make recipes containing them.

There is such a wide assortment of edible plants from around the world containing varieties of health-giving substances that it would be difficult, or impossible, to include them all in one book. But, it would be beneficial to know which ones you can include in your diet so that you may experience vibrant health.

While we can speak of the relatively few antioxidants that have been identified and named, humans don't actually know how many chemicals are found in plants, or how those chemicals benefit health. There are clearly many thousands of various plant chemicals in a simple raw vegan meal – such as a salad or green smoothie. Among the reasons so many plant chemicals have not been identified is that many of them have been identified by those working for or funded by companies interested making synthetic copies of the chemicals in the form of patented pharmaceutical drugs. Many of the drugs that are out there are synthetic versions of some substance identified in a plant. But, drugs do not contain beneficial co-substances that may be in the plant. It is interesting that people that take patented drugs but don't clean up their diet don't do as well as people who clean up their diet and don't take patented synthetic pharmaceutical drugs. Coincidence? I don't think so. The most basic things that you need for health are not found in pill form, or in a syringe, but they are in plants – including biophotons, amino acids, fiber, enzymes, essential fatty acids, and an unknown variety of antioxidants and unidentified phyto chemicals.

The brain is over 50% fat and benefits from healthful unheated oils naturally present in raw fruits, vegetables, sprouts, nuts, seeds, and seaweeds. Oil in raw hemp seeds, grape seeds, flax seeds, sunflower seeds, sesame seeds, and pumpkin seeds are often used in the raw food diet. Instead of purchasing the oil from these seeds, purchase the actual raw seeds, and use those as food. Eating these whole raw plant substances, or including them as ingredients in raw recipes, especially if the raw seeds and raw nuts have been soaked in water to enliven them, also provides the beneficial brain nutrients of amino acids, enzymes, vitamins, and minerals, including magnesium, which is important for brain health.

Scientists have discovered that pregnant women who consume healthful quantities of high quality essential fatty acids are more likely to have babies with higher IQs and that possess better language comprehension and eye-hand coordination. This reveals that it is especially important that pregnant women, and women planning on becoming pregnant, to totally eliminate low quality fats from their diet, including fried and sautéed oils, and also lard, mayonnaise, margarine, shortening, corn oil, other bottled oils, and heated tropical fats. They would benefit by making sure to include raw fruits and raw vegetables, especially raw green vegetables, in their daily food choices.

Raw nuts are beneficial to both heart and brain health. Raw nuts contain monounsaturated fats, which can lower LDL (bad) cholesterol levels while boosting HDL (good) cholesterol levels. It is good to soak raw nuts in water for an hour or so to deactivate their enzyme inhibitors, and activate their enzymes. After they become dry, store them in bottles and refrigerate.

Raw walnuts contain high quality dietary oils. Walnuts also contain a substance called uridine, which has been found to improve memory retention. Uridine also aids in the growth of the branches on brain cells called neurites, improving the connection between neurons. Many people make note of the similarities between the shape of the walnut and the shape of the human brain.

Nuts only become damaging to health when they have been heated, such as broiled, roasted, sautéed, fried, or otherwise exposed to high temperatures, and/or when they are coated with unhealthful substances, such as processed salt; sugar, artificial dyes, flavors, or preservative; milk chocolate, or other low quality chocolate; or candy substances, such as caramel.

Because nuts contain a lot of calories, it is best to limit your intake of nuts to less than one-third cup, per day. Some people completely avoid nuts, and that is absolutely fine. Dr. Caldwell Esselstyn advises patients with cardiovascular disease to avoid all nuts. If you are on a weight-lowering program, aim for consuming fewer nuts and more vibrant fruits and also fresh greens, such as kale, broccoli, chard, celery, dandelion, spinach, purslane, collards, cilantro, and parsley, which all contain some essential fatty acids. All raw fruits, including citrus fruits, avocados, and raw olives are also sources of essential fatty acids. Figs are another source because their tiny seeds are rich in quality fat, are rich in fiber, and contain a number of vitamins, minerals, and antioxidants (avoid figs that have been treated with sulfur, other drying agents, or preservatives, or that are cooked, such as in fig cookies – which usually also contain corn syrup or other unhealthful ingredients).

Essential fatty acids act as doorways on the cell membranes to exchange nutrients, enzymes, and electrical currents. They also allow for the output of cellular waste. Healthful cellular membrane function is one of the many reasons it is good to maintain a diet rich in raw fruits and vegetables to obtain fresh essential fatty acids.

The white matter in the brain is a fatty substance that plays a role in the speed of information processing. The nerves are coated with a fatty material called myelin.

The quality of nutrients in your diet plays out in the level of your thinking, including in your reasoning, judgment, and decision-making.

To get your brain to function at its highest level, avoid cooked and other low quality fats.

Again, to stress the issue of fat in the diet: You do not need a large amount of oil in your diet. Less oil is better. It is beneficial to brain health to follow a diet rich in natural, plant-based omega-3 fatty acid sources. This is to say: not fish, and not eggs, or other animal protein advertised as rich in omega-3s. While it is true that meat from grass-fed cattle is five times higher in omega-6 fatty acids than meat from grass-fed cattle, because meat contains other substances not good for human health, it isn't meat that should be considered as a good dietary source of essential fatty acids. Unlike plants, meat, eggs, and dairy, contain no fiber, but are rich in free radicals that negate health. Unlike meat, dairy, and eggs, plants are rich in antioxidants that fork against free radicals and promoted health. Unlike meat, plants do not contain arachidonic acid (AA), which is found in animals, is source of omega-6 fatty acids, and can trigger mood swings. Omega-3 fatty acids help to combat the effects of AA.

Some people say that you need to eat fish and other animal products to get essential fatty acids. This is not true. Excellent sources of essential fatty acids exist in the plant sources mentioned above, and in sea vegetables. There is no need to kill and eat fish or sea creatures, or oils derived from killed sea creatures, to obtain essential fatty acids.

Some people will say they need the long-chain omega-3 fatty acids from fish, including docosahexaenoic acid (DHA) and eicosapentaenoic acid (EPA). Like other omega-3s, which are long-chain fatty acids, DHA and EPA help to combat the effects of arachidonic acid (AA), protecting the brain and nerves from what can play out as mood swings and stress symptoms. But, consuming fish does not guarantee that the body will function at a better level with the benefit of the DHA and EPA in the system.

"The proportions of plasma long-chain n–3 fatty acids were not significantly affected by the duration of adherence to a vegetarian or vegan diet. This finding suggests that when animal foods are wholly excluded from the diet, the endogenous production of EPA and DHA results in low but stable plasma concentrations of these fatty acids."

– *American Journal of Clinical Nutrition*, Vol. 82, No. 2, 327-334; August 2005

The human system makes EPA and DHA from alpha-linolenic acid (ALA), an omega-3 fatty acid found in all raw fruits, vegetables, sprouts, germinates, nuts, and seaweeds. As mentioned elsewhere in this book, purslane, which is a common weed, is a source of eicosapentaenoic acid. But, because the body makes DHA from ALA and EPA, it doesn't mean that you need to include purslane, or fish oils, in the diet. A vegan diet rich in raw fruits and vegetables manufactures what the body needs to function healthfully, including through protecting the brain and nerves.

Today much of the fish on the planet live in water contaminated by industrial pollution, such as mercury, which is damaging to human health. Mercury is particular damaging to brain function. In addition to mercury, the oil from fish contains many other heavy metals and industrial pollutants. This is because the oil is typically from the liver of the fish, and the liver is the detox center of the body.

Mercury occurs naturally in the environment, but the increase in mercury in the tissues of waterlife is largely the result of industrial pollution, and much of that consists of pollution from coal-burning electric generating plants and from kilns used to process concrete that is used in construction of buildings, walls, sidewalks, and roads.

The high levels of mercury and other heavy metals in sea life are among the many reasons it is unhealthful to eat fish. Sea creatures are exposed to all sorts of toxins in the water. The toxins are also the result of poisoned rivers emptying into the lakes, marshes, and oceans; of pollution directly flowing into the oceans from coastal cities, military operations, and industries; from toxic chemical fertilizers and "pest control" chemicals spread on the greens of golf courses, lawns, farms, schools, and corporate campuses; from the shipping and oil industries; from cruise ships; and from air pollution, including from cars, trucks, airplanes, restaurants, coal-fueled electric generating plants, and cement kilns. Human exposure to the toxins in seafood can lead to nerve damage, miscarriages, learning disabilities, birth deformities, and various types of cancer.

Another problem with fish liver oil is that when people are taking more that 5 grams or 5,000 milligrams per day, it can cause excessive bleeding from simple skin wounds.

While fish is not a good source of omega fatty acids, water plants, such as chlorella and spirulina, are good sources.

Chlorella is a fresh water algae. It is often consumed in small amounts by raw foodists as a supplement, such as in compressed tablets, or in powder form added to salads, smoothies, and as an optional ingredient in other dishes. In addition to the nutrients B-6, beta-carotene; the minerals iron, magnesium, phosphorus, and potassium; and a variety of amino acids, chlorella contains porphyrins and sporopollenim, which bind with heavy metals, including mercury, and help remove them from the body.

While fish and crustaceans do contain substances that are damaging to health, they *do not* contain something necessary to maintain health, which is fiber.

The soluble fiber in a live food diet consisting largely of fruits and vegetables is excellent for protecting the brain and heart. This is so because soluble fiber helps to prevent heart disease and strokes.

A raw food diet may include plant substances containing soluble and insoluble fiber. These include raw oats, germinated quinoa, germinated buckwheat, soaked millet, sprouted barley, and whole non-gluten grains; fresh or dried apples, pears, figs, and other fruits, including fresh citrus; germinated beans and germinated bean and vegetable patés; soaked raw nuts; and a variety of fresh vegetables including cucumbers, broccoli, celery, fennel, and Brussels sprouts. Fiber helps to maintain a healthful balance of cholesterol in the system, which is important for brain health.

Some raw food recipes contain psyllium seed husks, which are also an excellent form of soluble fiber. Psyllium husk collects moisture, and it is best accompanied by adequate water or other hydration to help move it through the digestive tract.

Many people take psyllium husk for its beneficial impact on cholesterol levels. A healthy level of cholesterol is beneficial to brain health.

Because the body makes the cholesterol that it needs, there is no need to include cholesterol in the diet, such as from meat, dairy, or eggs. For those who have high cholesterol, it would be beneficial for them to eliminate all animal protein from their diet, and to include a variety of fresh fruits, vegetables, whole grains, and sprouted beans in their diet. These edible plants will help to remove excess cholesterol. This is because, in the intestines, soluble fiber attaches to cholesterol and bile acids, and then carries them out of the body through the natural digestive process.

"Typical high-protein diets are extremely high in dietary cholesterol and saturated fat. The effect of such diets on blood cholesterol levels is a matter of ongoing research. However, such diets pose additional risks to the heart, including increased risk for heart problems immediately following a meal. Evidence indicates that meals high in saturated fat adversely affect the compliance of arteries, increasing the risk of heart attacks. Adequate protein can be consumed through a variety of plant products that are cholesterol-free and contain only small amounts of fat."

– Physicians Committee for Responsible Medicine, PCRM.org; Citing Nestel PJ, Shige H, Pomeroy S, Cehun M, Chin-Dusting J. Post-prandial remnant lipids impair arterial compliance. *Journal of the American College Cardiology*. 2001;37:1929-1935.

Bile acids are made from cholesterol and are necessary for fat digestion. When the digestive system needs more bile acids, the body will take cholesterol from the blood stream to form more bile acids, thus lowering cholesterol levels.

A plant-based diet helps to remove cholesterol plaque from the body. This is why a raw diet is particularly beneficial for those who have experienced serious health problems, such as a heart attack or stroke.

"My message is clear and absolute: coronary artery disease need not exist, and if it does, it need not progress. It is my dream that one day we may entirely abolish heart disease, the scourge of the affluent, modern West, along with an impressive roster of other chronic illnesses."

– Dr. Caldwell B. Esselstyn, author of *Prevent and Reverse Heart Disease*; HeartAttackProof.com

The sterols and stanols (phytosterols and phytostanols) found in a plant-based diet provide additional benefits to maintaining heart and brain health. This is because these natural plant chemicals help maintain cholesterol levels.

In the intestines, sterols and stanols block the reabsorption of cholesterol that has been removed from the digestive tract by soluble fiber. They do this by replacing cholesterol, or filling in for cholesterol in mixed micelles, which are composite molecules containing substances that are fat- and water-soluble. When the stanols and sterols end up in the micelles, the cholesterol instead gets put out of the body through the regular digestive process.

Micelles exist in the blood stream, where they carry beneficial fats transporting nutrients, including fat-soluble vitamins. Sterols and stanols are in unheated plant oils. Lower amounts of them are in whole plant foods, such as raw fruits, vegetables, nuts, seeds, and seaweeds.

In a person following a sunfood diet the micelles are healthful because they contain stanols and sterols. But in a person following an unhealthful, meat-, dairy-, and egg-laden diet, the micelles contain cholesterol that ends up as plaque throughout the body.

If you are a person who shops at typical supermarkets, you may notice that some processed food products contain information on the labels that sterols and stanols have been added to the food, and thus the food companies have labeled the food as "heart healthy." But, what the processed foods may also contain are cooked fats; bleached grains; processed salts; clarified and processed sugars, such as corn syrup; synthetic chemical preservatives, dyes, flavors, and scents; MSG (monosodium glutamate), which is a neurotoxin; and traces of fossil-fuel-based farming chemicals from low quality, non-organic farming processes. The better choice would be to stick with a low-fat, raw or mostly raw, vegan diet. The plant substances will provide the heart healthy nutrients that are truly beneficial to maintaining vibrant health.

Because a sunfood diet does not contain trans fats, fried foods, heated nuts, processed salts, processed sugars, or MSG or other excitotoxins, it is all that more beneficial for protecting the heart and brain.

Raw fruits and vegetables containing the B vitamin folate also feed the brain. Folate improves brain memory and also appears to reduce the occurrence of Alzheimer's disease. Folate is found in oranges, dark greens, and in legumes. (Sprouted or germinated [slightly sprouted for two or three days] legumes, such as lentils, are used in a variety of live food recipes.) Other B vitamins help to protect the neural cell sheaths. So it is important to eat foods containing B vitamins. Raw, fermented foods, such as sauerkraut, kimchi, and fermented non-dairy seed cheeses, especially those containing nutritional yeast, are sources of vitamin B vitamins, enzymes, and amino acids (see the B-12 section in this book for more information about B-12). Those concerned with not getting enough B-12 can put their worries to rest by simply taking a vegetarian B-12 supplement.

Many people have heard that wine is particularly beneficial to brain health. Red wine and the skins of red grapes contain substances called polyphenols. The polyphenol that has been recognized as most beneficial in the skin of red grapes is resveratrol. This chemical has been found to lower cholesterol while also improving blood circulation to the brain. Because resveratrol brings more nutrients into the brain, it has a positive effect on memory. Resveratrol has been found to prevent the formation of the plaques in the brain that interfere with neural communication. Resveratrol may help to prevent Alzheimer's disease because it prevents the formation of beta-amyloid protein, an ingredient in the plaque found in the brains of Alzheimer's patients. Within plants, resveratrol helps to ward off fungal growth and bacterial infection.

Wine happens to be a raw food. But you don't have to drink red wine to get resveratrol. It is also found in berries and peanuts. Some stores and Internet sites that sell raw food products also sell raw "jungle peanuts" which do contain resveratrol. I have grown peanuts in my garden, which is one way to get fresh, raw peanuts.

To those who drink wine to obtain the health benefits, such as from resveratrol, I suggest that they seek out wine that is made from organically grown grapes, and preferably from the continent where you live on, or are closest to, so that you are supporting local organic farmers. Pinot noir seems to be the most beneficial wine in the health-benefits category, and white wine is the least.

Some people have a problem with alcohol, so they should stay completely away from it, as it can become an addictive and ruinous substance. Many people also stay away from alcohol because they consider it to be a neurotoxin.

Snacking on fresh seeded grapes, or blending whole seeded grapes into orange and apple juice with hemp seed and flax seed powders provides a variety of brain nutrients. If you don't have access to seeded grapes, find a place where you can grow some. You may also want to contact a local organic farm that may be growing seeded grapes, or encourage them to do so. A local food co-op or CSA may also carry or have access to seeded grapes.

There are a variety of nutrients found in live foods that the brain and nerve cells rely on. Vitamin C, which is in oranges, tomatoes, strawberries, dandelion greens, and other fruits and vegetables, works in combination with vitamin E as antioxidants that prevent the oxidation of cells. Vitamin E is found in green leafy vegetables, raw nuts, and raw vegetables and their oils.

Vitamin C also works in combination with iron in a number of ways, including in transporting oxygen to the tissues, including the brain.

Most animals form vitamin C in their bodies. Some animals don't, including fruit eating bats, humans and other primates, guinea pigs, and certain birds. Many foods that modern people consume have been so processed through canning, cooking, fermenting, pickling, milling, clarifying, and frying that they contain no or very little vitamin C. A plant-based diet that is rich in variety and mostly or all raw contains plentiful amounts of vitamin C.

When you consume fruits and vegetables, consider that what you use on your foods, including any oils, salts, sweeteners, or condiments should also be of high quality. Consider not using any oils, salts, sweeteners, or condiments.

Processed salts are not good for brain health. In the live food diet, those who use salt use unprocessed sea salt, pink salt, and powdered sea vegetables, such as dulse and kelp. Processed salts have been heated to temperatures that change their structure, may contain additives, and are harsh and damaging to the body tissues, including nerve cells, the kidneys and liver, and the walls of the veins, arteries, and capillaries. Processed salts can help cause varicose veins.

Dietary minerals are essential to the brain's ability to function, including the ability to memorize and recall. The sunfood diet includes highly mineral-rich foods, including sea vegetables, which are particularly abundant in both minerals and the nutrients that help transport the minerals in the body.

Minerals work in combination with other nutrients, such as vitamins, amino acids, essential fatty acids, antioxidants, and trace nutrients. If you don't have a wide spectrum of nutrients in your diet, other nutrients can't be metabolized, and truly vibrant health is less likely to blossom.

In other words, when selecting food, use your brain – especially if you want your brain and heart to function at the highest level.

> "Convenience foods are recipes for obesity, usually containing large amounts of fat, sugar, and salt and insufficient amounts of fiber. While 'convenience foods' save time in the kitchen, they may wind up stealing years from your life. Double this disaster with the efficiency of fast food restaurants to deliver all these fattening foods."
>
> – Dr. John McDougall, DrMcDougall.com

> "Tell me what you eat, and I will tell you what you are."
>
> – Anthelme Brillat-Savarin

> "The goal of life is living in agreement with nature."
>
> – Zeno

• Energy, Oxygen, and Breathing

> "Psyche depends on body and body depends on psyche."
>
> – Carl Gustav Jung

> "Every disorder and condition can be helped by learning how to breathe.
>
> Most of us take shallow breaths in and out, leaving us with little oxygen and too much CO_2.
>
> Inhaling deeper belly breaths not only brings in more oxygen to cleanse our system, but releases CO_2 from our systems and creates calming chemicals to offset fight or flight responses."
>
> – Dr. Barbara Foley

"Trees shade our ground, create topsoil, clean the air and help the land attract, hold, and filter water. The trees and their roots purify the water as the rains fall. Clean streams keep millions of aquatic and other species alive."

– Tim Hermach

"Destruction of forests is a leading cause of global environmental breakdown, including global warming."

– AncientTrees.Org

"Taking care of our planet – environment – is something like taking care of our own home. This blue planet is our only home."

– Dalai Lama

"God has cared for these trees, saved them from drought, disease, avalanches, and a thousand tempests and floods. But he cannot save them from fools."

– John Muir

"Too old to plant trees for my own gratification, I shall do it for my posterity."

– Thomas Jefferson

"The creation of a thousand forests is in one acorn."

– Ralph Waldo Emerson

"Trees are sanctuaries. Whoever knows how to speak to them, whoever knows how to listen to them, can learn the truth. They do not preach learning and precepts, they preach undeterred by particulars, the ancient law of life."

– Hermann Hesse

"Someone's sitting in the shade today because someone planted a tree a long time ago."

– Warren Buffet

"He that plants trees loves others besides himself."

– Thomas Fuller

"Trees outstrip most people in the extent and depth of their work for the public good."

– Sara Ebenreck

"As today's science has made clear, we take in the whole cosmos with each breath; the stuff of our lungs and of our cells and of the air we share with other creatures. With every breath, we take in molecules from other creatures and other humans who lived and breathed over hundreds of thousands of years."

– Matthew Fox

"To know even one life has breathed easier because you have lived. This is to have succeeded."

– Ralph Waldo Emerson

> "There's so much pollution in the air now that if it weren't for our lungs there'd be no place to put it all."
>
> – Robert Orben

> "It wasn't the Exxon Valdez captain's driving that caused the Alaskan oil spill. It was yours."
>
> – Greenpeace ad, *New York Times*, Feb. 25, 1990

> "There are no passengers on Spaceship Earth. We are all crew."
>
> – Marshall McLuhan, 1964

• YOGA

> "In this very breath that we take now lies the secret that all great teachers try to tell us."
>
> – Peter Matthiessen

> "Lack of activity destroys the good condition of every human being, while movement and methodical physical exercise save it and preserve it."
>
> – Plato

YOGA has been practiced for thousands of years and requires no fancy equipment. All you need to do yoga is your body, mind, and breath.

If there is one type of movement that is beneficial to do every day, it is yoga.

People who regularly do yoga call it "practicing yoga." This relates to the way yoga gets better with practice, and also how the intention learned while practicing carries over into their life.

Yoga is the skill of intellect and intention put into action. You may hear of it referred to as the "union of the principle of self."

> "We don't stop playing because we grow old; we grow old because we stop playing."
>
> – George Bernard Shaw

The practice of yoga is play, relaxation, and exercise for both the mind and body. It is low impact and is meditative while it works to teach a person that they are capable of getting better at doing a task. Yoga builds and improves physical and mental strength and agility.

A person practicing the physical exercises of yoga learns how to do the moves, poses, transitions, and breathing techniques with clearer intention. The concentration on intention can be brought into their daily thoughts and actions. They learn to act and think more intentionally to bring about what they want in their life.

Some may use fancier words than what I am using here. I am no yoga master, and I am using wording accessible to those less knowledgeable about yoga.

Many people today practice yoga strictly for the physical and other health benefits. In the U.S., most people who practice yoga strictly do it for the exercise, movement, and stress relief that it provides.

> "The outward freedom that we shall attain will only be in exact proportion to the inward freedom to which we may have grown at a given moment. And if this is a correct view of freedom, our chief energy must be concentrated on achieving reform from within."
> – Gandhi

Some people who are into doing yoga also study the books that teach the philosophy of yoga, such as the text of the *Bhagavad Gita*, which is known as "the song of the Lord," and the "immortal dialogue between soul and spirit." They may focus on the science of the mind, and what some call the "royal science of God-realization."

> "Movement is a medicine for creating change in a person's physical, emotional, and mental states."
> – Carol Welch

Stretching, holding poses, practicing a full and healthful flow of the breath, and working with your body weight as a workout tool – such as is done in yoga – increases your strength, flexibility, and endurance, while releasing stagnant energy and tension. This clears and strengthens the neural system in the brain and throughout the body. Yoga also improves the movement of blood to all of the tissues, reduces stress hormones, and helps to build a healthful appearance.

> "Those who think they have no time for bodily exercise will sooner or later have to find time for illness."
> – Edward Stanley

Scientists using medical technology have measured the stress relief that yoga induces. Yoga has a positive influence on the autonomic nervous system, which regulates the internal organs, such as the liver, heart, and digestive tract. Relieving stress through regular yoga practice increases the sense of wellbeing; strengthens the immune system and the muscular and skeletal systems; regulates blood pressure; and improves cholesterol, hormonal, and blood sugar levels.

Yoga can be especially beneficial for those who suffer migraines and insomnia, and for those with heart disease, diabetes, multiple sclerosis, and cancer.

Because it reduces stress while regulating the body system as it strengthens and works the body, regular yoga practice is beneficial to brain function, helps the brain rewire and grow new neural pathways, and increases the brain's release of hormones conducive to healthy body chemistry. Because stress and unhealthful levels of sugar and cholesterol can damage brain cells and brain function, daily yoga is particularly healthful for the brain. The cardiovascular workout that can be attained through yoga also increases the volume of the brain's frontal lobes, which improves alertness and memory.

Those who are unfamiliar with yoga can easily learn about it from magazines, books, videos, the Internet, and by attending yoga classes.

As a person begins practicing yoga, it is best to start out with an open mind and learn as the body becomes open to the poses. Many people try to hurry into yoga and fail to learn it in ways that are most beneficial. In yoga it is good to focus on the breath, to take time to learn the poses, and to work with the intention.

While there are a wide variety of yoga poses with each providing a benefit, there are an even wider variety of yoga teachers. There are some yoga instructors who are more beneficial to their students than others. Some are perhaps teaching classes before they are ready. Others are well informed and educated about the practice, and are helpful in guiding and inspiring their students.

When people ask me if I know of a good yoga teacher, I often advise people to ask around about the yoga teachers in their community. Then visit more than a few different yoga instructors to find what it is that feels most natural and beneficial. Some yoga teachers are into aggressive workouts, and others hold classes at different levels of learning. There are yoga teachers who hold classes outside, some who choose to work one-on-one, and some who only work with certain age groups, with recovering addicts, or with the handicapped. Some yoga teachers play no music during class, and others may play classical music, or even country, folk, jazz, hip hop, trance, world, jungle, or rock. Some will play their own instruments during class, and some may sing and encourage their students to sing along.

Because yoga is meditative, a person involved in teaching yoga influences the student's mind. This is a concept that some yoga teachers don't seem to understand: what a yoga teacher says during the time they are teaching a yoga class can touch a person deeply. Yoga teachers would benefit their students by focusing their thoughts and words on healing, positive, uplifting, kind, encouraging, and loving energy.

Any music played during a yoga class, be it playful or serene, loud or soft, should be of an uplifting, encouraging, life-affirming nature.

Many people credit yoga with helping them recover from various physical, mental, spiritual, and life ailments. While you are around those who practice yoga, it is not uncommon to hear people tell stories of how yoga has greatly benefited their lives.

Yoga is affective in improving health on all levels.

If there is not a yoga studio near you, start one! Make it affordable to all by establishing the classes as donation-only, with a suggested cost, but with only a box where people can donate after class. Yoga should not be about making money, it should be about enlightenment. Deny no one.

> "Yoga is a divine gift offered to all, unconditionally, by a nameless creator.
>
> Having engineered the human and animal form, the creator then planted a potent seed inside our bodies, a seed that may lay dormant for one lifetime or even hundreds, until enough intelligence, playfulness, curiosity, and desire for service brings this seed to life.
>
> By eating a diet replete in unprocessed, nutritious, enzyme rich raw food we give ourselves a greater opportunity to readily receive this gift. The body is purified, the mind centered, and the spirit energized.
>
> Furthermore, as eating is one of the few things that all of us do every day, by choosing to eat close to Earth we can make a personal, yet powerful statement. Each day we cast a vote for the type of world that we wish to live in and leave to our children. A life inspired by the combination of yoga and living food gives back to the planet rather than stripping it of all precious resources. In essence this lifestyle is nothing more than an expression of nature itself and the key to its practice is simplicity."
>
> – Michael Stein and Angela Starks, YogaInTheRaw.com

Acro Yoga, AcroYoga.com
Alchemical Yoga, Chavah Aima, Austin, TX; AlchemicalYoga.com
Aquarian Times **magazine**, AquarianTimesMagazine.com
Bhakti Yoga Shala, Santa Monica, CA; bhaktiyogashala.com. Govindas and Radha.
Bhakti Nove, BhaktiNove.com
Childrens' Yoga, ChildrensYoga.com
International Association of Yoga Therapists, Prescott, Arizona; IAYT.org
International Kundalini Teachers Assoc., KundaliniYoga.com
LA Yoga Magazine, LAYogaMagazine.com
Lygia Lima, Brazil; lygialimayoga.com.br
Rainbeau Mars, RainbeauMars.com
Off the Mat: OffTheMatIntoTheWorld.org
Power Yoga, PowerYoga.com
Radiantly Alive, RadiantlyAlive.com
Matthew Sanford, MatthewSanford.com
Shiva Rea, ShivaRea.com
Ashley Turner, California, New York, Brazil; AshleyTurner.org
Yoga in the Raw, Upstate New York; YogaInTheRaw.com
Yoga Movement, YogaMovement.com

• DANCE

> "And those who were seen dancing were thought to be insane by those who could not hear the music."
>
> – Friedrich Wilhelm Nietzsche

Dance is healing and a form of expression that releases pent-up energy. It is one way of getting exercise, engaging all of the muscles in combination with exploration of movement and freedom of thought.

Find the ecstatic dance events with live drumming and non-electric instrumentation in your community, or begin one.

> "Movement and dance to me is a spiritual practice that connects me to what is real and helps me to feel happy and very alive!"
>
> – Gary Olsen

> "Every dancer knows her goal to get to that point where the body no longer stands in the way but becomes the instrument of the soul's expression, the body and the psyche working together."
>
> – Iris Stewart

> "Perhaps dance's most important gift to us lies in its ability to unify us and make us whole by uniting our inward life with our outward expression."
>
> – Carla DeSola

> "For me, dance is an opportunity to dive into a place where I allow previous blocks to dissolve, joys to become present with full force, heart-breaks to be revealed and ecstasy to be tasted - it is a space to explore and taste my full authentic self, in all it's dimensions and forms, beyond my previous limitations."
>
> – Tzadik

Drum Circle Finders on the Internet,
drumcircles.net/circlelist.html;
drumcircles.net/internationalcirclestext.html
drumcirclefinder.com/drumcirclefinder/Drum_Circle_Finder.html
drumconnection.com
Ecstatic Dance, ecstaticdance.org

• ARTISTS

TODAY we need a whole new set of artists dedicated to designing all levels of society to establish a more environmentally sustainable culture.

> "Art enables us to find ourselves and lose ourselves at the same time."
>
> – Thomas Merton

> "I think raising consciousness, helping people see and understand how they're connected to these larger systems in the

world around us, is an incredibly important thing. I think art can do this in ways that are provocative, meaningful and inspirational, deeply moving, beautiful, connected with history and culture and resonant. I think that's a big part of it. There's another part of it where I think artists have the opportunity to more than call attention to problems and preach, to really help solve problems. To help create things that work better, that are just more beautiful and right."

– Sam Bower

"The creative individual has the capacity to free himself from the web of social pressures in which the rest of us are caught. He is capable of questioning the assumptions that the rest of us accept."

– John W. Gardener

"A musician must make music, an artist must paint, a poet must write, if they are to be ultimately at peace with themselves. What a man can be, he must be."

– Abraham Maslow

"To the artist is sometimes granted a sudden, transient insight which serves in this matter for experience. A flash, and where previously the brain held a dead fact, the soul grasps a living truth! At moments we are all artists."

– Arnold Bennett

"We rely upon artists to articulate what most of us can only feel in joy and sorrow. Whenever I feel my courage wavering I rush to them. They will give me the wisdom of acceptance, the will and resilience to push on."

– Helen Hayes

"In art and dream may you proceed with abandon. In life may you proceed with balance and stealth."

– Patti Smith

If you are an artist, please become a part of the movement to create a more healthful, environmentally sustainable society that protects Nature and wildlife while following a plant-based diet.

"At the deepest level, the creative process and the healing process arise from a single source. When you are an artist, you are a healer; a wordless trust of the same mystery is the foundation of your work and its integrity."

– Rachel Naomi Remen

• POLITICIANS

"Mistrust those in whom the urge to punish is strong."

– Nietzsche

"A lot of times in politics you have people look you in the eye and tell you what's not on their mind."

– George W. Bush

"Political language is designed to make lies sound truthful and murder more respectable."

– George Orwell

"It is difficult to get a man to understand something when his salary depends upon his not understanding it."

– Upton Sinclair

"Don't expect politicians, even good ones, to do the job for you. Politicians are like weather vanes. Our job is to make the wind blow."

– David Brower

"I have always held firmly to the thought that each one of us can do a little to bring some portion of misery to an end."

– Albert Schweitzer

DON'T wait around for politicians to change the world and make it into a better place. Start with yourself, working in your community to change things for the better, and spread it from there.

"I cannot control the wind. But I can adjust my sails."

– An optimistic sailor

"We must be silent before we can listen. We must listen before we can learn. We must learn before we can prepare. We must prepare before we can serve. We must serve before we can lead."

– William Arthur Ward

"In every community, there is work to be done. In every nation, there are wounds to heal. In every heart, there is the power to do it."

– Marianne Williamson

Do you want to change the world? Be your own revolution. Start with what you eat and how you spend your time, energy, and resources. Collectively, the more people who live a certain way has more of an impact on society than the mindset of a politician. The choices of the people are what lead.

"A lot of people are waiting for Martin Luther King or Mahatma Gandhi to come back – but they are gone. We are it. It is up to us."

– Marian Wright Edelman

"Self-realization is not a matter of withdrawal from a corrupt world or narcissistic contemplation of oneself. An individual becomes a person by enjoying the world and contributing to it."

– Francine Klagsbrun

"It is the greatest of all mistakes to do nothing because you can only do a little. Do what you can."
– Sydney Smith

Get involved in your community. Work for a more environmentally safe and sustainable culture that doesn't use fossil fuels, does work to protect and restore nature, does value the welfare of the environment above corporate interests, and does not put up with politicians who support environmentally damaging, pro-fossil fuel, pro-nuclear energy, and pro-war laws, subsidies, and regulations.

"Our tendency to create heroes rarely jibes with the reality that most nontrivial problems require collective solutions."
– Warren Bennis

Get involved in supporting environmental groups that work to protect and restore forests, meadows, deserts, rivers, and wildlife habitat.

"It's a little arrogant to say, there's nothing you can do. You know there are people who say, 'Who am I to be fabulous and powerful?' To that I say, 'Well, who are you not to be?'"
– John Robbins

Some people get involved in politics because they are seeking power. At the start of their goal they are already losing. Being involved in politics shouldn't be about self-promotion, it should be about doing what is right for the people, the environment, wildlife, and Earth.

"When the power of love overcomes the love of power, the world will know peace."
– Jimi Hendrix

"A good leader inspires others to have confidence in the leader, a great leader inspires people to have confidence in themselves."
– Groucho Marx

"The lust for power is not rooted in strength, but in weakness."
– Erich Fromm

The politician of the new generation should have their success measured by what they do that is right for Earth, and not what is right for corporations, for the prison industry, for war contractors, for the fossil fuel industries, for the growth of the nuclear energy industry, for money making, or for hoarding ownership of substances.

"The whole course of human history may depend on a change of heart in one solitary and even humble individual – for it is in the solitary mind and soul of the individual that the battle between good and evil is waged and ultimately won or lost."
– M. Scott Peck

The way I view it, we are all politicians. We are all involved in making changes in society. And we are doing it every day with our personal choices, and with how sustainable our lives are. We are doing it through how we are, or are not, working to make change for the better, to make society better for the health of the web of life on Earth.

> "The next major advance in the health of the American people will be determined by what the individual is willing to do for himself."
>
> – John H. Knowles

As you go about each day, know that what you do is impacting others. What you choose to eat, accumulate, dispose of, and enjoy is part of the big picture. What we are doing every day is in answer to something, or the opposite.

> "Person to person, moment to moment, as we love, we change the world."
>
> – Samahria Lyte Kaufman

Be aware of which societal questions you are answering through your thoughts, actions, choices, and ways of communicating. And be aware that your answers in all of these are not only defining your future, but the future of many other forms of life on this planet.

> "Everybody can be great because everybody can serve. You only need a heart full of grace, a soul generated by love. And you can be that servant."
>
> – Martin Luther King Jr.

> "In the truest sense, freedom cannot be bestowed, it must be achieved."
>
> – Benjamin Franklin

> "We can all be angels to one another. We can choose to obey the still small stirring within, the little whisper that says, 'Go.' 'Ask.' 'Reach out.' Be an answer to someone's plea. You have a part to play. Have faith."
>
> – Joan Wester Anderson

> "Freedom is when the people can speak, democracy is when the government listens."
>
> – Alastair Farrugia

> "I have one life and one chance to make it count for something… I'm free to choose what that something is, and the something I've chosen is my faith. Now, my faith goes beyond theology and religion and requires considerable work and effort. My faith demands – this is not optional – my faith demands that I do whatever I can, wherever I am, whenever I can, for as long as I can with whatever I have to try to make a difference."
>
> – Jimmy Carter

"I am a believer in nonviolence and I say that no peace or tranquility will descend upon the people of the world until nonviolence is practiced, because nonviolence is love and it stirs courage in people. There is advantage only in construction. I want to tell you categorically I will not support anybody in destruction."
– Abdul Ghaffar Badshah Khan

"The Right would return to an ideal past that never was. The Left would legislate an ideal future that can never be. The Wise say it's here and now that we practice kindness; grow in peace."
– Tom Mahon

"A man's true wealth is the good he does in the world."
– Muhammad

"We have come to rely on the notion that we need authorities to fix everything for us. That they are our symbols of hope.

When it seems that in reality, they are the ones tearing this world apart and forcing us to work at jobs we don't love so we can buy stuff we've been deceived into wanting.

You (we) are directly responsible for the reality we create, and we must empower ourselves to live that truth every day of our lives. When we finally give the power back to ourselves, we can begin to re-create the paradise that has been destroyed."
– Anthony Anderson

"Every great dream begins with a dreamer. Always remember you have within you the strength, the patience, and the passion to reach for the stars to change the world."
– Harriet Tubman

• Self Reliance

RATHER than relying on restaurants and stores to supply all of your food, grow some of your own.

Growing your own organic food is one of the most powerful things you can do to live a more sustainable and environmentally friendly life. It will also help to disconnect you from corporate food, and from participating in the carbon- and resource-heavy diet that is described in the book *Tomatoland: How Modern Industrial Agriculture Destroyed Our Most Alluring Fruit*, by Barry Estabrook. Most people in industrial society are consuming food that has traveled thousands of miles, and that has been grown using a variety of chemicals and low-paid workers.

The news is continutally reporting record heat waves that are impacting large areas of the planet. Increasing temperatures bring drought, fires, the loss of wildlife, the collapse of crops, stress to small communities, and higher food prices.

Pay attention! Know this: It is wise to be involved in growing some or all of your food.

Learn to compost your food scraps to build healthy soil. Gather seeds. Read up about organic gardening techniques. Become educated about edible plants and helpful bugs that are native to your region. If possible, have a greenhouse in which you can grow food in colder months. Use biodegradable cleansers and convert your household to a graywater system to use the water from your sinks and laundry as irrigation water for your garden. Learn about humanure (humanurehandbook.com).

Book: *The Edible Front Yard: The Mow-Less, Grow-More Plan for a Beautiful, Bountiful Garden*, by Ivette Soler.

Baker Creek Heirloom Seeds, RareSeeds.com

Community Garden, CommunityGarden.org

Council for Responsible Genetics, 5 Upland Road, Suite 3 Cambridge, MA 02140; councilforresponsiblegenetics.org. Founded in 1983, the CRG is comprised of scientists, lawyers, public health advocates and citizens concerned about the social, ethical and environmental impact of new genetic technologies. They have influenced a group of seed companies to sign a "safe seed pledge," committing to preserving the integrity of seeds from genetic engineering. For a list of the seed companies that have signed the pledge, please contact the Council.

Eat the View, Kitchen Gardeners International, 3 Powderhorn Dr., Scarborough, ME 04074; eattheview.org. This organization got thousands of people to sign a petition to encourage the Obama family to plant an organic garden at the White House. On March 20, 2009, work on the garden began, with Michelle Obama digging in.

Eat the Weeds, eattheweeds.com

Edible Forest Gardens, edibleforestgardens.com

Fallen Fruit, fallenfruit.org. Fruit share site.

Food is Power, FoodIsPower.org

Food Not Lawns, FoodNotLawns.net

Fruit for Our Children, New Zealand, fruitforourchildren.com.

Gardenerd, gardenerd.com

Goode Green, goodegreennyc.com. Green rooftop design and installation.

Green Grid Roofs, greengridroofs.com

Green Roofs, greenroofs.org

Guerilla Gardening, guerrillagardening.org

High Mowing Organic Seeds, highmowingseeds.com/blog

Island Seed and Feed, Goleta, CA; IslandSeed.com

Karma Kitchen, Berkeley, CA; KarmaKitchen.org. This is a restaurant that makes meals and gives bills amounting to zero with the encouragement that the customer will pay what they can so that the kitchen can keep running.

KitchenGardeners.org

Neighborhood Fruit, neighborhoodfruit.com. Fruit- and vegetable-sharing site for those who have home grown produce they can share with others.

The Organic Gardener, Chicago, IL; theorganicgardener.net. Jeanne Pinsof Nolan helps families, schools, and businesses create organic gardens.

Path to Freedom, PathToFreedom.com

Permaculture, Permaculture.net

Rare Seeds, RareSeeds.com

Roof Meadow, roofmeadow.com
Rooftop Farms, rooftopfarms.org
Saving Our Seed, SavingOurSeed.org
Seed Alliance, SeedAlliance.org
Seed Savers, SeedSavers.org
Square Foot Gardening, SquareFootGardening.com
Urban Homestead, UrbanHomestead.org
Veggie Trader, veggietrader.com.
Victory Seeds, VictorySeeds.com
Yards to Gardens, y2g.org

Find food that is more healthful, safer for the environment, and less connected to the corporate food giants.

The number one way you interact with the planet is through your food choices. Start now by recognizing ways in which you can become more sustainable through what you consume.

> "The soil is the great connector of our lives, the source and destination of all."
> – Wendell Berry

> "We forget that the water cycle and the life cycle are one."
> – Jacques Cousteau

> "Learn from the lowliest in the earth, in the birds, in the trees, in the grass, in the flowers, in the bees – likewise listen to the birds, watch the blush of the rose, listen to the life rising in the tree."
> – Edgar Cayce

• Inventors of a Sustainable Culture

> "I do know that craft, if you pursue craft, will return you again and again to this creative state. To pursue the craft means to endeavor to bring together the intention of the mind to the hand, and an invitation to feeling – an invitation to a new kind of feeling."
> – Nicholas Hlobeczy

> "Every storm must begin with a single drop of rain. And so it is with every worthwhile movement."
> – Marco Caceres

> "For most of a century, idealistic people have been encouraged to use anger, protest, lobbying, and legal action in order to make the world a better place. While most certainly some of these behaviors and activities were necessary, we have reached the point at which the social benefit of such behaviors is decreasing. We have reached the point at which creation, rather than attack, ought to be the first obligation of reformers. The social entrepreneurship movement is the first tip of this iceberg."
> – Michael Strong

> "You never change something by fighting the existing reality. To change something, build a new model that makes the existing model obsolete."
>
> – Richard Buckminster Fuller

> "We cannot live by the past; the present is so transient that is almost does not exist. As a matter of fact, we live by the future; or more accurately, we are unceasingly preparing ourselves toward it, trying to anticipate it, and from this process flow all new ideas. It is impossible to be alive without the effort to create and bring something new into concrete manifestation."
>
> – Nicolai Fechin

> "It is not the strongest of the species that survives, nor the most intelligent, but the one most responsive to change."
>
> – Charles Darwin

HUMAN culture needs a new set of experimenters, inventors, and envisionists, including on the smallest scale. Creativity is a key to all of this.

> "Creativity requires the courage to let go of certainties."
>
> – Erich Fromm

There are many jobs that will be created to help form a sustainable culture within all societies around the planet. There will be jobs that never existed, but there will also be jobs that are in fields that have been around for many years.

> "Innovation seldom depends on discovering obscure or subtle elements but in seeing the obvious with fresh eyes. Billions of tea drinkers observed the force of steam escaping from water boiling in a kettle before James Watt realized that this vapor could be converted into energy."
>
> – Richard Farson

> "U.S. consumers and industry dispose of enough aluminum to rebuild the commercial air fleet every three months; enough iron and steel to continuously supply all automakers; enough glass to fill New York's World Trade Center every two weeks."
>
> – Environmental Defense Fund ad, *Christian Science Monitor*, 1990

The opportunities within a new sustainable culture include carpentry. In addition to using hemp fiber and bamboo for building materials, which saves trees and protects wildlife and the environment, there is the opportunity to use the huge amounts of all sorts of used wood being discarded every day. This includes the finest wood available. Instead of carpenters going to the lumber yard to purchase new wood for building materials and furniture making, woodworkers should consider the sources of free wood made up of discarded furniture and of buildings that are about to be demolished.

> "To think creatively, we must be able to look afresh at what we normally take for granted."
>
> – George Kneller

> "To raise new questions, new possibilities, to regard old problems from a new angle, requires creative imagination and marks real advance in science."
>
> – Albert Einstein

> "I only feel angry when I see waste. When I see people throwing away things we could use."
>
> – Mother Theresa

> "Dig a trench through a landfill and you will see layers of phone books like geographical strata or layers of cake. During a recent landfill dig in Phoenix, I found newspapers dating from 1952 that looked so fresh you might read one over breakfast."
>
> – William Rathje, *The Economist*, 8 September 1990

> "A man should look for what is, and not for what he thinks should be."
>
> – Albert Einstein

An idea of inventiveness for a sustainable culture includes looking at what there is a lot of, and figuring out ways of dealing with these things that is more sustainable than the way they have been dealt with. For example, most bottles end up either as trash, or are thrown into recycling bins, which results in them being crushed to make new bottles. Why can't they be divided and reused, saving the energy, time, and resources to destroy them and make them anew? For instance, most wine bottles now end up in landfills. This amounts to hundreds of millions of wine bottles being "thrown away" every year. That is not sustainable. There is no "away," there is only here, on Earth, where we are. A solution to the wine bottle problem would involve something like collecting the discarded boxes from wine stores, and collecting the discarded wine bottles from restaurants, hotels, and homes. Then cleaning these bottles and selling them back to the wineries for less than what the wineries pay for new bottles. Recycling one bottle saves enough energy to power a light bulb for four hours.

> "Every time I see an adult on a bicycle, I no longer despair for the future of the human race."
>
> – H. G. Wells

Inventiveness for a sustainable culture involves getting people to stop using cars and petroleum. One solution includes what is going on with people creating bike rental stops in towns and cities where people can rent bikes instead of renting or using cars. It includes what is going on with people starting up local donation-only or low-cost bike repair service stations to support bike culture. It involves redesigning towns and cities to be more accessible to bikes and less reliant on fossil fuels. And it involves reducing the amount of land used for parking lots, roads, gas stations, and petroleum drilling and refining. We have covered way too much of Earth with roads and parking lots. And we have destroyed tremendous areas of the planet to get and make the fuel needed to run cars. And we have damaged enormous parts of the planet to get the resources to build all of those cars.

> "That which is lacking in the present world is a profound knowledge of the nature of things."
> – Frithjof Schuon

Inventiveness for a sustainable culture includes providing access to healthful ways of growing food, especially among disadvantaged people. This includes teaching people how and where to grow food on the land where they live. This will get them away from depending on corporate food, stores, and restaurants while improving their nutrition by eating a more natural diet, and that will lower medical costs.

> "There is a sufficiency in the world for man's need but not for man's greed."
> – Mohandas K. Gandhi

Inventiveness for a sustainable culture includes second hand stores and creating things out of damaged and discarded items. An example of this is creating insulation from discarded clothing, which would save money while also reducing the use of heating, which would save resources, reduce pollution, and otherwise help the environment.

> "The earth laughs in flowers."
> – Ralph Waldo Emerson

Inventiveness for a sustainable culture includes ways of making dwellings more in tune with the local environment. An example of this is by converting barren rooftops into landscapes of native flowers, which would in turn support local bee and bird populations while also insulating the buildings. This would save on heating and air conditioning costs while also reducing the use of fossil fuels. In some places, such as in Cuba, people have been growing culinary gardens on their rooftops. Doing this would add another set of benefits to landscaping rooftops, as it would save people money, provide fresh food, improve health, and localize communities.

> "Real generosity toward the future lies in giving all to the present."
> – Albert Camus

Inventiveness for a sustainable culture would involve rethinking the way we use land in the cities. This includes landscaping rooftops of buildings. It includes creating green spaces in parking lots where trees can grow, and creating shade that would reduce heat ponds while supporting local wildlife and absorbing air pollution. Sustainable landscaping could be supported by graywater systems, which is using water that goes down the drains of sinks, showers, and bathtubs. This would require the use of biodegradable soaps, which turn into fertilizer for the landscaping, and this reduces the use of toxic chemicals.

> "Sometimes, all you need to invent something is a good imagination and a pile of junk."
>
> – Thomas Alva Edison

Inventiveness for a sustainable culture would involve rethinking what trash is and what trash is not, and what to do with it. It would include collecting what is truly biodegradable, such as food scraps and expired food so that it can be turned into compost to improve soil conditions – and not sending vegetable food scraps into landfills. It would include collecting landscape clippings, which can be used as compost. Landscape clippings also can be used to create ethanol, reducing our use of fossil fuels while helping to eliminate the use of food crops to create ethanol. The number one crop in North America is landscape clippings. Nearly all of the landscape clippings go to the landfills or garbage dumps. They should be taken to ethanol plants and to compost piles.

> "Not all revolutionaries set out to change the world per se; some set out to change their own worlds. And in so doing, they often change the way one person, or a few people, or whole communities, or entire nations or the world thinks and operates in some significant way."
>
> – Anita Roddick

In each step of the way of converting our cities and towns into more sustainable places to live and work there are jobs that also support communities. And it can be done by using natural products, some of which need to be invented, and some that already exist, but which aren't being utilized.

> "Creativity, as has been said, consists largely of rearranging what we know in order to find out what we do not know. Hence, to think creatively, we must be able to look afresh at what we normally take for granted."
>
> – George Kneller

Tragically, humanity continues destroying Earth's forests. Much of it is done to obtain lumber for construction and tree pulp to make paper and cardboard.

Two sustainable plants that provide materials that can be used for building materials are bamboo and hemp.

While bamboo is growing in popularity for fabric, flooring, and other construction materials, hemp remains illegal to grow in the U.S. based on the misconception that it is a drug, which is based on its relationship to a sister plant, marijuana. While many state governments in the U.S. have agreed to allow farmers to grow hemp, the federal government refuses to allow hemp farming, which is absurd and criminal.

> "There is one thing stronger than all the armies in the world and that is an idea whose time has come."
>
> – Victor Hugo

Hemp can easily provide the pulp needed to make paper, eliminating the use of trees for paper. Hemp makes a higher quality paper than that of tree pulp, and hemp paper can be recycled more times than tree pulp paper. An acre of hemp trees provides more pulp than an acre of trees, and it does so on a yearly basis while absorbing more air pollution than an acre of trees. Hemp can also be used to make ethanol, and hemp seed oil can be used for diesel engines, greatly reducing the use of petroleum, oil imports, and drilling into Earth. Because hemp absorbs global warming gasses, it helps to reverse the problem that fossil fuels are causing. Hemp fiberboard made out of hemp resin and hemp fiber is four times stronger than plywood made from tree wood. Hemp easily grows without pesticides and intensive fertilization. Hemp fiber is excellent for making fabric, and it can be used to replace much of the cotton farming that uses tremendous amounts of water, fertilizer, and pesticides. Hemp seeds carry a complete profile of the essential amino acids our bodies need to form protein. This makes hemp seed powder a healthful ingredient to be used in a variety of foods. Hemp oil is more nutritious and has a better balance of essential fatty acids than oil from flax, olives, walnuts, or the seeds of grapes, and is a perfect nutritional oil to combine with flax and pumpkin seed or grape seed oil. Hemp oil is more healthful than oil from fish, and does not contain the toxins of fish oil that are now found in fish from all over the world as the world's lakes, rivers, and oceans have been polluted by industry and air pollution caused by the burning of fossil fuels. Hemp oil can be used to make biodegradable soaps, cosmetics, and skincare products. Hemp fiber can be used to make a form of concrete blocks that are stronger and lighter than standard concrete. The furnaces used to create concrete spew mercury into the atmosphere – which poisons our air, land, and water.

Hemp and bamboo can be grown in every region of the U.S. and many other countries. Allowing industrial hemp farming would localize economies by helping to provide materials for making various products, including fuel, paper, fabric, construction material, food oil, finishing oils, and paints, and insulation. Legalizing industrial hemp farming in the U.S. would be excellent for farmers and the environment.

> "A man has made at least a start in discovering the meaning of human life when he plants shade trees under which he knows full well he will never sit."
> – D. Elton Trueblood

We should not be cutting down any more forests. We should be planting trees, restoring forests, and allowing wildlife to return to its habitat. We should abolish laws that prevent farmers from growing industrial hemp.

Look around you and observe what has been and is being done and consider how it can be done in a more sustainable way. Consider what there is and what there may be. Factor the non-toxic and sustainable solutions for the toxic and non-sustainable problems. Be of the mind that is part of the solution.

> "Be not simply good. Be good for something."
> – Henry David Thoreau

Inventing a sustainable culture starts where you are and involves what you do and how you do it.

> "Once you've found your own voice, the choice to expand your influence, to increase your contribution, is the choice to inspire others to find their voice."
> – Stephen Covey

> "The next Buddha may take the form of a community, a community practicing understanding and loving kindness, a community practicing mindful living. And the practice can be carried out as a group, as a city, as a nation."
> – Thich Nhat Hanh

> "The free exploring mind of the individual human is the most valuable thing in the world."
> – John Steinbeck

> "You must give some time to your fellow men. Even if it's a little thing, do something for others – something for which you get no pay but the privilege of doing it."
> – Albert Schweitzer

"Nothing can withstand the power of the human will if it is willing to stake its very existence to the extent of its purpose."
– Benjamin Disraeli

"Many persons have a wrong idea of what constitutes true happiness. It is not attained through self-gratification but through fidelity to a worthy purpose."
– Helen Keller

"The return we reap from generous actions is not always evident."
– Francesco Guicciardini

"If you are not creating a legacy for the benefit of your grandchildren's grandchildren then you are wasting other people's oxygen!"
– Papa Joe, Maori Healer

"Live your beliefs and you can turn the world around."
– Henry David Thoreau

• Localizing Economies

INSTEAD of supporting businesses owned by multinational corporations, consider supporting businesses that are more localized.

Localizing economies includes choosing to shop at farmers' street markets rather than at large supermarkets; going to family-owned businesses rather than corporate chains; growing your own food; using the skills of local craftspeople; and even supporting local musicians and artists rather than generic, corporate-sponsored music and art events. Disconnect from celebrity culture, turn off your TV, and connect with your local culture.

Localizing cuts down on waste and pollution, builds local expression, and keeps resources in the community – rather than sending them to investors in distant cities and countries. Localizing includes creating local energy, such as with wind turbines and solar panels.

Walking and biking instead of driving helps communities localize because it reduces dependence on foreign fuel, and keeps money in the community.

When industrial hemp farming is legalized, it will provide a way for people to locally produce paper, fabric, fiberboard, insulation, oil, and fuel using hemp fiber, pulp, cellulose, and seeds. This will protect local forests and wildlife habitat, improve the water and air, and reduce dependence on imported fuel, paper, food, fabric, and building materials. See: VoteHemp.com.

Locavores, Locavores.com
Food Not Lawns, FoodNotLawns.com
KitchenGardeners.org
Slow Food, slowfood.com

John McCabe
Slow Money Alliance, slowmoneyallliance.org
Yards to Gardens, y2g.org

• The Cuba Solution

IN the present day United States we are seeing certain aspects of our economy collapsing. Fuel prices have fluctuated as much as over 100%, food prices have gone risen, and the cost of just about everything has climbed northward faster than we have seen in many decades. Prices of some products and services have risen faster than ever. Many thousands of people are losing their jobs as corporations and government departments cut costs. People are struggling to keep food on their tables. Many people have lost their homes. Unemployment claims are shooting skyward. College tuition has risen, college funding has been slashed, and enrollment has dropped. The U.S. is spending more on prisons than on schools. Large U.S. cities have tens of thousands of homeless living on the streets, under bridges, in parks, in camps, and in shelters.

Although not a perfect example of a solution, Americans can learn a lesson by looking to Cuba and considering how the people in that country responded to their economic collapse.

For many years the Soviet Union was supporting Cuba by purchasing Cuba-grown cane sugar for excessive prices, and often exchanging sugar for food, fuel, and other goods.

When the cold war ended and the wall fell in the 1980s, the Cuban economy collapsed with the disintegration of the Soviet Union. Most of Cuba's food and fuel had been imported. Suddenly they had less than one-third of what had become their normal flow of food, fuel, and cash. They couldn't afford imported goods. Many had no food, and some starved.

That is when Cubans got busy. They turned to home gardening, planting food in every available space. The government gave away plots of land to people who promised to use the land to grow food. Some people created food gardens on their rooftops, and on the roofs of commercial buildings. Plots of land that had become trash dumps were cleaned up and turned into neighborhood farms. The lawns of government buildings, schools, senior housing centers, and apartment complexes were turned into culinary gardens. The Ministry of Agriculture tore up its lawn and turned it into a culinary garden.

From the mid-eighties to the mid-nineties, Cuban food production increased several hundred percent. While they still import a large amount of their food, farmers' markets in Cuba are filled with a variety of homegrown foods and produce from local organic farms. Fresh food improved the health of Cubans. Malnutrition has been greatly reduced as food has become more plentiful. The infant mortality rate has decreased.

While Cuba still imports food products, many Cubans have no question about where they will get their next meal, they simply turn to the culinary gardens in their yards, in pots on their patios, on their rooftops, or in their community gardens.

While they still have much room for improvement, home gardening and localizing their economy benefited Cubans in ways they never considered. It saved people money and built strong communities that are less reliant on stores, distant corporations, foreign products, and foreign fuel. Pollution has decreased as economies have become localized, reducing packaging and fuel use. More money stays within the communities, and less of it is needed.

Because the people could not afford to purchase chemical fertilizers, they naturally learned how to grow food without chemicals, thus becoming organic farmers and gardeners by default. They compost their kitchen, restaurant, and food market scraps into garden soil, returning nutrients to the land. Today, 85% of the food in Cuba is organically grown.

In early 2010, there was some talk that the government would soon permit the operation of private farms on the fallow land previously used for sugar can fields. And the plan is to keep the farms organic. The aim is to reduce imports, making Cuba more self-sufficient. As of 2010, the country was still importing more than 60% of its food. With the new farms, the estimated that they could grow over 70% of the food uses in the largest cities.

At the same time, in the U.S. nearly all kitchen, restaurant, and food market scraps are not composted. Instead, they are sent to landfills and trash dumps.

Today, most U.S. food is grown using toxic farming chemicals that pollute the land, water, air, wildlife, and people.

Today, most children in the U.S. know little or nothing about growing food. Schools that do have gardening programs struggle to survive under budgetary cuts and lack of funding.

Today, nearly everyone in the U.S. relies on stores and restaurants to supply their food, which creates a tremendous amount of waste. The average meal in the U.S. travels over 1,400 miles from farm to plate. This uses enormous amounts of fuel and other resources for transporting, packaging, and marketing the food products. Compounding the problem is the issue of discarded food. In 2007, U.S. supermarkets threw away an estimated $20 billion worth of food. This includes food used for display rather than for sale, food that expires, and food that arrives spoiled or damaged. Even after purchasing food, many people end up throwing as much as half of it away after it expires, is never used, or they order more food than they can eat at restaurants.

The amount of food being imported into the U.S. continues to increase as the population grows and fewer people are involved in growing food. From 1973 to 2008, U.S. food imports rose 78%. The vast majority of that food was grown using synthetic farming chemicals. Some of the chemicals, including fertilizers, pesticides, insecticides, fungicides, and miticides, are so toxic that the U.S. will not allow them to be used within its borders. According to the U.S. Department of Agriculture, imported foods are three times more likely to carry infectious diseases.

People often think of Cuba as a shutoff country living in the dark ages. But their healthcare system, schools, libraries, and food production are all far better than many other countries.

Cuba is also advanced in alternative fuel sources. When the Soviet Union collapsed, so did Cuba's energy imports. Suddenly, they couldn't afford to run their cars, tractors, trucks, and bus systems. People started riding bikes, growing foods, and turned to alternative fuel sources, including solar energy, wind turbines, and biofuels.

> "The use of solar energy has not been opened up because the oil industry does not own the sun."
>
> – Ralph Nader, quoted in Linda Botts, ed., *Loose Talk*, 1980

To reduce electricity use, the Cuban government gave away many thousands of compact fluorescent light bulbs. Today they are turning to LED lights, which last longer, use less energy, and don't contain the toxic mercury that is in compact fluorescent bulbs. They are also beginning to use hybrid solar lighting, which uses a reflective dish and fiber optic cables to bring sunlight into homes and businesses, reducing the use of electricity.

There is no combination of alternative fuels that can sustain the current U.S. use of fuels and energy in an environmentally safe manner. But there are combinations of alternative ways of living that can transform our neighborhoods into more sustainable human communities.

Every step people take toward a more sustainable culture makes a difference in breaking away from the Earth-trashing toxemian culture. Localizing our foods; growing home culinary gardens; composting our kitchen, restaurant, food market, and food manufacturing waste; supporting organic family farms; cutting back on car culture; riding bikes; walking; building monorail systems instead of freeways and subways; using green products; legalizing industrial hemp farming; reducing electricity use and closing coal-fired power plants; using cloth bags instead of paper or plastic; reducing our use of petro-plastic and other petroleum products; using biodegradable botanical soaps; planting fruiting trees; planting and protecting trees and forests; refusing to pollute our land, rivers, lakes, oceans, and air; and protecting our environment and wildlife by turning away from petroleum, coal, and natural gas holds promise for a more sustainable and healthful planet.

In the 1940s Americans planted culinary "victory gardens" to become more independent. By doing this Americans produced nearly 40 percent of their food during that time of war. Today, one of the most effective ways of reducing our carbon footprint is to grow our own food. Because of this, it is time to revive the home food gardening movement, never to let it end. When Michelle Obama and a crew of workers, volunteers, and local school children planted an organic kitchen garden on the White House lawn, it was landmark in awakening a lot of people to what we should all be doing.

Relying on corporations, markets, and restaurants to supply most of our food fails us. The most basic need is for food. Today most Americans have never grown any of their food, and have instead relied on stores and restaurants for their supply. They don't know what most of the food plants look like in their natural environment. Many people hold an attitude that growing a food garden is something beneath them. They have no idea what they are missing out on. Schools would benefit the children by teaching culinary gardening, and parents would benefit their children even more by being involved in growing some food. Every household would benefit by being involved in some aspect of culinary gardening – be it growing food in pots on patios, porches, and rooftops, or replacing lawns with food gardens. All food scraps from every household, restaurant, food market, and food-processing plant should be turned into compost to grow local culinary gardens.

It should no longer be okay and normal to completely rely on corporations for our most basic needs while tossing compostable materials into the trash. It is clear that doing so weakens us, gives up our power, wastes resources, and damages every form of life on Earth.

The way the Cuban people responded to a rapidly collapsing economy by localizing their economy holds lessons for all of us, no matter where we live.

Let us all be involved in transforming our way of living to be sustainable, Earth-friendly, and healthful.

Grow an organic food garden.

> "The more you respect nature, the more she gives to you."
> – Vandana Shiva, author of *Soil Not Oil*

> "The Earth is what we all have in common."
> – Wendell Berry

• Landscaping Rooftops

EVERY product you use has something to do with natural resources and the stream of trash being produced on the planet. Everything from the substances used to produce the product to how the product is manufactured, packaged, shipped, and used impacts the planet.

According to Keith Agroada of Sky Vegetables, the grocery store chains of the U.S. contain over 32,000 acres of space that can be used to grow food. As the roofs sit barren of anything but roofing, the roofs and their accompanying parking lots create "heat islands" and contribute to global warming.

It is time for grocery store chains to get committed to sustainable buildings with green roofs, and parking lots with hanging gardens from their lamps, which can also support solar panels.

Earth Pledge Green Roofs Initiative: EarthPledge.Org
Emory Knoll Farms: GreenRoofPlants.Com
Green Grid Roofs: GreenGridRoofs.Com
Green Roof Directory: GreenRoofs.Com
Green Roofs for Healthy Cities: GreenRoofs.Org
Greening Gotham: GreeningGotham.Org
RoofScapes Inc.: RoofMeadow.Com

• Gardening and Farming

> "Let's not dissect the evils of corporate food – let's feed ourselves! The creation of a garden is as simple as you make it. Be it a barren patch of Earth newly liberated from the smothering embrace of concrete, a rooftop or a porch smattering of five-gallon buckets, it can take any form you desire. Be resourceful! Imagination can manifest square-foot primitive horticulture just about anywhere… Free yourself from wage slavery by eliminating the need to buy some or most of what you eat. Grow enough to feed the nomads among us. Ingesting fresh, native, seasonal plants gives us vibrant health. And how delicious it is to sink our fangs into a succulent squash that we first knew as a seed!"
>
> – The Moment is Ripe, aleksandra, *Earth First! Journal*, Dec.-Jan, 2002

IN addition to wild foods, the best way to get fresh food bursting with nutrients is to grow your own organic food garden.

Growing a food garden is good for the soul, for the mind, for the body, and for your life. Growing and harvesting your own food gives you exercise; connects you with nature; tunes you into the seasons; raises your your frequency; bonds you with your environment; and provides you with the freshest food you can possibly have.

If you live in nearly any town or city you are living on land that was once farmland of some sort. Cities now cover most of the ancient farmland. This is because people originally settled on land that was good for growing food. As the settlements grew into towns and cities, houses, stores, schools, churches, jails, office buildings, streets, and parking lots covered the farmland. By planting food gardens in your area you are bringing back an ancient culture of growing and harvesting food.

> "Today, 58 million Americans spend approximately $30 billion every year to maintain over 23 million acres of lawn. That's an average of over a third of an acre and $517 each. The same-size plot of land could still have a small lawn for recreation, plus produce all the vegetables needed to feed a family of six. The lawns in the United States consume around 270 billion gallons of water a week – enough to water 81 million acres of organic vegetables all summer long.
>
> Lawns use ten times as many chemicals per acre as industrial farmland. These pesticides, fertilizers, and herbicides run off into our groundwater and evaporate into our air, causing widespread pollution and global warming, and greatly increasing our risk of cancer, heart disease, and birth defects. In addition, the pollution emitted from a power mower in just one hour is equal to the amount from a car being driven 350 miles. In fact, lawns use more equipment, labor, fuel, and agricultural toxins than industrial farming, making lawns the largest agricultural sector in the United States. But it's not just the residential lawns that are wasted on grass. There are around 700,000 athletic grounds and 14,500 golf courses in the United States, many of which used to be fertile, productive farmland that was lost to developers when the local markets bottomed out.
>
> Turf is big business: $45 billion-a-year big. The University of Georgia has seven turf researchers studying genetics, soil science, plant pathology, nutrient uptake, and insect management. They issue undergraduate degrees in Turf. The turf industry is responsible for a large sector of the biotech (GMO) industry, and much of the genetic modification that is happening in laboratories across the nation is in the name of an eternally green, slow-growing, moss-free lawn."
>
> – Heather Coburn, author of *Food Not Lawns: How to Turn Your Yard into a Garden and Your Neighborhood into a Community*; FoodNotLawns.org

By growing your food, you reduce pollution because you will be reducing the use of shipping, packaging, marketing, and all of the fuel, paper, plastics, and other resources and processes used to otherwise bring commercial food to your plate.

By maintaining your own organic garden you can feel assured that there are no toxic farming chemicals on your food. Not only will you experience the benefit of getting food as fresh as possible, you will also benefit from food that is nutritionally and energetically stronger than food available at the store.

Chemically grown food is weaker in electrical frequency and has diminished nutritional properties. Studies have shown that organically grown food has a denser reserve of vitamins, minerals, and other nutrients than food that has been grown chemically. Perhaps this is because the organically grown plants have to fend for themselves, and don't rely on chemical fertilizers for nutrients, or depend on chemicals to protect them. Like people who become weak when they are pampered, plants also can become weak if they are grown in an atmosphere where too much is done for them.

In America today about 35 percent of all household water goes to tend lawns. Because there are so many lawns, including those on school campuses, golf courses, cemeteries, and around government buildings and office buildings, and even prisons, the number-one crop being produced in the U.S., and many other countries, is landscape clippings.

> "When you use a manual push mower, you're cutting down on pollution and the only thing in danger of running out of gas is you!"
> – Grey Livingston

It is amazing how much time, energy, money, and water is spent in the U.S. and other wealthy countries to try to keep home lawns green. The people get nothing out of it but a green lawn. They don't have food gardens, even though they have the land to grow them, but instead buy all their food at grocery stores, snack shops, and restaurants. This scenario has helped create the situation that exists today where, on average, the typical meal in the U.S. has traveled 1,250 miles from farm to consumer. This is a terrific waste of resources and causes enormous amounts of pollution.

According to Ted Steinberg, author of *American Green: The Obsessive Quest for the Perfect Lawn*, there are 25 million acres of lawn in America, more land than what is used to grow cotton. To care for those lawns, there are more than 35 million gas-powered lawn mowers, over 25 million leaf blowers, and tons of lawn-treatment chemicals. And all this produces landscape clippings and polluted air, soil, and water. The leaf blowers alone produce more air pollution per engine cylinder than automobiles.

Think of how much better people would be if, instead of spending time, energy, water, and money, and using toxic fertilizers and weed killers to try to keep their lawns green and hedges perfectly trimmed, they would plant organic food gardens, including fruiting trees – and let the rest of the land grow wild and free. Not only would they not spend money and time on landscaping, they would save money on food as well. They would pollute less: A typical lawnmower can use enough gas in an hour to operate a small car for over 50 miles.

The products commonly used to keep a residential lawn green and weed-free contain many toxic chemicals. Glyphosate, a chemical in weed killer, which is poisonous to a variety of plants and wildlife, has been linked to non-Hodgkin's lymphoma, a cancer that is becoming more common. Other lawn chemicals are known to cause breast cancer, birth deformities, and learning disabilities. Lawn chemicals also cause health problems in pets and wildlife. Ironically, the companies that manufacture these toxic chemicals are often the same companies that manufacture cancer drugs.

When used as a well-organized food garden, a small plot of land the size of a common U.S. household lawn can produce more food in a season than a family of four can consume. The result would be that people would be sharing their food with neighbors, family, and friends. The people, their environment, and their community would be healthier.

Growing your own food may be a new concept for those who have lived their lives relying on commercial and restaurant food. It isn't new to a large percentage of the world's population that has always grown some or all their own food. Some countries that have relied on commercial food are now encouraging their citizens to grow more food gardens. Venezuela and Cuba are two countries that have been promoting self-sufficiency through home food gardens. The U.S. hasn't been involved in this type of program since the 1940s. At that time the government encouraged its citizens to grow "victory gardens." That was a revival of what went on during WWI when the U.S. encouraged people to grow "liberty gardens."

Even if you don't grow part, or all, of your own food, you can at least get involved with purchasing foods that have been grown locally. You can find these at your nearest farmers' markets.

You may also obtain locally grown food through "community supported agriculture" (CSA) co-ops that prepay local farmers for produce. This is an idea that began in the 1970s, and has been growing in popularity in Europe, the U.S., and other regions of the world.

Some people have the idea of moving the CSA and organic farming movement into the restaurant food sector. They want to gather people to gather the finances to open co-op vegetarian restaurants that use locally grown produce.

If you live in a city you may find that growing a garden in an abandoned lot to be an awarding experience. Many people have done this throughout the years and it has spurred activism to create and maintain food gardens in the largest cities. The city or other government department may own the land, or it may be privately owned. Many communities have grown food on such land for many years without any problem from the landowner.

When New York's Mayor Giuliani announced that more than 100 city-owned lots where gardens had been planted were to be auctioned off to land developers in the spring of 1999, a citizen's campaign was organized to save the gardens. It was only a last minute arrangement by entertainer Bette Midler and some others that the gardens were saved as they were purchased by the Trust for Public Land.

In Los Angeles a plot of land that contained garden plots maintained by hundreds of families was bulldozed in 2006. The South Central Community Farm was planted with an enormous variety of food and medicinal plants and trees. It came into existence after the riots that took place after the 1992 Rodney King verdict. Originally purchased by the city through the eminent domain process, the city had planned to build trash incinerators on the site. The local community spoke out against this plan. The Concerned Citizens of South Central organized protests and the city eventually canceled their plan to build the incinerators. After the riots the city offered the land as space for community gardens. Many of the farmers were people who had moved to Los Angeles from Central and South America. As the years went by the farming gardens became a center of community with generations of families involved in planting and maintaining their gardens. Then, the person who originally owned the land wanted it back. In 2003 the land was transferred back to the original owner, who had plans to build warehouses on the property. As time passed, lawsuits were filed and the community organized protests. By the spring of 2006 the future of the farm was dismal. Community activists gathered to maintain a 24/7 presence. Julia Butterfly Hill, who once famously lived in a redwood tree for two years to save it from a lumber company, joined Darryl Hannah and other activists who camped in the farm. Finally, on a June morning hundreds of riot police were brought in to evict the protestors. Some, including Darryl Hannah, who were camping in a tree, were handcuffed and taken away. In the end the landowner won, bulldozing the gardens and placing people back in line at the supermarkets to purchase their food.

Wherever you are, get involved in growing some of your own food. If you don't have land, borrow some, or use pots, a roof, or window boxes. Be sure to plant some native flower species so that your garden attracts native bees and other helpful insects.

When you look for plants and seeds to plant in your garden, seek out those that have been organically grown, and that have not been genetically altered. You also may want to try "open pollinated" "heirloom" seeds, which have not been hybridized, and that can provide a better variety of food plants. Look into planting some food plants that you have never heard of.

There are many organizations involved in getting people to grow their own food. From the Slow Food movement that started in Italy to protest McDonald's opening at Rome's Spanish Steps in 1986, to city farming activists and organizations like Food Not Lawns, to EdibleSchoolyard.org, there is likely an organization that is near you and/or can help you get into growing food – and start your disconnect from total reliance on stores and restaurants.

Acres: The Voice for Eco-Agriculture, Austin, TX, 78709; 512-892-4400; AcresUSA.com. Sells books on organic gardening and farming.

Alternative Farming Systems Information Center, Community Supported Agriculture, NAL.USDA.gov/AFSIC/CSA

American Community Gardening Association, Council on the Environment, 51 Chambers St., Ste. 228; New York, NY 10007; CommunityGarden.org

American Farmland Trust, 1200 18th St., NW, Washington, DC 20036; Farmland.org

AppleLuscious Organic Orchards, AppleLuscious.com

Australian Community Gardens Network, communitygarden.org.au.

Avant Gardening, Avant-Gardening.com

Barefoot Farmer, BarefootFarmer.com

Big Barn, BigBarn.co.uk

Bio-Integral Resource Center, IGC.org

Black Farmers and Agriculturists Association, POB 61, Tillery, NC 27887; BFAA-US.org

Bountiful Gardens, 18001 Shafer Ranch Rd., Willits, CA 95490-9626; 707-459-6410; BountifulGardens.org

California Certified Organic Farmers, POB 8136, Santa Cruz, CA 95061; CCOF.org

California Rare Fruit Growers, CRFG.org

Canadian Organic Growers, COG.ca

Center for Food and Justice, 323-341-5099; Departments.Oxy.edu/UEPI/CFJ

Center for Informed Food Choices, InformedEating.org

Center for Rural Affairs, POB 136, Lyons, NE 68038-0136; CFRA.org

Center for Vegan Organic Education, POB 13217, Burton, WA 98013; 206-463-4520; VeganOrganicEd.org

City Farmer, Canada's Office of Urban Agriculture, Box 74561, Kitsilano RPO, Vancouver, BC V6K 4P4; Canada; CityFarmer.org

City Food Growers, Australia; cityfoodgrowers.com.au

City Repair Project, POB 42615, Portland, OR 97242; CityRepair.org

Coalition of Immokalee Workers, POB 603, Immokalee, FL 34143; CIW-Online.org

Common Ground Garden Program, CELosAngeles.UCDavis.edu/Garden

Community Farm Alliance, 614 Shelby St., Frankfurt, KY 40601; CommunityFarmAlliance.org

Community Food Security Coalition, Venice, CA; FoodSecurity.org. Site contains listings of community gardening and urban farming resources.

The Cornucopia Institute, POB 126, Cornucopia, WI 54827; Cornucopia.org

CSA California, csacalifornia.org. Community Supported Agriculture is one way of supporting local farmers. Some may provide boxes or bags of locally-grown produce that you pick up once a week at your farmers' market, at another location, or that gets delivered to you.

Desert Harvesters, DesertHarversters.org

Dirty Girl Produce, Santa Cruz, CA; dirtygirlproduce.com. An organic produce farm.
Eat Grub, EatGrub.org
Earth Works Gardens, 1820 Mount Elliot, Detroit, MI 48207; Earth-Works.org
Eat the View, England, Countryside.gov.UK/LAR/Landscape/ETV/Index.asp
Ecological Farming Association, Watsonville, CA; Eco-Farm.org
Edible Estates Initiative, FritzHaeg.Com/Garden/Initiatives/EdibleEstates/Main.html
Edible Forest Gardens, EdibleForestGardens.com
Edible Schoolyard, EdibleSchoolyard.org
Environmental Working Group, 1436 U Street NW, Ste. 100, Washington DC 20009; EWG.org
Fair Trade Resource Network, POB 33772, Washington, DC 20033-3772; FairTradeResource.org
Family Farm Defenders, POB 1772, Madison, WI 53701; FamilyFarmDefenders.org
Farm Aid, 11 Ward St., Ste. 200, Somerville, MA 02143; FarmAid.org
Farmers' Legal Action Group, 360 N. Robert St., Ste. 500, St. Paul, MN 55101; FLAGInc.org
Farming Solutions, FarmingSolutions.org
Farm Labor Organizing Committee, 1221 Broadway St., Toledo, OH 43609; FLOC.com
Farm to Consumer Legal Defense Fund, FarmToConsumer.org
Farm Worker Justice Fund, 1010 Vermont Ave., NW, Ste. 915, Washington, DC 20005; FWJustice.org
FedCo Co-op Garden Supplies, POB 520, Waterville, ME 04903; 207-873-7333; fedcoseeds.com
Food First, Institute for Food and Development Policy, 398 60th St., Oakland, CA; FoodFirst.org
Food Not Bombs, POB 424, Arroyo Seco, NM 87514; 800-884-1136; FoodNotBombs.net
Food Not Lawns, POB 42174, Eugene, OR 97404; FoodNotLawns.com
The Food Project, POB 705, Lincoln, MA 01773; TheFoodProject.org
Free Wheelin Farm, Santa Cruz, CA; freewheelinfarm.com/home.html
The Future of Food, TheFutureOfFood.com
Garden Project, GardenProject.org
Garden Valley Seed Trust, GardenValleySeedTrust.org
Global Exchange, 2017 Mission St., 303, San Francisco, CA 94110; GlobalExchange.org
Going Organic, GoingOrganic.com
Goode Green, goodegreennyc.com. Green rooftop design and installation.
Green Earth Institute, Illinois; greenearthinstitute.org
Green Grid Roofs, greengridroofs.com
Green Guerillas, New York, NY; GreenGuerillas.org. Helping establish community gardens.
Green People, GreenPeople.org. Site contains a list of companies that sell organic seeds.
Green Roofs, greenroofs.org
Growing Gardens, 2003 NE 42nd Ave., #3, Portland, OR 97213; Growing-Gardens.org
Growing Power, 5500 W. Silver Spring Rd., Milwaukee, WI 53218; GrowingPower.org
Guerrilla Gardening, GuerrillaGardening.org. A group of people in London who have late night planting parties to enliven previously neglected small plots of city land.
Heirloom Gardening Newsletter, 203-354-8756; HeirloomGardening.com
Home Orchard Society, HomeOrchardSociety.org

Institute for Community Economics, 57 School St., Springfield, MA 01105; ICECLT.org

International Confederation of Autonomous Chapters of the American Indian Movement, AmericanIndianMovement.org

International Culinary Tourism Association, 4110 SE Hawthorne Blvd., #440, Portland, OR 97214; CulinaryTourism.org

International Society for Ecology & Culture, ISEC.org.uk

Island Seed and Feed, Goleta, CA; IslandSeed.com

Kings Hill Farm, Wisconsin; kingshillfarm.com. An organic produce farm.

KitchenGardeners.org

The Land Institute, 2440 E. Water Well Rd., Salina, KS 67401; LandInstitute.org

Land Stewardship Project, 2200 4th St., White Bear Lake, MN 55110; LandStewardshipProject.org

Land Trust Alliance, 1331 H St., NW, Ste. 400, Washington, DC 20005; LTA.org

Leopold Center for Sustainable Agriculture, Iowa State University; Leopold.IAState.edu

Linking Environment and Farming, England; LeafMarque.com/LEAF

Local Harvest, LocalHarvest.org

Local Harvest, Santa Cruz, CA; LocalHarvest.org. Searchable database of farmers' markets, small farms, and related groups and businesses.

Lost Valley Educational Center, LostValley.org

Maine Organic Farmers and Gardeners Association, POB 170, Unity, ME 04988; MOFGA.org

Mindfully, Mindfully.org/Farm

Mindfully, Mindfully.org/Food

More Gardens Coalition, 376 E. 162nd St., #2, Bronx, NY 10451; MoreGardens.org

Mountain Gardens, MountainGardensHerbs.com. A botanical garden featuring the largest collection of native Appalachian and Chinese medicinal herbs in the eastern U.S.

Mycorrhizal Applications, Mycorrhizae.com. Information on beneficial fungi that improves soil health, plant health, and crop yields.

National Coalition for Pesticide-Free Lawns, BeyondPesticides.org/PesticideFreeLawns/DoorHanger/Index.htm. This organization offers door tags you can put on your neighborhood doors encouraging people to stop using pesticides on their lawns. The first 50 are free, and they ask only for a donation to handle the postage. You can also purchase more.

National Family Farm Coalition, 110 Maryland Ave., NE, Ste. 307; Washington, DC 20002; NFFC.net

National Farm to School Program, Center for Food and Justice, Occidental College, Los Angeles, CA; FarmToSchool.org

National Farm Transition Network, FarmTransition.org

National Immigrant Farming Initiative, 88 Atlantic Ave., #8, Brooklyn, NY 11201; ImmigrantFarming.org

Native Seeds, NativeSeeds.org

New England Small Farm Institute, 275 Jackson St., Belchertown, MA 01007; SmallFarm.org

New Farm, NewFarm.org. Sponsored by the Rodale Institute. Community Supported Agriculture information.

New World Publishing, Auburn, CA 95602; NWPub.net. Books on small-scale farming.

North American Fruit Explorers, NAFEX.org

North American Native Plant Society, NANPS.org

Northeast Organic Farming Association, Barre, MA; NOFA.org
Northern Nut Growers Association, ICSERV.com/NNGA/Index.html
Oakhill Organics, Dayton, OR; oakhillorganics.org. A 17-acre certified organic produce farm,
Organic Volunteers, OrganicVolunteers.org
Oregon Tilth, Tilth.org
Organic Gardening **magazine**, OrganicGardening.com
Osborn International Seed Co., osbornseed.com
Pennsylvania Association for Sustainable Agriculture, POB 419, Millheim, PA 16854; PASAFarming.org
Permaculture Institute, PortlandPermaculture.com
Pesticide Action Network, San Francisco, CA; PANNA.org
Planet Natural, 1612 Gold Ave., Bozeman, MT 59715; 800-289-6656; 406-587-5891; PlanetNatural.com
Plan Organic, PlanOrganic.com
Plants for a Future, 1 Lerryn View, Cornwall, United Kingdom; PFAF.org
Portland City Repair Project, CityRepair.org
Portland Permaculture Institute, PortlandPermaculture.com
Pro Active Ecology, ProActiveEcology.org
Real Goods RealGoods.com
Resource Centres on Urban Agriculture and Food Security, RUAF.org
Robin Van En Center for Community Supported Agriculture; Center for Sustainable Living, Wilson College, Chambersburg, PA; CSACenter.org
Roof Meadow, roofmeadow.com
Rooftop Farms, rooftopfarms.org
Sacred Earth Institute, SacredEarthInstitute.org
Safe Food and Fertilizer, SafeFoodAndFertilizer.org
Salt Springs Seeds, SaltSpringsSeeds.com
San Francisco League of Urban Gardeners (SLUG), Grass-Roots.org/USA/Slug.shtml
Seasonal Chef, SeasonalChef.com
Seattle Tilth Association, 4649 Sunnyside Ave. North, Rm. 120, Seattle, WA 98103; SeattleTilth.org
Seeds of Change, POB 15700, Santa Fe, NM 15700; 888-762-7333; SeedsOfChange.com
Seeds of Diversity, Seeds.ca/EN.php
Seedsaving and Seedsavers' Resources, Homepage.Eircom.net/%7Emerlyn/SeedSaving.html
Seed Savers Australia, seedsavers.net
Seed Savers Exchange, SeedSavers.org
Seed Savers Network, Australia; SeedSavers.net
Seeds Trust, Seedstrust.com
The School of Self Reliance, Los Angeles, CA; Self-Reliance.net
Slow Food, SlowFood.com
Slow Food USA, SlowFoodUSA.org
Small Farm Association, England, Small-Farms-Association.co.uk
Snow Seed Organic, 831-758-9869; SnowSeedCo.com
Soil and Health Library, SoilAndHealth.org
Soil Food Web, Inc., SoildFoodWeb.com
South Central Farmers, SouthCentralFarmers.com
Sow Organic Seed, POB 527, Williams, OR 97544; 888-709-7333; OrganicSeed.com

Spiral Gardens Community Food Security Project, 2880 Sacramento, St., Berkeley, CA 94702; SpiralGardens.org
SunFowFarm, SunBowFarm.org
Sustainable Food, SustainableFood.com
Sustainable Table, New York, NY; SustainableTable.org
Sustain: The Alliance for Better Farming and Food, London, UK; SustainWeb.org
Tilth Producers, Washington; tilthproducers.org. Organic and sustainable farming association.
Toledo Garden, ToledoGarden.org
True Food Now Campaign, Greenpeace USA, TrueFoodNow.org
Trust for Public Land, 116 New Montgomery St., 4th Flr., San Francisco, CA 94105; TPL.org
United Plant Savers, UnitedPlantSavers.org
Via Comesina, ViaCampesina.org
Virginia Association for Biological Farming, Lexington, VA, VABF.org
Virginia Independent Consumers and Farmers Association, POB 915, Charlottesville, VA 22902; VICFA.net
Washington State University's Organic Agriculture Program, 888-468-6978; World-Class.WSU.edu/2006/Organic/Index.html. In 2006 Washington State University became the first university in the U.S. to offer a major in organic agriculture.
White Earth Land Recovery Project, 32033 E. Round Lake Rd., Ponsford, MN 54575; NativeHarvest.com
Wild Food Adventure, WildFoodAdventures.com
Willing Workers on Organic Farms, OrganicVolunteers.org
Women, Food, and Agriculture Network, 59624 Chicago Rd., Atlantic, IA 50022; WFAN.org
World Social Forum, Rua General Jardin, 660, 8th Flr., Sao Paulo, SP 01223-010; Brazil; WorldSocialForum.org
Worldwide Opportunities on Organic Farms, WWOOF.org
Worm Digest, POB 2654, Grants Pass, OR 97528; WormDigest.org
Yards to Gardens, y2g.org
Zenger Farm, ZengerFarm.org

• THE PLIGHT OF THE FAMILY FARMERS

> "Family farms are an important part of the American tradition of self-sufficiency, forming the bedrock for communities across the U.S.
>
> Since 1935, the U.S. has lost 4.7 million farms. Fewer than one million Americans now claim farming as a primary occupation.
>
> Farmers in 2002 earned their lowest real net cash income since 1940. Meanwhile, corporate agribusiness profits have nearly doubled (increased 98 percent) since 1990.
>
> Large corporations increasingly dominate U.S. food production. … Encourage your local grocery store and area restaurants to purchase more of their products from local farmers."
>
> – FoodRoutes.Org, 2006

THERE was once a time when families ran the farms. They would work the land, grow a variety of fruits and vegetables, rotate the crops to manage a healthy soil, maintain seed supplies, and sell their produce to the markets.

More recently, farms in the U.S., as well as an increasing number of farms in other parts of the world, have been and are being taken over by multinational corporations worth billions of dollars and that control many levels of the food manufacturing and distribution processes. These monolithic companies take over land, demolish forests, and turn what were once may family polycrop (a variety of crops) farms into one massive, intensive monocropping (single crop) complex. They also contract with land-owning farmers and dictate that farmers grow crops using GMO seeds and toxic chemicals, and also determine how much farmers get for the harvest.

This has created a nightmare for family farmers, some of whom find themselves dealing with depression, life-threatening stress-related illnesses, and suicidal tendencies as they witness multigenerational farm life come to an abrupt halt. The family farm may have been all they and generations before them had ever known. A farmer can experience deep anguish when the farm is taken away instead of it being handed on to the next generation.

In the U.S., one reason the destruction of the farm community has taken place is because the government has been foreclosing on farmer loans and because laws formed under the influence of lobbyist pressure have made it easier for corporations to take over. The result is that several multinational corporations, such as Cargill, Continental Grain, Archer Daniels Midland, Bayer CropScience, and Monsanto now control much of the global food supply.

Mental depression related to economic stress among farmers is such a problem that one of the leading causes of death among farmers has been suicide. In 2003, the U.S. farmer suicide rate was five times the national average. Farmers sometimes make their deaths appear accidental so that their families can collect insurance to pay off family farming debts. Other countries have also been experiencing large numbers of farmer suicides. In India there have been thousands of suicides among farmers.

Kyung-Hae Lee, a farmer who was president of the Korean Advanced Farmers Federation, killed himself with a knife as a form of protest at the World Trade Organization's convention held in Cancun, Mexico on September 10, 2003. He had written about the plight of the family farm and how "undesirable globalization" of multinational corporations is ruining the environment and killing farmers.

Farming in the U.S. changed rapidly starting in the Depression and Dustbowl periods. The government drew up a plan to help farmers by paying subsidies to those involved in growing corn, cotton, wheat, soybeans, and other crops under the farm subsidy program. Part of this involved paying farmers not to grow crops, or to destroy crops rather than to flood the market.

While the farm subsidy program may have been designed to keep family farmers in business, it quickly switched gears to benefit large industrialized agricultural businesses. These corporations began creating large, single-crop farms consisting of thousands of acres. This robbed the soil of nutrients, creating weaker plants susceptible to infestation. To improve crop harvests farms began using tremendous amounts of synthetic pesticides, fertilizers, and other chemicals made out of toxic substances developed during the World Wars.

The farm subsidy program turned into what is referred to as "corporate welfare" for the large agribusinesses. Today about 75 percent of the subsidies go to large corporate agribusinesses. These corporations rely on billions of dollars in U.S. government subsidies every year to support their damaging business practices. The huge amounts of food they produce flood the world market, putting the food on the market for less than it took to grow it, and less than what farmers in other countries can get for their own crops – ruining the livelihood of farmers globally.

The glut in American-produced grains and cottons has a negative impact on farmers and farm communities throughout the world that would be doing much better if this U.S. farm subsidy program were not so abused by corporate agriculture. Because of these subsidies, the corporations flourish, but the family farmers suffer, as does the environment from corporate farming practices relying on chemicals.

In another way industrial agriculture subsidies also affect people of the inner cities of the U.S. When ways of cutting the budget of the U.S. Department of Agriculture are considered, often it isn't the farm subsidies that are the focus, but another part of the USDA, the school lunch programs – which largely serve corporate-farmed food.

Cities around the world are affected by the industrialization of agriculture. When farmers lose their farms, they often move to larger communities, such as large cities. Often they travel to other countries to find a better way of life than what they are presented with in their local towns, where many often end up working in factories producing products sold to wealthier countries. In the cities the immigrants become members of the working poor. In the country they often end up working as laborers for the industrial farms, for the factory animal farms, and for slaughterhouses. Some join the military to gain citizenship.

The corporate agribusinesses have a big influence on what the government does because these businesses often give donations to politicians and to political parties favoring the corporations. These corporations feed off and perpetuate the lie that writer George Pyle talks about in his book, *Raising Less Corn, More Hell: The Case for the Independent Farm and Against Industrial Food.* It is the lie that the industrial agribusiness corporations are going to save the world from a food shortage. In truth, it is those corporations involved in industrial farming and the genetic engineering of food plants that are playing a major role in the world food problems, and especially in the problems being faced by family farmers and the environment surrounding them.

Rather than flooding the Third World countries with an overabundance of crops from American corporate farms, it would be better for the farmers to grow their own crops. If you give a person a piece of food, that person can eat for a day. If they are able to grow it, they can eat for a lifetime. The USDA doesn't seem to support this idea and keeps on promoting the idea that we need to bring more money into big business agriculture by exporting more and more crops.

On multiple levels the U.S. government has been no friend to family farmers – both domestically and internationally.

Historically, African-American farmers have had a rougher time of it than their lighter-skinned neighbors. The promise of land and a mule that was made when the slaves were freed never materialized. Throughout the years African-American farmers have been much less likely to benefit from government programs set up to help farmers. In 1999 a lawsuit was settled between the USDA and a group of African-American farmers in which a history of discrimination was acknowledged. But few have received any part of that settlement.

For many years, Japanese-Americans couldn't even own farmland. If they wanted to farm they had to rent land. Compounding the deprivation, many of them had lost the rented farmland they were operating when they were forced into internment camps during World War II.

Not to be overlooked are the Native peoples, not only in what is now the U.S., but indigenous peoples on every continent, and on many islands. Indigenous peoples the world over have been forced from their lands, which was then given to or sold to others, or kept by the new government. Some who have been allowed to keep their land have been taxed at stiff rates and/or subject to laws and regulations that create unreasonable hardship. Others who have had their prime farmland taken away have been moved to land difficult or impossible to farm.

More recently, many U.S. farmers went into debt to the federal government because the Farm Home Administration counseled farmers to take out loans in the 1970s when the value of the farms was inflating faster than the interest rates. Then the government raised interest rates on the farmers and foreclosed on family farms at record levels.

Under the massive takeover of farms by multinational corporations, family farmers are struggling to maintain and update equipment to pay for water, to keep up with packing fees, to pay for labor and transportation, and to compete with pricing. This is a driving force in the formation of rural groups that have found good reason to mistrust the government.

In addition to losing their farms to the corporate farming industry takeover, farmers have been selling out to housing developers who offer more money for the farmland than the farm can make in several years of operating at a tight budget. So the housing tracts get built on the farmland and the streets are given pleasant country names like Wildflower Lane, Cherry Orchard Court, and Apple Blossom Road.

Some U.S. farmers have moved to other countries, including Brazil where they have started *fazendas* (Portuguese for farms). They arrive with the belief that the land there will be the next leader in world produce. What they are finding is land that costs a fraction of the farming land in the U.S. There, among the tens of millions of acres in Brazil's interior, with a long and favorable season, farmers can grow a wide assortment of crops, including bananas and tropical fruits as well as coffee and sugar. While corn is being used to make ethanol in the U.S., sugar cane in Brazil is a common crop used in producing the fuel. Brazil is the world's second-largest producer of soybeans, much of which goes to feed livestock in Brazil, and is exported to feed livestock in other countries. Animal farming is huge business in Brazil, which has about 70 million cattle and an even larger population of chickens. The country exports about three billion dollars worth of beef per year to countries around the world, much of it raised on illegally-cleared rainforest land. It is a country that has an enormous export industry supplying the world food market. Unfortunately, the farmers relocating from the U.S. also are finding the same multinational farming companies working their way into the Brazilian farming industry, promoting their toxic farming chemicals, and making big plans for expansion with mechanized mono-crop farming that employs very few people. Much of this farming is being done on land that was bulldozed, chainsawed, burned, or otherwise cleared of pristine rainforest – displacing indigenous peoples, fragmenting the land, drying out surrounding forests, inducing droughts, and decimating wildlife. Cultural and language differences can require some adjustment and learning for farmers moving to new lands. Other problems include people illegally harvesting crops; labor contracting problems; squatters; hired guns; illegal logging operations; an unreliable infrastructure; a different tax structure; dishonesty in suppliers, processors, and land sales and leasing; and government bureaucracy.

Those considering a move to distant lands to start a farm may want to stay put and move toward a different way of doing business.

Some U.S. farmers have found that cooperative selling and food processing organizations are a way to do business and increase income security. Under NGCs (New Generation Cooperatives), farmers join in and own food processing and marketing associations. Under CSA (Community-Supported Agriculture), member consumers, often from nearby towns and cities, buy into the upcoming season of vegetables and fruits grown on particular farms. It is "subscription farming," and it is helping small farmers, localizing what people eat, improving nutrition, reducing pollution, and creating sustainable agriculture. More and more farmers are finding the growing demand for organically grown produce to be a way to create a brighter future for their small farms.

When you purchase organic foods, purchase non-GMO foods, purchase locally grown produce, and shop at farmers' markets, you are more likely to be supporting small farms, and less likely to be supporting the companies that have taken over family farms.

Becoming a member of a CSA is one sure way to support family farmers as well as to get food that is both locally and organically grown.

While traveling I spoke with some residents of Eugene, Oregon, who were planning to organize themselves into an organic CSA by turning the yards of at least a dozen homes into food gardens growing a variety of produce. They planned on selling their produce to local residents and restaurants as well as at farmers' markets. That is a wonderful idea, and a great way to both eliminate wasteful lawns and become independent from corporate farms. By creating a local CSA and growing their own food, they will improve their environment, their health, and their community.

• Farmers' Market Locators

FARMERS' street markets provide direct access to produce grown on family farms in your region.

By shopping with a biodegradable cloth bag and purchasing whole, locally-grown foods, you are eliminating packaging and the use of global food transportation, which uses enormous amounts of fossil fuels and other resources.

Australian Farmers' Markets Association, farmersmarkets.org.au. Lists farmers' markets throughout Australia.

CSA California, csacalifornia.org. Community Supported Agriculture is one way of supporting local farmers. Some may provide boxes or bags of locally-grown produce that you pick up once a week at your farmers' market, at another location, or that gets delivered to you.

Farm Direct Co-op, FarmDirectCoop.org. A Massachusetts cooperative of three hundred fifty members who receive locally grown produce. Their example of how to run a farm co-op can be duplicated in other regions.

Farmers' Market, FarmersMarket.com

Farmers' Market Finder: search.ams.usda.gov/farmersmarkets

Food Routes, FoodRoutes.org

Local Foods, localfoods.org.uk/local-food-directory. For finding farmers' markets in the UK.

Local Harvest, LocalHarvest.org

London Farmers' Markets, lfm.org.uk

Pick Your Own, PickYourOwn.org. Lists farms in a growing number of countries where you can harvest your own produce. Blake2007 (at) PickYourOwn.org

> "One of the problems is that the government supports unhealthy food and does very little to support healthy food. I mean, we subsidize high fructose corn syrup. We subsidize hydrogenated corn oil. We do not subsidize organic food. We subsidize four crops that are the building blocks of fast food. And you also have to work on access. We have food deserts in our cities. We know that the distance you live from a supplier of fresh produce is one of the best predictors of your health. And in the inner city, people don't have grocery stores. So we have to figure out a way of getting supermarkets and farmers markets into the inner cities."
>
> – Michael Pollan

• NATURAL FOODS STORE LOCATORS

Australian Farmers' Markets Association, farmersmarkets.org.au. Lists farmers' markets throughout Australia.

CoOpDirectory.org

FoodRoutes.org

Organic Consumers Association, OrganicConsumers.org. For a list of natural foods stores, including co-ops and buying clubs, click on "find organics."

Veg Project, 4547 E. 16yth Ave., Denver, CO 80220; 303-399-6479; kindle (at) vegproject.org; VegProject.org. Veg restaurant collective. The site contains listings of vegetarian restaurants. It was started by Kindle Fahlenkamp-Morell. Also runs veggietrip.com, which contains information about vegetarian restaurants around the world.

• VEGETARIAN RESTAURANT LOCATORS

IN addition to the restaurants and cafes listed below that are serving raw cuisine, the following Web sites provide information about vegetarian restaurants around the planet:

Happy Cow, HappyCow.net

Mercy for Animals' vegetarian restaurant guide, VegGuide.org

Raw Food Planet, RawFoodPlanet.com

Soy Stache, SoyStache.com

Vegan Steven, VeganSteven.com

Vegetarian Resource Group, VRG.Org

Vegetarian Restaurants, Vegetarian-Restaurants.Net

Veggie Trip, veggietrip.com

• Organic Foods

"We are witnessing a massive corporate genocide - the killing of people for super profits. To maintain these super profits, lies are told about how, without pesticides and genetically modified organisms (GMOs), there will be no food. In fact, the conclusions of International Assessment of Agricultural Science and Technology for Development, undertaken by the United Nations, shows that ecologically organic agriculture produces more food and better food at lower cost than either chemical agriculture or GMOs."

– Vandana Shiva, *The Killing Fields Of Multi-National Corporations*, The *Asian Age*, July 14th, 2010. VandanaShiva.org

"Organic farming and ranching not only uses less fossil fuel and emits fewer climate-disrupting gases, but can actually clean greenhouse gas pollution from the atmosphere; while at the same time feeding the world, improving public health, and restoring biodiversity. If we can move the world's 12 billion acres of farm and ranch lands into a transition to organic, and preserve and restore our 10 billion acres of forests, at least 50ppm of CO_2 can be drawn down from the atmosphere and stored naturally and safely in the soil. This is literally the difference between present and future climate stability or climate hell. Organic soil and land management can and must be scaled up now in order to buy us the time we need to make the long-term transition to radical energy efficiency and solar, wind, and geothermal power.

Obviously this Great Organic Transition is not going to be easy. Our energy-, chemical-, and GM-intensive food and farming system needs to shift from one where 125,000 megafarms produce 75% of the food, to a mass movement of millions of farmers, ranchers, and urban gardeners growing organic food for their local communities. Factory farms and feedlots belching methane and nitrous oxide must be phased out. Twenty-four billion pounds of synthetic nitrogen fertilizer needs to be replaced with organic compost and compost tea derived from food and yard waste.

This Great Transition will require a massive shift in public consciousness to wake up the majority of the population who are being force-fed a nutrition-poor diet of genetically engineered junk food and animal products."

– Organic Consumers Association; OrganicConsumers.org

MANY studies have found that organically grown foods contain more nutrients than what is in the same foods that are grown using farming chemicals. A study by the University of California, Davis found that organic tomatoes contain two times the amount of flavonoids. Organically grown fruits and vegetables also grow stronger, and are less likely to be susceptible to pest infestation. In other words, conventionally grown foods are weaker, less vibrant, and provide fewer nutrients.

Every minute enormous quantities of toxic pesticides, fertilizers, fungicides, insecticides, miticides, and other agricultural chemicals are being spread over farmland throughout the world. These chemicals are known to cause birth defects, hormonal imbalances, learning disabilities, cancers and other diseases in both humans and wildlife. Farming and industrial chemicals also accumulate in water, poisoning it, and resulting in large areas of the seas that are void of natural life. Inland, there are people who are told not to drink the tap water because it contains such high levels of chemical fertilizers that drinking the water can cause brain damage.

Low-paid farm laborers are exposed to toxic farming chemicals, and often get sick from them. Many farm workers have no idea what the dangers are of the chemicals they are being exposed to. For example, the fumigant chloropicrin that is used on farms contains the same active ingredient as tear gas. A chemical called Nemagon had been used for decades on sugar cane, pineapple, and banana farms. It caused cancers and a variety of terrible ailments in the farm workers. Women repeatedly exposed to it had miscarriages and stillbirths, and their babies that lived often were born with horrible deformities. Today there are similar chemicals being used that are poisoning workers on farms around the planet. When farm workers who are exposed to toxic chemicals do get sick they may not know what caused it. If they are able to visit a nurse or doctor they may be misdiagnosed, or their concerns are dismissed or become lost in translation. Long-term exposure can result in numerous health problems in the workers and in their children.

Farming chemicals damage soil organisms, such as mycorrhizal soil fungi, which play a major role in soil health and help plant root systems obtain nutrients and water from the soil. There are many hundreds of trillions of natural chemical reactions taking place in a handful of soil as various forms of microorganisms live and interact through their life processes. If the genetically engineered plants and/or various toxic chemicals produced by industries begin to kill soil organisms or lead to a bacteria that largely damages or kills soil organisms, it could stop all plants from growing. If the obscene development of genetically engineered food plants isn't bad enough, there are companies that are developing genetically engineered bacteria. This should be stopped.

> "The amount of pesticides and non-organic fertilizers used in farming today is shocking, and it is being ingested by us and Earth

and damaging us both – for example, conventional strawberries use 300 pounds of synthetic pesticides, herbicides, fertilizer, and fungicides per acre."

– Terces Engelhart, co-author with Orchid of *I Am Grateful: Recipes & Lifestyle of Café Gratitude*; CafeGratitude.com

"Many new studies prove we can grow more food per acre on small organic farms than big chemically addicted agribusiness farms and that organic food is more nutrition than industrial food, so a lot of what we know instinctively is now backed by science. Which is great. What is good for our bodies and our communities is good for the planet."

– Deborah Koons Garcia, director of the documentaries *The Future of Food* and *In Good Heart: Soil and the Mystery of Fertility*

"GMOs (genetically modified organisms = genetically engineered foods) can't beat the capacity of organics for restoration, resilience, and abundance. Organic agriculture is the best way to remove billions of tons of greenhouse gases from the atmosphere and safely sequester them for centuries in the living soil of organic farms, pastures, and rangelands. If all the world's cropland were transitioned to organic, it would sequester 40% of current greenhouse gas emissions. Organic systems also produce higher yields than GMOs and are more resistant to droughts, floods, diseases and pests.

The organic solution to the climate crisis is threatened by contamination from GMOs. Organic agriculture relies on the diversity and resilience of the thousands of varieties of crops and food animals that humans have cultivated for every soil and climate on Earth. GMOs, also known as "recombinant DNA." are bizarre combinations of foreign genes forcefully inserted into "host organisms" from different species. Once you insert foreign genes into a food crop or animal, these mutant varieties breed and reproduce. These GE mutations are likely permanent, meaning that it is only a matter of time before natural and organic varieties are contaminated with GMO traits."

– The Organic Consumers Association

Beyond Pesticides, BeyondPesticides.org
Bioneers, Bioneers.org
Co-op Directory, coopdorectory.org
Food Consumer, foodconsumer.org
Farm to Consumer Legal Defense Fund, FarmToConsumer.org
Gardenerd, gardenerd.com
Local Harvest, localharvest.org/store/local-csa.jsp
Monsanto Watch, MonsantoWatch.org
Non-GMO Shopping Guide, nongmoshoppingguide.com
Occupy Monsanto, OccupyMonsanto360.org

Organic Consumers Association, OrganicConsumers.org
Organic Foodee, OrganicFoodee.com
Organic Its Worth It, organicitsworthit.org
Organic Seed Alliance, SeedAlliance.org
Pesticide Action Network, PANNA.org
Real Food Challenge, RealFoodChallenge.org
Rodale Institute, RodaleInstitute.org
Say No to GMOs, SayNoToGMOs.org
The War on Bugs, TheWarOnBugsBook.com
Worldwide Opportunities on Organic Farms, WWOOF.org

• FAIR TRADE

"The Organic Consumers Association (OCA) launched the Fair World Project (FWP) in September 2010 to promote fair trade in commerce, especially in organic production systems in developing countries as well as at home, and to protect the term 'fair trade' from dilution and misuse for mere PR purposes. The OCA's new project fills the critical need for a watchdog of misleading fair trade claims, and a cheerleader for dedicated fair trade mission-driven companies. Through FWP, OCA will focus on promoting projects that connect the environmental and health benefits of organic agriculture with the social benefits derived from fair trade.

'As demand from conscious consumers expands the market for fairly traded products we must ensure that claims made by companies hold up to fair trade standards and that marketing and labeling of these products are accurate,' says Dana Geffner, Executive Director of the Fair World Project. 'With new fair trade certifiers joining the movement, seasoned certifiers enabling questionable opportunistic fair trade claims and 'fair-washing' practices more common, the Fair World Project aims to discuss and dissect,' adds Geffner.

The FWP intends to encourage critical thinking rather than blind faith regarding fair trade claims and certification schemes. Through publications, events, and targeted campaigns the group articulates and advances the issues involved in fair trade, with the goal of helping consumers, business owners, employees and activists make informed decisions about where and on what to spend their money and resources - to build a better and more just world. The FWP's new website provides a space and forum where consumers can discuss issues within the Fair Trade movement, ask tough questions and share information.

According to Ryan Zinn of the OCA, 'OCA's Fair World Project will highlight corporations that are truly implementing fair trade practices, but at the same time hold 'fair-washers' accountable and insist on safeguarding fair trade's integrity. We will put pressure on schools, institutions, and businesses, especially in the organic and natural products sector, to walk their talk and guarantee fair labor practices throughout the supply chain.'"

– Organic Consumers Association, OrganicConsumers.org

"Fair Trade supports some of the most bio-diverse farming systems in the world. When you visit a Fair Trade coffee grower's fields, with the forest canopy overhead and the sound of migratory songbirds in the air, it feels like you're standing in the rainforest."

– Professor Miguel Altieri, Leading expert and author on agroecology

Fair World Project, FairWorldProject.org

• Grow Food

"The glory of gardening: hands in the dirt, head in the sun, heart with nature. To nurture a garden is to feed not just on the body, but the soul."

– Alfred Austin

THE absolute number one cause of greenhouse gas emissions is related to food production, packaging, shipping, marketing, and cooking – and especially to diets that include meat, dairy, and junk food.

"Lead with your fork, not your mouth."

– Bernie Wilke

Eat regionally: it uses at least 50 times less fossil fuel. Eat organic: It uses 50% less fossil fuels. Eat a vegan diet that is all or mostly raw: it uses over 15 times less water, over 25 times less land, and over 30 times less petroleum than the typical American diet.

Disconnect from the corporate food train that has guided the majority of people to rely on stores and restaurants for food. Grow food using heirloom and non-genetically modified seeds. Aim for variety in your garden. There are 7,000 species of edible plants.

Educate yourself about *veganic* gardening, which uses no bone meal or blood fertilizers. However, soil isn't vegan, and consumes animal protein.

Creating an amazing culinary garden doesn't have to cost much. Books and magazines about gardening are available at libraries. There are many places from where you can get free seeds, cuttings, vines, and fruiting bushes and trees. Some of the Web sites listed below provide information about this. Many people who own land, including people with empty backyards, will allow people to plant there.

Nurture wild edible plants native to your region. Include wildflowers to support local bee colonies. Plant berry bushes and fruiting trees in nearby wildland. Learn how to identify edible plants in your local environment, including what you may think of as weeds, such as dandelion, purslane, young fiddlehead ferns, watercress, milkweed shoots, lambs quarters, chickweed, and sorrel. Also, learn the difference between edible and non-edible mushrooms.

Learn about the Dervaes family of Pasadena, California. They turned their small yard into a garden that produces thousands of pounds of fruits and vegetables every year: PathToFreedom.com.

> "We live off of what comes out of the soil, not what's in the bank. If we squander the ecological capital of the soil, the capital on paper won't much matter... For the past 50 or 60 years, we have followed industrialized agricultural policies that have increased the rate of destruction of productive farmland. For those 50 or 60 years, we have let ourselves believe the absurd notion that as long as we have money we will have food. If we continue our offenses against the land and the labor by which we are fed, the food supply will decline, and we will have a problem far more complex than the failure of our paper economy. Remember, if our agriculture is not sustainable then our food supply is not sustainable... Either we pay attention or we pay a huge price, not so far down the road. When we face the fact that civilizations have destroyed themselves by destroying their farmland, it's clear that we don't really have a choice."
>
> – Wes Jackson, co-founder of The Land Institute, LandInstitute.org

> "Thoughtful and informed people realize that local is the answer. Local seeds which grow well in a certain area need fewer chemicals, practices like crop rotation, composting, and green manure-ing (using crops, especially nitrogen-fixing plants like beans, to return nutrients to soil). All these techniques create a healthier soil which needs fewer chemicals. That creates healthier people."
>
> – Deborah Koons Garcia, director of the documentaries *The Future of Food* and *In Good Heart: Soil and the Mystery of Fertility*

Get away from giving your food dollars to multi-national corporate food companies. Grow some of your own food!

Used and discount gardening supplies can be found at garage sales, second hand stores, and though Websites such as craigslist.org.

Local vegan restaurants and juice bars may be more than happy to give you buckets-full of quality food scraps you can use in composters and to build up healthful soil.

Book of interest:
The Forager's Harvest: A Guide to Identifying, Harvesting, and Preparing Edible Wild Plants, by Samuel Thayer

American Community Gardening Association: CommunityGarden.org
Australian Community Gardens Network, communitygarden.org.au.
Bay Area Seed Interchange Library, EcologyCenter.Org/BASIL
Bioneers, Bioneers.org
Bountiful Gardens, BountifulGardens.org

City Food Growers, Australia; cityfoodgrowers.com.au
Community Alliance with Family Farmers: CAFF.org
Community Gardening Association: CommunityGarden.org
Earth Garden Magazine, POB 2, Trentham, VIC 3458, Australia; earthgarden.com.au. Magazine for sustainable living
Edible Estates, EdibleEstates.org
FedCo Co-op Garden Supplies, POB 520, Waterville, ME 04903; 207-873-7333; fedcoseeds.com
Food Empowerment Project, POB 7071, San Jose, CA 95150-7071; 530-848-4021; FoodIsPower.org
Food Not Lawns: FoodNotLawns.com
Gardenerd, gardenerd.com
Gardening at the Dragon's Gate, gardeningatthedragonsgate.com
Garden Project, GardenProject.org
Growing Organic, GrowingOrganic.com
Harmony Hikes, HarmonyHikes.com. Sergei Boutenko's wild food foraging adventure hikes. Sergei is part of the Boutenko family of Ashland, Oregon. They have hiked hundreds of miles in the wild while surviving on wild plants. With his sister, Valya, he is also the author of the recipe book, *Fresh*. Access: RawFamily.com.
Hollygrove Market and Farm, New Orleans, hollygrovemarket.com
Institute for the Study of Edible Wild Plants and Other Forageables, WildFoodAdventures.com
Island Seed and Feed, Goleta, CA; IslandSeed.com
Kids Gardening, kidsgardening.com.
KitchenGardeners.org
The Learning Garden, TheLearningGarden.org. Venice, California location. Often have raw food gatherings on weekends.
Mid-City Community Garden, New Orleans, midcitycommunitygarden.com
Montview Neighborhood Farm, 38 Henry St., Northampton, MA 01060; montviewfarm.org. A CSA (community supported agriculture) food forest located on three acres of land near downtown Northampton.
National Farmers Union Seed Saver Campaign, 2717 Wentz Ave., Saskatoon, SK S7K 4B6, Canada; NFU.CA/SeedSaver.html
National Gardening Association, garden.org.
National Plant Germplasm Service, ARS-Grin.Gov/NPGS
Native Seeds: NativeSeeds.org
New Orleans Food & Farm Network, noffn.org
Organic Gardening Magazine, organicgardening.com
Oregon Tilth: Tilth.org
Organic Seed Alliance: SeedAlliance.org
Osborn International Seed Co., OsbornSeed.Com
Theodore Payne Foundation, TheodorePayne.Org. Promotes the preservation and use of native plants. Sells native fruiting trees and bushes.
Peoples' Global Action, AGP.Org
Permaculture, Permaculture.co.uk
Planting Seeds Project, New City Institute, Vancouver, CA; NewCity.CA/Pages/Planting_Seeds.html
Primal Seeds, PrimalSeeds.Org
Rare Seeds, RareSeeds.com
Ray Mears, RayMears.com
Real Food Challenge, realfoodchallenge.org
Restoring Our Seed, POB 520, Waterville, ME 04903; GrowSeed.Org

The Rhizome Collective, Austin, TX; rhizomecollective.org
Save Our Seed: SavingOurSeed.org
Scatterseed Project, POB 1167, Farmington, ME 04938; GardeningPlaces.Com/ScatterSeed.htm
Seed Alliance, SeedAlliance.org
Seed and Plant Sanctuary for Canada, Salt Spring Island, BC; SeedSanctuary.Org
Seed Savers Australia, seedsavers.net
Seed Savers Exchange: SeedSavers.org
Seed Savers Network, SeedSavers.Net
Seeds of Change, SeedsOfChange.com
Seeds of Diversity, POB 36, Stn. Q, Toronto, ON M4T 2L7, Canada; Seeds.CA
SeedSave.Org
Seeds Trust, Seedstrust.com
Snow Seed Organic, 831-758-9869; SnowSeedCo.Com
Sow Organic Seed Co., POB 527, Williams, OR 97544; OrganicSeed.Com
Square Foot Gardening, SquareFootGardening.com
Synergy Seeds, synergyseeds.com
Tilth, Tilth.org
Tilth Producers, TilthProducers.org
Underwood Gardens, Maryann Underwood, 1414 Ximmerman Rd., Woodstock, IL 60098; UnderwoodGardens.Com. Maryann Underwood's company sells endangered and heirloom seeds; works to preserve genetic diversity of food plants; teaches people the ancient practice of saving seeds; and publishes books and videos on how to save seeds. The Web site features a forum where gardeners can share gardening tips, ask questions, and receive feedback.
United Plant Savers, POB 400, East Barre, VT, 05649; UnitedPlantSavers.Org
Victory Seeds, VictorySeeds.com
Wild Man Steve Brill, WildManSteveBrill.com.
Willing Workers on Organic Fams (WWOOF), WWOOF.org
Yards to Gardens, y2g.org

• Fruit & Veggie Sharing Organizations

"Doing things for free encourages people to share. It encourages people to be community, to be family. It provides people the chance to be generous with each other."

– Tree

"When you reap the harvest of your land, you shall not reap all the way to the edges of your field, or gather the gleamings of your harvest. You shall not pick your vineyard bare, or gather the fallen fruit of your vineyard; you shall leave them for the poor and the stranger."

– Leviticus 19:9-10

Eat the Weeds, eattheweeds.com
Fallen Fruit, fallenfruit.org. Fruit share site.
Food Not Bombs, foodnotbombs.net.
Food Not Lawns, foodnotlawns.com.
KitchenGardeners.org
Neighborhood Fruit, neighborhoodfruit.com. Fruit- and vegetable-sharing site.
Veggie Trader, veggietrader.com. People sharing homegrown and wild harvested produce.

• SPROUTING

"Scientists have studied sprouts for centuries to better understand their high levels of disease-preventing phytochemicals, and how they contribute to better health, from prevention to treatment of life-threatening diseases. Major organizations including the National Institutes of Health, American Cancer Society and Johns Hopkins University have reinforced the benefits of sprouts with ongoing studies that explore various sprout varieties for their nutritional properties and to validate health claims.

According to Paul Talalay, M.D., in the American Cancer Society *NEWS*, 'broccoli sprouts are better for you than full-grown broccoli, and contain more of the enzyme sulforaphane which helps protect cells and prevents their genes from turning into cancer.' His findings are consistent with several epidemiologic studies that have shown that sprouts contain significant amounts of vitamins A, C and D. Sprouts are widely recognized by nutrition-conscious consumers and health care professionals as a 'wonder food.'"

– *Good Sprout News* of the International Sprout Growers' Association; ISGA-Sprouts.Org

EATING fresh sprouts is an excellent way to get phytonutrients (plant nutrients), such as enzymes (vital to all life), amino acids (for building protein), chlorophyll (abundant in greens, especially baby greens), biophotons (vital nutrients that are tiny specs of light in living cells, and often referred to by sunfoodists as "vital life-force energy"), anti-oxidants, high-quality oils (including omega 3 fatty acids, which we need for brain and nerve health), fiber, and other nutrients.

Sprouting is also one of the least expensive ways, besides growing your own garden, to get raw greens, and all of their beneficial components, into your diet, which is important for anyone wanting to experience vibrant health.

The magic of a seed is that it is a plant-making kit. Seeds are amazing in that they can be eaten by an animal, pass through the digestive tract, and start to grow only after they have left the animal's digestive tract. Magically, what seeds need to grow is provided in the nutrient-rich feces. That is how many plants are spread through nature, by being eaten by animals, who then unknowingly provide themselves as a vehicle to transfer the seed to a new location, where it grows.

Exposing seeds to moisture takes the seed out of its dormant state, shutting off the enzyme inhibitors, which mostly exist in the skin or shell, and igniting the nutrient factories that build the structure from a seed into a plant. The first few days of a plant's life is a time of exuberant energy and a microscopic storm of nutrient-making activity. By consuming the sprouts, you are transferring the concentrated vibrant nutrients of the young plant into your body.

> "What is the great secret that has been eluding the investicgations of scientists and lives of laypersons for centuries? Enzymes. You are only alive because thousands of enzymes make it possible. Every breath you take, thought you think, or sentence you read, is a result of thousands of complex enzyme systems and their functions operating simultaneiously."
>
> – Ann Wigmore, author of *The Hippocrates Diet*

Some of the beneficial components of sprouts include antioxidants. These are natural plant chemicals that work in the plant to both protect it from various stressors, such as the invasion of bacteria and fungi. When we consume the sprouts, the substances that work to protect the sprouts then work inside of us to protect our health.

Because some of the chemicals that form in sprouts specifically fight the invasion of harsh bacteria, sprouts can also help to improve digestion and rid the digestive tract of certain types of bacteria that can cause illness.

As long as you have an area that is between about 50 to 100 degrees Fahrenheit, and that has indirect sunlight, you can grow sprouts anywhere on the planet (although some seeds are more likely to grow when in the temperature range of between 60 and 90 degrees Fahrenheit). You don't need anything special to grow sprouts. All it takes is something like a big glass jar and a screen to cover the top. You can also use a bowl covered with a screen, or a sheer cloth. Of course, you also need clean water to first soak the seeds, then to rinse them. I often germinate seeds in a bowl covered by a plate, which also makes it easy to rinse as I put water in the bowl, then hold the plate on with my thumbs as I tip the bowl over the sink or outside in the garden, and let the water seep out.

Probably the most common method of growing sprouts is to use a big jar covered by a screen, keeping the jar tilting almost upside down at an approximate 45° angle in a big bowl to drain excess water.

Some people use mesh bags to sprout seeds. This also makes it easy to rinse the seeds.

There are a variety of sprouting trays and machines on the market that can make it easier to sprout seeds. Some sprouters automatically spray and rinse the sprouts so that you don't have to. I've never owned one of those fancy gizmos. Some people like them. I do fine with bowls and jars.

There are a variety of seeds that are good for sprouting. Seek those that are from organic sources.

Make sure your soaking and sprouting bowls, jars, screens, and/or mesh bags are clean, or else you may also find that you will be growing some unwanted bacteria – turning your germinates rancid.

During the soaking time remember that seeds can die if they remain in water too long. The soak times listed below vary according to the temperature of the room and water. If it is cold, you may want to soak for the longer period; if it is warm you want to sprout for the shorter period. In warmer weather the seeds will also need to be rinsed more often. As you get more familiar with sprouting, you will learn what works best for the types of seeds you are using, and the environment of the room.

Unless you have an automatic sprouting machine that regularly mists the sprouting seeds, you will need to rinse them one to three times per day with clean water to keep them clean, fresh, and hydrated (moist). It is good to have a screened strainer for rinsing the smaller seeds, and a colander with smallish holes for rinsing the larger seeds/beans.

Sprouting takes place faster in warm weather, and also in a brighter location.

Also, people often use the word *sprout* when they really mean *germinate*. But that is a technicality. For instance, you may hear people say *sprouted garbanzo hummus*, which is really germinated garbanzo hummus. The difference between a *germinate* and a *sprout* is that a germinate is only when the root has appeared, such as *germinated* garbanzo beans used to make raw hummus, and a *sprout* is when the leaf has started to appear, or is in full form, such as alfalfa sprouts, sunflower sprouts, bean sprouts, and sprouted wheatgrass. But, people seem to have a thing against the word *germinate*, and maybe because it reminds them too much of the word *germ*. So, they will continue to use the word *sprout* for both sprouted and germinated seeds. Commonly some of the seeds that are only germinated rather than sprouted include buckwheat, garbanzo, chia, and quinoa.

There are also a lot of raw recipes that call for *soaked* seeds or nuts, such as *soaked* macadamia nuts or *soaked* sunflower seeds. Soaking seeds and nuts for a time (usually less than a few hours) turns off the enzyme inhibitors, ignites the factory of the seed in making enzymes, amino acids, essential fatty acids, biophotons, and other nutrients, including vitamins and antioxidants. Soaking makes nuts and seeds more nutrient-rich and easier to digest. Commonly, some of the seeds that are soaked rather than sprouted include nuts, including almonds, macadamias, cashews, Brazil nuts, and other nuts (yes, nuts are seeds).

People who are into the *Living Foods* diet commonly will soak their seeds and nuts before eating them so as to make them truly living foods, rather than dormant seeds and nuts.

Most types of grain germinates are sweetest when the tail on the seed has just started to grow. The longer the tail grows, the less sweet it will become.

Once seeds have passed the germination stage, and start to develop leafs, they are then sprouts.

Sprouts benefit from exposure to light, such as indirect sunlight, as this will trigger the development of chlorophyll in the sprouts.

Within a plant, chlorophyll transforms sunlight and CO_2 into sugar and oxygen. Chlorophyll is molecularly very similar to human blood plasma. There are strong nutritional qualities in chlorophyll as it helps strengthen the immune system in fighting off infections, and helps rid the body of toxins, especially those that gather in the liver. Because chlorophyll helps generate new cell growth, it also is important in healing from wounds and illnesses.

Some sprouts are more chlorophyll-rich than others. With a content of about 70 percent chlorophyll, wheatgrass is perhaps the richest sprout of all.

If you are not going to use the sprouts right away, you can slow their growth by putting them in the refrigerator, or in a cold room (not freezing). Rinse and drain once a day with clean water and you should be able to keep them in a cold, slowed growing state for two to four days, or more.

You can also slow soaked seeds from sprouting fully by keeping them in the refrigerator. Then, when you are ready to sprout them, remove them from the refrigerator, rinse, and let them grow in the room temperature.

Sprouts are living, breathing plants. They need air. Don't put them into a sealed container. A screened jar or a casserole dish with a glass top left slightly open work well because they both allow for air to enter the container. A jar with a screen fastened around the top and turned almost upside down at an angle in a jar works best for many seeds because it prevents them from sitting in water while also letting in air. As they sprout at room temperature, remember to rinse them two or three times a day to keep them from rotting.

One way of keeping sprouts fresh in the refrigerator is to store them in a bamboo bowl covered by a second bamboo bowl that has a dozen or more small holes drilled into it. This also provides an easy way to rinse them once a day by pouring water into the bowl, covering with the top bowl, and tilting upside down over the sink or outside to eliminate excess water before putting them back into the refrigerator.

The amount of time listed below for soaking can often be reduced to a few hours, or less. Some seeds can be soaked a lot longer, up to a day, but you risk killing the seeds.

Some people will drink the soak water as it contains enzymes that are released by the seeds.

Just as long as the soaked seeds are kept moist and you don't let them dry out, you break down the enzyme inhibitors, and nurture the seed to turn into a plant.

Again: Sprouts must be rinsed, and most are best if they are rinsed two times per day, although some may only require rinsing once per day. The more you get used to sprouting, the more you will learn which seeds require more attention, and which require less.

When the sprouts have reached the size you want them, put them in direct sun for an hour or more. By doing this you will ignite the chlorophyll and nutrient-making factory within the sprouts, greatly increasing their nutritional value. Make sure not to allow sun to bake them or let them dry out. Keep them covered with a screen or sheer cloth to keep little buggy friends away.

Popular seeds used in sprouting:

Seed:	Soak for:	Sprout for:
• **Adzuki**	6 to 7 hours	3 days
• **Alfalfa**	5 to 6 hours	2 to 4 days
• **Almond**	2 to 3 hours	Freshly soaked to 2 days

Toss into salads. Use as ingredient in smoothies, and desserts.

• **Black-eyed peas**	7 to 9 hours	2 to 4 days
• **Broccoli**	5 to 6 hours	3 to 4 days

Strong taste. Use sparingly in salads, sandwiches, dressings.

• **Buckwheat**	5 to 6 hours	2 to 3 days to germinate

If you are to use the grain in only its soaked form, without sprouting them, you may want to put them through a process to activate the phytase enzyme. This breaks down the phytic acid, which is phosphoric, exists in the outer layer/bran of grains, and binds with minerals, preventing them from being absorbed into the digestive tract. After draining the water, soak the seeds in vinegar or lemon juice for about 30 minutes. Raw sauerkraut juice or kimchee juice also work in activating the phytase.

• **Cabbage**	5 to 6 hours	2 to 4 days
• **Cashew**	2 to 3 hours	Freshly soaked to 2 days

Toss into salads. Use as ingredient in smoothies, and desserts.

• **Chia**	20 minutes to 1 hour to germinate, use soon after	

Amazingly quick to germinate. Rich in amino acids, essential fatty acids, and trace nutrients. Stir into cut fruit bowl for a breakfast treat.

• **Clover**	5 to 6 hours	2 to 4 days
• **Corn**	7 to 9 hours	2 to 4 days
• **Dill**	5 to 6 hours	2 to 3 days
• **Fenugreek**	6 to 7 hours	2 to 4 days
• **Flax**	2 to 5 hours	Freshly soaked to 3 days

Not the easiest to germinate. It is good to use a large, wide-mouthed jar with a screen cover. This way the seeds can be rinsed by pouring water through the screen, and the upside-down jar kept at an angle to drain.

Time to use them depends on what you are using them for. If you are going to use them in raw dehydrated crackers, you may want to soak them only for several hours to ignite the enzymes. But for soft dehydrated breads and crusts you may want to sprout them a while longer. Also good for adding crunch to guacamole, salsa, and gazpacho.

- **Garbanzo** 8 to 10 hours 2 to 4 days

Make a germinated garbanzo bean salad with olive oil, salt, lemon juice, chopped red bell pepper, chopped red onion, and pepper powder.

Blend into hummus after germinating for two to four days (lemon juice, salt, raw tahini, garlic, olive oil. You can also add fresh Italian herbs, raw olives, chopped red bell pepper, and/or dried tomatoes).

- **Kamut** 5 to 6 hours Freshly soaked to 3 days
- **Lentil** 6 to 8 hours 2 to 4 days
- **Macadamia** 2 to 3 hours Freshly soaked to 3 days

Use as ingredient in smoothies, deserts, crusts, and fruit salads.

- **Millet** 7 to 9 hours 2 to 4 days

You can also make rejuvelac fermented water using sprouted millet soaked in water for 12 to 24 hours in a clean, warm place out of direct sunlight.

It is best to soak a small amount of millet in a big, screened jar to make them easier to rinse.

Raw, unsoaked millet can also be tossed into salads to add crunch.

- **Mung beans** 6 to 8 hours 2 to 4 days

Mung bean sprouts will remain white if they are kept in the dark. If you expose them to light, they become green, but they also become bitter.

- **Mustard** 5 to 7 hours 2 to 4 days

Strong taste. Use sparingly in salads, sandwiches, and dressings.

- **Oat groats** 5 to 6 hours Freshly soaked to 2 days

Use in crusts, or in breakfast bowl with berries and/or cut fruit, a bit of lemon juice, vanilla, shredded coconut, and soaked macadamia.

If you are to use the grain in only its soaked form, without sprouting them, you may want to put them through a process to activate the phytase enzyme. This breaks down the phytic acid, which is phosphoric, exists in the outer layer/bran of grains, and binds with minerals, preventing them from being absorbed into the digestive tract. After draining the water, soak the seeds in vinegar or lemon juice for about 30 minutes. Raw sauerkraut juice or kimchee juice also work in activating the phytase.

- **Onion** 5 to 7 hours 2 to 4 days
- **Peas** 6 to 9 hours 2 to 4 days
- **Pine nuts** 2 to 3 hours freshly soaked
- **Pumpkin** 3 to 5 hours Freshly soaked to 4 days

Toss onto salads. Blend into smoothies. Use soaked pumpkin seeds as an ingredient in raw dehydrated crackers.

- **Quinoa** 1 to 2 hours 1 to 3 days

Amazingly quick to germinate, it will often start forming a root in a few hours. Some people will use them after germinating for several hours, such as with cutup vegetables as a salad.

Use in fresh or dehydrated crusts.

You can also make rejuvelac fermented water using germinated quinoa soaked in water for 12 to 24 hours in a clean, warm place out of direct sunlight.

- **Radish** 5 to 7 hours 1 to 5 days
- **Red clover** 5 to 7 hours 3 to 5 days
- **Rye** 7 to 9 hours 2 to 4 days

Use in fresh or dehydrated crusts.

- **Sesame** 4 to 6 hours Freshly soaked to 3 days

- **Spelt** 5 to 6 hours Freshly soaked to 3 days
- **Sunflower** 5 to 7 hours Freshly soaked to 3 days

Toss into salads. Use soaked seeds in dehydrated raw crackers.

You can also grow sunflower sprouts in a flat of organic soil, then after a few days, harvest them, including the roots, rinsing off the soil (or cutting off the roots), and using them in salads and as garnish for raw burgers (see raw vegan recipe books).

- **Triticale** 5 to 7 hours 2 to 3 days
- **Wheat berries** 5 to 7 hours 2 to 3 days, or for grass

Use in mixed sprouted grain salad.

Make rejuvelac, fermented water from the enzyme-rich soak water.

Use to grow wheat grass for juicing.

If you are to use the grain in only its soaked form, without sprouting them, you may want to put them through a process to activate the phytase enzyme. This breaks down the phytic acid, which is phosphoric, exists in the outer layer/bran of grains, and binds with minerals, preventing them from being absorbed into the digestive tract. After draining the water, soak the seeds in vinegar or lemon juice for about 30 minutes. Raw sauerkraut juice or kimchee juice also work in activating the phytase.

- **Wild rice** 6 to 8 hours 2 to 4 days

Use in germinated grain salad mixed with chopped soaked almonds or walnuts, raw oil, a little lemon juice, and Himalayan salt.

Eat Sprouts, EatSprouts.Com
International Sprout Grower's Association, ISGA-Sprouts.Org
Mumm's Sprouting Seeds, Sprouting.Com
Sprout Man, SproutMan.Com
Sprout People, SproutPeople.Com
Tim Tyler's Sprout Farm, Sprouting.Org

• Genetically Engineered Food

"Genetically modified foods are less nutritious, more likely to trigger an allergy, and contain higher levels of growth hormones and pesticides.

Common genetically modified food ingredients include corn syrup from GM corn, sugar from GM sugar beets, vegetable oils from GM soy, cotton and canola, and cheese, eggs, milk and meat from animals given GM feed or shot up with GM growth hormones and vaccines.

The same foods that are making people fat, sick, and undernourished are the ones that Monsanto has genetically engineered. High fructose corn syrup, trans-fats, fryer grease, chicken nuggets, and bacon cheeseburgers all contain GMOs.

The industrial-scale mono-crop farms, factory farms and slaughterhouses that are abusing workers and animals, destroying the soil, poisoning the water, polluting the atmosphere with climate-destabilizing greenhouse gases, and creating a breeding ground for mad cow disease, E. coli, salmonella, and swine flu, are the best customers for Monsanto's RoundUp Ready and Bt-spliced crops. Agribusiness thrives off feeding taxpayer subsidized GMO crops, especially corn, soy and cotton seeds, to the chickens, pigs and cows they keep confined in cesspools of their own waste.

Companies like Monsanto and AquaBounty (the Frankenfish inventor), claim that GMOs are "sustainable" because they're going to feed the world as the global climate crisis accelerates. But genetic engineering companies' business model - mass-marketing techno-fixes for the industrialized food system - only perpetuates the waste and pollution that have already made agriculture the source of at least one-third of global greenhouse gas emissions.

GMO contamination could lead to the collapse of the industrialized food system. GMOs have the capacity to break the species barrier. Weeds that plague row crops have adopted the RoundUp Ready trait, creating super-weeds that are forcing farmers to turn to greater amounts of super-toxic herbicides and pesticides. The overuse of RoundUp, the most widely-used pesticide in the history of agriculture, enhances the virulence of pathogens such as Fusarium and may have dire consequences for agriculture such as rendering soils infertile, crops non-productive, and plants less nutritious."

– The Organic Consumers Association

PLEASE, read and learn about farmer Percy Schmeiser, who has been sued by Monsanto. Access his Web site: PercySchmeiser.com.

"The companies that are genetically engineering and parenting seed are chemical companies. They have interest in selling more chemicals. They don't do genetic engineering to reduce chemical use; they do genetic engineering to increase chemical use."

– Vandana Shiva, author of *Soil Not Oil*

"We are facing the ultimate takeover bully – genetic engineering on the cellular level and corporate control on the global scale – and, of course, there is a relationship. Corporate control of the genetic material of the planet by buying up the planet's seed supply and patenting everything they can patent has a major impact on the basic security of every person who eats. After all, having access to seeds and food is the foundation of security."

– Deborah Koons Garcia, director of the documentaries *The Future of Food* and *In Good Heart: Soil and the Mystery of Fertility*

"In 1992, Monsanto successfully lobbied President George H.W. Bush's administration to deregulate its controversial and untested technology of genetic engineering or genetic modification. Vice President Dan Quayle made the announcement, saying, 'We will ensure that biotech products will receive the same oversight as other products, instead of being hampered by unnecessary regulation.'

The official policy is based on industry propaganda rather than peer-reviewed science; it claims that genetically engineered food, crops, and animals "substantially equivalent" to conventional food and crops. No safety testing or labels are required.

The result is that genetically engineered foods are everywhere. Nobody knows that they're eating them, and there isn't any scientific research that could tell us what effect this is having on human health. Study after study indicating serious damage to animals fed GMOs have been downplayed or ignored. Links to human hazards, such as the genetically engineered L-tryptophan disaster of 1989, which killed scores of Americans and permanently injured thousands more, or experiments in 1999 in the UK by renowned scientist Arpad Pusztai, have been literally suppressed."

– Organic Consumers Association, July 2010; OrganicConsumers.org

"Four Simple Ways to Avoid GMOs

1. Buy organic - organic producers are not allowed to use GMOs
2. Look for "Non-GMO" labels
3. Avoid risky ingredients: corn, soy, vegetable oil (canola, cottonseed, and soybean), sugarbeet sugar
4. Buy products listed in the Non-GMO Shopping Guide"

– Organic Consumers Association, OrganicConsumers.org

"Top 10 Reasons to Label Geneticall Engineered Food

10. Almost all non-organic processed food or animal products in the U.S. today contain ingredients that come from genetically engineered crops or from animals given genetically engineered feed, vaccines or growth hormones.
9. Genetically engineered foods have not been tested to determine whether they are safe for human consumption.
8. Genetically engineered foods ARE different from conventional and organic foods.
7. A single serving of genetically engineered soy can result in "horizontal gene transfer," where the bacteria in the human gut adopts the soy's DNA.
6. Animals fed genetically engineered feed ARE different from animals fed conventional and organic feed.
5. The third generation of hamsters fed genetically engineered soy suffered slower growth, a high mortality rate, and a bizarre birth defect: fur growing in their mouths. Many also lost the ability to have pups.
4. The more genetically engineered corn fed to mice, the fewer babies they had and the smaller the babies were.
3. Biotech's scattershot technique of spraying plant cells with a buckshot of foreign genes that hit chromosomes in random spots would trigger the expression of new allergens and change the character of plant proteins.

2. Scientists reviewing data from Monsanto's own studies "have proven that genetically engineered foods are neither sufficiently healthy or proper to be commercialized."
1. The Convention on Biodiversity recognizes that genetic engineering is a threat to amount and variety of life on the planet."

– Organic Consumers Association, OrganicConsumers.org

Watch the documentary, *The World According to Monsanto*, by accessing: FreeDocumentaries.org.

"Q. Hasn't research shown GM foods to be safe?

A. No. The only feeding study done with humans showed that GMOs survived inside the stomach of the people eating GMO food. No follow-up studies were done.

Various feeding studies in animals have resulted in potentially pre-cancerous cell growth, damaged immune systems, smaller brains, livers, and testicles, partial atrophy or increased density of the liver, odd shaped cell nuclei and other unexplained anomalies, false pregnancies and higher death rates.

Q. But aren't the plants chemically the same, whether or not they are GM?

A. Most tests can't determine the differences at the level of the DNA. And, even if they appear to be the same, eyewitness reports from all over North American describe how several types of animals, including cows, pigs, geese, elk, deer, squirrels, and rats, when given a choice, avoid eating GM foods.

Q. Haven't people been eating GM foods without any ill effect?

A. The biotech industry says that millions have been eating GM foods without ill effect. This is misleading. No one monitors human health impacts of GM foods. If the foods were creating health problems in the US population, it might take years or decades before we identified the cause.

Q. What indications are there that GM foods are causing problems?

A. Soon after GM soy was introduced to the UK, soy allergies skyrocketed by 50 percent.

In March 2001, the Center for Disease Control reported that food is responsible for twice the number of illnesses in the U.S. compared to estimates just seven years earlier. This increase roughly corresponds to the period when Americans have been eating GM food.

Without follow-up tests, which neither the industry or government are doing, we can't be absolutely sure if genetic engineering was the cause.

Q. What about GM hormones in milk?

A. Milk from rbGH-treated cows contains an increased amount of the hormone IGF-1, which is one of the highest risk factors associated with breast and prostate cancer, but no one is tracking this in relation to cancer rates.

Q. Why do genetically engineered foods have antibiotic resistant genes in them?

A. The techniques used to transfer genes have a very low success rate, so the genetic engineers attach "marker genes" that are resistant to antibiotics to help them to find out which cells have taken up the new DNA. That way scientists can then douse the experimental GMO in antibiotics and if it lives, they have successful altered the genes. The marker genes are resistant to antibiotics that are commonly used in human and veterinary medicine. Some scientists believe that eating GE food containing these marker genes could encourage gut bacteria to develop antibiotic resistance."

– NonGMOShoppingGuide.com. Excerpted from Jeffrey Smith's book *Genetic Roulette: The Documented Health Risks of Genetically Engineered Foods*

Ban Terminator Seeds, BanTerminator.org
Bioneers, Bioneers.org
The Center for Food Safety, TrueFoodNow.org/Campaigns/Genetically-Engineered-Foods/
The Corporation, TheCorporation.com
Earthlings, Earthlings.com
EarthSave, EarthSave.org
Farm to Consumer Legal Defense Fund, FarmToConsumer.org
Food Inc., FoodIncMovie.com. Please watch the documentary.
The Food Revolution, FoodRevolution.org
The Future of Food, TheFutureOfFood.com
GE Food Alert, GEFoodAlert.org
Genetically Engineered Food Dangers, HolisticMed.com/ge
Institute for Responsible Technology, ResponsibleTechnology.org
King Corn, KingCorn.net. Please watch the documentary, King Corn.
Monsanto Watch, MonsantoWatch.org
Mothers for Natural Law, Safe-Food.org
Non-GMO Shopping Guide, nongmoshoppingguide.com
Occupy Monsanto, OccupyMonsanto360.org
Organic Consumers Association, OrganicConsumers.org
Percy Schmeiser, PercySchmeiser.com
Rodale Institute, RodaleInstitute.org
Say No to GMOs, SayNoToGMOs.org
Seeds of Deception, SeedsOfDeception.com
Via Organica, Mexico, ViaOrganica.org

• Food Irradiation

"A chest x-ray gives about 0.01 rad of energy. The average dose of radiation from background radiation (radiation due to cosmic rays and natural radioactivity such as radon in rocks) annually is 0.1 rad. On the other hand, the dose of radiation from gamma rays applied to food during irradiation is 100,000 to 1 million rads (1-10 kGy). The amount of radiation being applied to food during irradiation is therefore massive, 10 million to 100 million times the dose of a chest x-ray... Food irradiation creates nuclear waste just like a nuclear power plant."

– Citizen.org/CMEP/FoodSafety

"Food irradiation is a process in which food is exposed to high doses of radiation. Food is irradiated using radioactive gamma sources, usually Cobalt 60 or Cesium 137, or high-energy electron beams. The gamma rays break up the molecular structure of the food, forming free radicals. The free radicals react with the food to create new chemical substances called 'radiolytic products.' Those are known as 'unique radiolytic products.' (URPs) because they can only be found in irradiated products."

– The European Food Irradiation Campaign, Irridation.info

IRRADIATION of food is a form of pasteurization. It uses high doses of radiation to kill microbes in food. Specifically, irradiation is meant to kill bugs that can make humans sick, including (Escherichia coli) E. coli 0157, salmonella, shigella, and listeria.

Radiating food kills what may or may not cause human illness. It also kills enzymes, and damages other nutrients, including thiamin, and vitamins E and A. It also exposes food to radiation.

Food irradiation is a technology developed by the U.S. Department of Energy's Byproduct Utilization Program. The word "byproduct" in this case refers to leftovers of the nuclear industry. Specifically, cesium 37 and cobalt 60.

Many foods in supermarkets and in school, hospital, corporate, prison, military, and government cafeterias are irradiated, or "cold-pasteurized." Many foods being imported and exported are also irradiated. This is done even though it is known that irradiation creates health-altering free radicals and radiolytic substances in the foods.

The E. coli outbreaks that have been used as an argument for radiating food are directly related to animal farms and factory animal farms polluting farmland, water, and farm and food processing equipment. The spinach that triggered the recall across the U.S. in 2006 was contaminated with a strain of E. coli that originates in the intestines of cattle treated with antibiotics. Giving cattle antibiotic-treated grain creates a particularly hazardous strain of bacteria resistant to common antibiotics.

"In the unsanitary conditions typical of confined feedlots, animals are given continual low doses of antibiotics in their feed to prevent sickness, promote faster growth, and boost profits. This contributes to increased antibiotic resistance in the bacteria that infect people – a serious threat to public health. In 2009, 80 percent of all antibiotics used in the U.S. were given to livestock."

– Environmental Working Group, July 2011

At first the USDA said it was organic spinach that was contaminated with the E. coli. This was front-page news, got lots of people to stop eating organic spinach, and was financially damaging to organic farmers and natural foods stores. After weeks, the USDA finally admitted that organic spinach wasn't the culprit. This was after the damage had been done to the organic farming industry. Many people never heard the news that it wasn't organic spinach, because the latter news stories largely didn't make front-page news.

Many of the people who work for the USDA have worked for, or eventually work for, the large corporate farming companies, for some branch of the animal farming industry, for the industrialized food industry, and/or for the companies that produce farming chemicals that cause illness.

Do you really want to be eating foods exposed to radiation, which accumulates in tissues? I don't.

Because irradiated foods are not labeled as such, ways of *avoiding* irradiated foods include eating organically grown, locally grown, home-grown, and wildharvested foods.

"What Irradiation Does To Food

Ionizing radiation reduces the number of disease causing organisms in food by disrupting their molecular structure, thereby killing potentially harmful bacteria and parasites. But not all pathogens are destroyed, and irradiated meat must be cooked as thoroughly as non-irradiated meat. Irradiated meat can be re-contaminated from improper handling and storage.

Irradiated food does not itself, become radioactive, but the ionizing radiation creates new radiolytic chemicals implicated as carcinogens, while destroying the vitamins A, B complex, C and E. It increases the trans fatty acids in meat, which have been linked to higher levels of "bad cholesterol." The watchdog organization, Public Citizen, indicates research has found a wide range of health problems in laboratory rats fed irradiated food, including genetic damage and cancer. Additional research shows that cyclobutanones, a new class of chemicals created by irradiation, cause genetic damage to human cells.

As for flavor, Consumer Reports trained tasters noted a slight, but distinct off-taste and smell in most of the irradiated beef sampled, likening it to singed hair.

An Experiment on Children

The federal government has recently acknowledged the unique vulnerability of children as more likely than adults to get cancer from exposure to toxic chemicals, and has drawn up new guidelines for the US Environmental Agency (EPA) to evaluate dangers posed by pesticides and other cancer-causing chemicals. But the entire issue of irradiation destroying nutrient content of food, while creating a whole new class of chemicals that cause cancer and genetic damage is being completely ignored by all three federal regulatory agencies the EPA, USDA, and FDA. Opponents to irradiation believe this is an unprecedented and dangerous experiment on the nations children."

– Rose Marie Williams, Townsend Letter for Doctors & Patients, Oct. 2004

"Why do we oppose food irradiation?

• Irradiated food is dangerous for human health.
• Food irradiation can be used as a substitute for good sanitary prac-tices in food production.
• Irradiation plants and transportation of nuclear materials to them create environmental threat to workers and surrounding communities.
• Food irradiation is used to lengthen the food shelf life. By doing so, it encourages globalization of production, which proves detri-mental to small family farmers around the world and to the envi-ronment."

– The European Food Irradiation Campaign, Irradiation.info

"Who's responsible for irradiation policy?

The FDA is responsible for evaluation of the existing scientific evidence on whether or not irradiation is harmful (as it does for new drugs). It is also responsible for writing the policy on the permitted doses and labeling of irradiation for nonmeat products, and the enforcement of that policy.

The USDA is responsible for writing the policy on the permitted doses and labeling of irradiation for meat, poultry and their products, and the enforcement of that policy.

No law prevents states from passing their own labeling laws, but in practice their right to label (under Amendment X to the Constitution) has consistently been overturned IF the labeling 'impeded' interstate commerce. Only in unusual cases should we expect a state-level labeling law to survive legal challenges from businesses that operate interstate.

The most powerful players: Congress and the food industry (which influences Congress):

CONGRESS: Congress tells the FDA what to do. The FDA must carry out the will of Congress. So if Congress passes legislation that says, "Invent a new word for irradiation that won't scare people, and also make sure that all irradiated products which must be labeled use that new word by March 2002," the FDA has to carry out that policy. Depending on the type of policy, the FDA may or may not ask for public comments on its decision before actually putting it into action.

The public tends to ignore food issues, unless they are from farm states. Large agricultural businesses have a great deal of influence over farm-state and Western Senators as well as some Representatives. As a result, agribusiness and food processors tend to set the agenda in Congress, because Members from urban and suburban districts often vote on food issues without having to pay for their votes politically. Also, urban and suburban Members can easily pay back a campaign contributor with a vote that benefits the food industry rather than the public. For urban and suburban Members, votes on food issues can be 'traded' without much expectation of consumer backlash."

– Organic Consumers Association, 2002; OrganicConsumers.org

European Food Irradiation Campaign, Irradiation.info
FactoryFarm.org, FactoryFarm.org/Topics/Irradiation
Farm to Consumer Legal Defense Fund, FarmToConsumer.org
Food and Water Watch, FoodAndWaterWatch.org
Food Irradiation Watch, FoodIrradiationInfo.org
Organic Consumers Association, organicconsumers.org/irrad/status.cfm
No Cobalt 4 Food, NoCobalt-4-food.org

• Cooked Food

NOBODY knows where or when the first cooked meal was made. On every continent there is evidence that ancient humans used fire to cook food, including meals consisting of both plant matter and animal flesh. But like the belief that sun revolves around earth, or that air causes infections in wounds, the idea that cooked plant substances are better for you should go the way of the other two beliefs.

The way nature provides food is already in its best form. You can't improve nutrients in fruits, vegetables, herbs, nuts, seeds, or sea vegetables by cooking them. While certain nutrients in some vegetables, such as tomatoes, broccoli, and carrots, may become more bioavailable when the vegetables are heated, it doesn't mean they should be cooked at temperatures higher than it takes to boil water. Heating does destroy or degrade some of the nutrients in the plants, but there are beneficial substances that remain, such as certain vitamins, minerals, atioxidants, and fiber. So, for that reason, some otherwise raw foodists may consume some steamed foods or simmered soups.

Heating plant substances alters their molecular structures, placing them outside of the way nature formed them. When you consume those altered molecules, they become part of your body tissues. In this way eating cooked food changes your body in the most basic way. Consuming a diet that is largely cooked and lacking in unheated botanical nutrients sets the stage for other unnatural things to take place within your body, such as disease and illness of all sorts.

You are what you eat. Either you can be eating living, vibrant foods as nature grows them, or you can be eating cooked food that has been degraded by heat and chemical additives. The higher the heat, the more nutrients are destroyed, and the higher the heat, the more harmful chemicals form within the foods, such as glycotoxins, acrylamides, polycyclic aromatic hydrocarbons, and heterocyclic amines.

Cooked foods are no longer alive. Cooking kills their enzymes, eliminates their life energy biophotons, and damages nutrients. Just as a cooked seed will not sprout into a plant, a cooked food diet will not provide for vibrant health. Eating deadened food deadens your life force, your spirituality, and your thought processes.

Cooking foods at high temperatures creates chemicals that do not naturally exist in plants. The substances also have no place in the human body. When you are eating cooked food you are eating substances that your body would not naturally have to deal with. They are foreign, useless, and damaging. I write about this in my other books, *Igniting Your Life* and *Sunfood Diet Infusion.*

Eating cooked food triggers an immune response in the body called leukocytosis. When someone eats food cooked at high temperatures, the body responds as if it is being invaded, and there is an increase in the white blood cells. This confuses the immune system, is wearing on the system, and results in fatigue.

Eating a diet of cooked and processed foods leaves residues in the tissues that inflame and damage the tissues, decrease vitality, cause mood swings and grogginess, clog the system, and make each cell work harder to maintain health. Ultimately this leads to a body that is overweight, discolored, plaqued with residues the body has trouble getting rid of, and that is not functioning at the level it would be if the person would simply eat a diet consisting of a variety of vibrant, living foods.

When you consider that an addiction is a craving for something that is void of the true needs of the person, and that satisfying the craving takes time and energy, and that the craving is often related to substances that are liable to have damaging effects on the person, then cooked food is addictive in every sense of the word. Cooked food causes a chemical change within the body. The consumption of cooked food leads to a physio-chemical pattern that alters the body and limits the ability of the body and mind to function at their best level, leading to diseased organs and to traumatic health events like heart attacks, strokes, organ failure, and cancers.

Not only is a diet consisting largely of cooked foods unhealthful to the human body, it is also damaging to the environment of Earth.

Governments around the planet spend tremendous amounts of money to manage the trash their citizens produce from eating processed foods. Typical packaged foods cause more solid pollution by bulk than any other product. At least one-fourth of the plastic used in the U.S. is used for toss-away packaging, and much of this is used for packaged food. Most of this packaging is from foods that are cooked or otherwise processed, and especially those that contain animal products, such as meat, eggs, and milk. These forms of pollution are spreading around the world as more countries adopt the “American way” of food processing, marketing, and consumption.

The U.S. has only about 5 percent of the world’s population, but uses an estimated 30 percent of the world’s resources, emits over 28 percent of the world’s greenhouse gasses, and consumes 20 percent of the world’s beef. Taking that into account, it is clear to see why it is important to change our ways.

Besides requiring the use of millions of ovens the world over, which use enormous amounts of fuel, cooked food is wasteful in another way.

Cooking food destroys or damages many nutrients in the food. If a large amount of the nutrients are destroyed, then so is a large amount of the time, energy, and resources used to grow and handle the food before it is cooked.

The cooking of food causes a lot of damage to the forested areas of the planets. Some areas of the world where there are few trees are that way because people have cut down the trees to cook food. Much of Haiti has been deforested not because the trees were used for building houses, but because people used the trees to create fire for cooking. This sort of thing continues to happen on all of the continents and islands of the world, especially in areas that are not using electricity or gas to cook food.

According to a study conducted by a team of researchers from around the world and that was published in the March 2005 issue of the journal *Science*, the number one source of climate-changing black carbon pollution in the air of south Asia is from cooking fires. In addition to wood, the people of that region also use agricultural waste and animal manure to cook their food. The study concluded that 42 percent of black soot was the result of cooking fires, and 25 percent was the result of burning fossil fuels. The result is that pollution in the air collects the heat of sunlight, warming the atmosphere and altering weather patterns.

In addition to the pollution caused by burning wood to cook food, a tremendous amount of air pollution is caused by people using other types of fuel to cook. From restaurants to delis, resorts, schools, prisons, military bases, and hospitals, hotels and homes, enormous amounts of fuel are used to cook food. This is done in the form of natural gas, coal, and in the use of electric stoves and ovens and microwaves. A mile from my home there is a restaurant that is famous for its cheap (and very unhealthful) lunch menu consisting of large hamburgers, barbecued meat, and beef chili. The place is usually packed, and the chimney pumps out so much smoke that the surrounding area sometimes smells of animal flesh being cooked. If you magnify this one restaurant by millions of restaurants around the world that are spewing cooking fumes into Earth's atmosphere, you begin to get an idea of how much pollution is the result of cooking food.

Food cooking is a major source of air pollution, and in many regions of the planet ovens, stoves, grills, and microwaves cause more pollution than that caused by engines.

In Los Angeles the number-one cause of air pollution is not automobiles, but is the result of cooking food with gas, electricity, barbeque, wood, and microwaves. Not everyone drives a car, but nearly everyone in Southern California eats cooked food during every meal.

Cooks working in busy restaurants are more likely to experience asthma attacks. This is because they are exposed to gasses being emitted by the ovens and stoves. Cooking food creates pollution that causes lung damage, global warming, and harms all life forms on Earth.

The sunfood diet results in less pollution and trash. While you may have been subsisting on an unhealthful diet that consisted of a lot of processed foods that were in all sorts of plastics, boxes, and other type of packaging, on the sunfood diet you will basically be eating fruits and vegetables, nuts, seeds, and things made of them. These can be grown by you, wildharvested, purchased at a farmers' market, or bought in the bulk or produce sections of your local natural foods market, through a food co-op, or a CSA (community supported agriculture food delivery subscription service). Thus you will be causing less pollution. If you shop with a cloth bag that you bring to the store every time you shop, you will also eliminate your need for "paper or plastic" bags.

• PROTEIN

"Plant protein can meet requirements when a variety of plant foods is consumed and energy needs are met. Research indicates that an assortment of plant foods eaten over the course of a day can provide all essential amino acids and ensure adequate nitrogen retention and use in healthy adults, thus complementary proteins do not need to be consumed at the same meal."

– American Dietetic Association, 2009

PEOPLE who are vegetarian often get asked if they eat a lot of soy products. The assumption is that because vegetarians don't eat animal tissues they need to have soy protein in their diet. But what many people don't seem to understand is that you don't need to eat protein-dominant plants to get protein into your system.

Some vegetarians and vegans also get caught up in the belief that they need soy in their diet as a sort of replacement for meat. They do this by eating all sorts of soy bean products – soy milk, soy ice cream, soy yogurt, tofu everything, soy burgers, soy powders, soy cheese, and soy custards and puddings.

The structures of our bodies are made of protein. The enzymes, blood, and lymph also consist of protein. People tend to think that we need to eat protein in the form of flesh, eggs, and milk to build our tissues. This is a huge misconception that drives people to focus on eating protein-rich diets, which are rough on the system and trigger degenerative diseases. The misconception helps to fuel the animal farming industry with its slaughterhouses and monocropped GMO grains; the colon, prostate, and breast cancer indusrties; the diabetes industry; the heart attack industry; the hospital and pharmaceutical industries; the fast food industry; deforestation; and cruelty to animals on a massive scale.

You do not need to eat animal flesh to get protein.

If you don't eat animal flesh, you don't need to eat soy products to get protein.

Your body needs amino acids to build protein. Proteins are made out of chains of amino acids. There is an abundance of amino acids in fresh fruits, vegetables, sprouts, nuts, and seeds. The body makes the protein it needs out of the amino acids obtained through the foods you eat.

There are amino acids in all plants.

> "The old ideas about the necessity of carefully combining vegetables at every meal to ensure the supply of essential amino acids has been totally refuted."
>
> – Charles Attwood, M.D.

Even when a person eats animal protein, the body does not simply transfer that protein into the tissues of the body. The body takes the individual amino acids from the protein to form the type of amino acid chains it needs.

> "You may have heard that vegetable sources of protein are incomplete and become complete only when correctly combined.

Research has discredited that notion so you don't have to worry that you won't get enough usable protein if you don't put together some magical combination of foods at each meal."

– Andrew Weil, M.D.

Amino acids that need to be obtained from food:

Isoleucine
Leucine
Lysine
Methionine + Cysteine
Phenylalaline + Tyrosine
Threonine
Tryptophan
Valine
Histidine

Those are the "essential amino acids" – known as such because they need to be obtained from food.

It is essential for children to obtain histidine from food. Adults synthesize it [their systems naturally create it].

In other words, there are nine essential amino acids that children need to obtain from food. But there are eight amino acids that adults need to obtain from food.

There are 22 proteinogenic amino acids in total, which your body uses to create protein. Other than those listed above, the human body synthesizes the others.

The non-essential amino acids are:

Alanine
Arginine
Aspartate
Cyeteine
Glutamate
Glutamine
Glycine
Proline
Serine
Asparagine

These amino acids are unclassified:

Pyrrolysine
Selenocysteine

All fruits and vegetables contain the essential amino acids your body needs to make protein. You will get all of the amino acids you need by eating enough calories of fruits, vegetables, nuts, and seeds.

You don't need to combine fruits and vegetables, or nuts and seeds, or legumes and rice, to get complete protein.

"Complementing proteins is not necessary with vegetable proteins. The myth that vegetable source proteins need to be complemented is similar to the myths that persist about sugar making one's blood glucose go up faster than starch does. These myths have great staying power despite their being no evidence to support them and plenty to refute them."

– Dennis Gordon, M.Ed, R.D.

"It is very easy for a vegan diet to meet the recommendations for protein, as long as calorie intake is adequate. Strict protein combining is not necessary; it is more important to eat a varied diet throughout the day."

– Reed Mangels, Ph.D., R.D.; Vegetarian Resource Group, VRG.org

A balanced live vegan diet provides an abundance of amino acids and other nutrients from a variety of live plant substances.

I use animals as examples of natural vegans. The natural diet of cows, horses, gorillas, giraffes, deer, moose, goats, hippopotamuses, and elephants consists of plants. Their bodies get protein out of the substances within the plants, and their diets chiefly consist of green leaves.

When I was in my 20s, I had a lot of kidney problems, to the point that doctors were telling me that I was going to die if I didn't go onto dialysis, and then get a kidney transplant as soon as possible. One of the many doctors told me that I should follow a strictly vegan diet, and I should be okay. Other doctors told me that following a vegan diet would be "difficult." As if having my body cut in half was going to be simple and low risk. Instead of having the kidney transplant, I began following a vegan diet. I have since learned very clearly that a high-protein diet is not good for the kidneys.

"When people eat too much protein, it releases nitrogen into the blood or is digested and metabolized. This places a strain on the kidneys, which must expel the waste through the urine. High-protein diets are associated with reduced kidney function. Over time, individuals who consume very large amounts of protein, particularly animal protein, risk permanent loss of kidney function. Harvard researchers reported recently that high-protein diets were associated with a significant decline in kidney function, based on observations in 1,624 women participating in the Nurses' Health Study. The good news is that the damage was found only in those who already had reduced kidney function at the study's outset. The bad news is that as many as one in four adults in the United States may already have reduced kidney function, suggesting that most people who have renal problems are unaware of that fact and do not realize that high-protein diets may put them at risk for further deterioration. The kidney-damaging effect was seen only with animal protein. Plant protein had no harmful effect.[1]

The American Academy of Family Physicians notes that high animal protein intake is largely responsible for the high prevalence of kidney stones in the United States and other developed countries and recommends protein restriction for the prevention of recurrent kidney stones.[2]"

– Physicians Committee for Responsible Medicine, PCRM.org. Citing 1. Knight EL, Stampfer MJ, Hankinson SE, Spiegelman D, Curhan GC. The Impact of Protein Intake on Renal Function Decline in Women with Normal Renal Function or Mild Renal Insufficiency. Ann Int Med. 2003;138:460-467; 2. Goldfarb DS, Coe FL. Prevention of Recurrent Nephrolithiasis. Am Fam Physician. 1999; 60:2269-2276.

I don't depend on soy, or any one particular plant, for protein in my diet. Soybeans are best consumed raw, such as directly out of the pod, or tossing them into a salad. I eat a variety of fruits, vegetables, herbs, nuts, seeds, and sea vegetables. My body gets more than enough protein-building properties in the form of amino acids from the variety of foods that I eat.

Mushrooms are a protein-dominant food. But they aren't a plant, they are a fungus. They are okay to eat in moderation. They contain the mineral potassium as well as nutritional compounds, including some glyconutrients, that improve the immune system, and that may help prevent cancer.

I have reservations about picking my own mushrooms from the wild, as I know that certain types of mushrooms can make you very ill, and others can kill you. Of course there are also mushrooms that can open your mind. Mushrooms that fall under the poisonous category make up only a small fraction of the variety of mushroom species. I prefer to purchase mushrooms from people who are educated about mushrooms – such as the family who have a stand at the local farmers' market.

Dietary protein can also be obtained from legumes, which are protein-dominant seeds. These include chickpeas (also known as garbanzo beans), kidney beans, lentils, mung beans, and soybeans. Protein-dominant foods can be harsh on the system. To increase the presence of amino acids and enzymes in legumes, soak them for several hours in water, or germinate them over three to six days by keeping them moist in a clean place (being sure to thoroughly rinse them at least once a day, and preferably two or three times). Soaking, germinating, or sprouting legumes increases their nutritional value, making them less heavy and harsh on the digestive system.

> "Modern researchers know that it is virtually impossible to design a calorie-sufficient diet based on unprocessed whole natural plant foods that is deficient in any of the amino acids. The only possible exception could be a diet based solely on fruit."
> – Jeff Novick, M.S., R.D.

Don't believe the nonsense put out by the meat, dairy, and egg industries that advise people to consume meat, milk, and eggs to get protein into their diet. Even the United States government programs that supposedly establish nutrition "requirements" – such as the food pyramid – are flawed.

The U.S. Recommended Daily Allowance (USRDA) standards, and the government's food triangle, were largely created using money from trade groups supported by the meat, dairy, and egg industries.

It is no secret that many of the people who work for the FDA and USDA are people who have worked or eventually work for some branch of the meat, dairy, and egg trade groups – often through employment with lobbying groups that work to get laws past to increase government welfare for the meat, dairy, and egg industries – and usually for large, corporate farming interests.

Much of the nutritional information presented to children in their classrooms is flawed, and is most often provided free to school systems from organizations supported by the meat, dairy, and egg industries. Included in this biased and flawed information is the advice that humans should eat a large amount of animal protein. Again, this information is propaganda financed by the meat, dairy, and egg industries.

What you won't hear in the advertising of meat, dairy, and eggs is that people who consume the largest amounts of animal protein also experience degenerative diseases, such as heart disease, diabetes, arthritis, obesity, macular degeneration, kidney disorders, osteoporosis, cancers, etc., in conjunction with the amount of animal flesh, milk, and eggs they consume.

Some people promote a high-protein diet as a way to become lean. A high-protein diet is clearly not healthful, and can lead to a variety of health problems. Dr. John McDougal, who is one of the few doctors I know of promoting true health, has some interesting things to say about the high protein diet. He has written a number of books, including about heart health. He promotes a vegan diet.

> "Our Creator designed us to run on carbohydrates. Glucose, one of the simplest, most basic carbohydrates, is our primary fuel. It is more easily converted into energy than fat or protein, and, therefore, our bodies will always burn it first. In addition, it is the cleanest-burning fuel of the body, creating fewer byproducts than

other nutrients. By our very design, the body needs carbohydrates to operate efficiently and provide ample energy. A testament to their importance is the fact that the brain tissues, red blood cells, and cells of the kidneys will only use glucose as fuel.

When you take the carbohydrates away, your body runs out of glucose and is forced to burn its secondary fuel - fat.

When your cells burn fat instead of glucose, byproducts known as ketones are produced. This creates a metabolic state called ketosis, which leads to a loss of appetite and a decrease in food intake, which results in weight loss. Ketosis also has a strong diuretic effect, resulting in significant water loss-and, again, weight loss. However, ketosis is also associated with fatigue, nausea, and low blood pressure."

– Dr. John McDougall

To obtain the high-grade protein your body needs to build healthy tissues, stick to eating a variety of edible plants, including fresh fruit, raw green vegetables, some sprouts, and some sea vegetables and soaked raw nuts.

For more information on the topic of nutrients for optimum body performance, read *Thrive Fitness: Mental and Physical Strength for Life*, by Brendan Brazier. Also, *Becoming Raw: The Essential Guide to Raw Vegan Diets*, by Brenda Davis, RD, Vesanto Melina, MS, RD, and Rynn Berry. For prevention of and reversal of common diseases, read Dr. Caldwell Esselstyn's book, *Prevent and Reverse Heart Disease: The Revolutionary, Scientifically-proven, Nutrition-based Cure*. Esselstyn's book also helps kill through the myth that we need to consume meat, dairy, and eggs to get protein, and how animal protein can degrade health.

"Some Americans are obsessed with protein. Vegans are bombarded with questions about where they get their protein. Athletes used to eat thick steaks before competition because they thought it would improve their performance. Protein supplements are sold at health food stores. This concern about protein is misplaced. Although protein is certainly an essential nutrient which plays many key roles in the way our bodies function, we do not need huge quantities of it. In reality, we need small amounts of protein. Only one calorie out of every ten we take in needs to come from protein. Athletes do not need much more protein than the general public. Protein supplements are expensive, unnecessary, and even harmful for some people."

– Reed Mangels, Ph.D., R.D., Protein in the Vegan Diet, Vegetarian Resource Group, VRG.org

"All proteins are made up of the same amino acids. All. No exceptions. The difference between animal and vegetable proteins is in the content of certain amino acids. If vegetable proteins are mixed, the differences get made up. Even if they aren't mixed, all you need to do to get the right amount of low amino acids is to eat more of that food. There is no 'need' for animal proteins at all."

– Dr. Marion Nestle, Professor, Department of Nutrition, Food Studies, and Public Health, New York University

The protein per calorie of legumes, vegetables, grains, fruits, and nuts and seeds.

Notice that, per calorie, lettuce contains more protein than fruits, nuts, seeds, and some legumes.

Legumes

54%	Soybean sprouts	29%	Lentils
43%	Mungbean sprouts	28%	Split peas
43%	Soybean curd (tofu)	26%	Kidney beans
35%	Soy flour2	23%	Garbanzo beans
35%	Soybeans2	6%	Lima beans
33%	Soy sauce	6%	Navy beans
32%	Broad beans		

Grains

31%	Wheat germ	15%	Buckwheat
20%	Rye	12%	Millet
17%	Wheat, hard red	11%	Barley
16%	Wild rice	8%	Brown rice
15%	Oatmeal		

Fruits

16%	Lemons	8%	Watermelon
10%	Honeydew melon	7%	Tangerine
9%	Cantaloupe	6%	Papaya
8%	Strawberry	6%	Peach
8%	Orange	5%	Pear
8%	Blackberry	5%	Banana
8%	Cherry	5%	Grapefruit
8%	Apricot	3%	Pineapple
8%	Grape	1%	Apple

Nuts and Seeds

21%	Pumpkin seeds	12%	Almonds
17%	Sunflower seeds	12%	Cashews
13%	Walnuts, black	8%	Filberts
13%	Sesame seeds		

Vegetables

49%	Spinach	26%	Green beans
47%	New Zealand spinach	24%	Cucumbers
46%	Watercress	24%	Dandelion greens
45%	Kale	26%	Green pepper
45%	Broccoli	22%	Artichokes
44%	Brussels sprouts	22%	Cabbage

43%	Turnip greens	21%	Celery
43%	Collards	21%	Eggplant
40%	Cauliflower	18%	Tomatoes
39%	Mustard greens	16%	Onions
38%	Mushrooms	15%	Beets
34%	Chinese cabbage	12%	Pumpkin
34%	Parlsey	11%	Potatoes
34%	Lettuce	8%	Yams
30%	Green peas	6%	Sweet potatoes
28%	Zucchini		

– Nutritive Value of American Foods in Common Units, USDA *Agricultural Handbook No. 456.*

• Make Your Diet Sustainable

"It is scandalous that at a time when an estimated 20 million people die annually worldwide of hunger and its effects, 70% of the grain produced in the US and over 40% of the grain produced worldwide is fed to animals destined for slaughter. Animal-based diets threaten to make global hunger worse in the future by contributing significantly to water shortages, global warming, and soil erosion. It takes up to 14-times as much water for an animal-based diet than for a plant-based diet. According to a 2006 UN FAO report, animal-based agriculture emits more greenhouse gases (in CO_2 equivalents) than all of the cars and other means of transportation worldwide combined (18% vs. 13.5%). Making matters worse, that same UN report projected a doubling of meat consumption in 50 years, worsening global warming and many other environmental problems. A major shift to plant-based diets is essential to move our imperiled planet to a sustainable path."

– Richard Schwartz

"It's phenomenal to me that groups come out with lists like '20 Things You Can Do to Change the Environment' and will list 'drive a fuel-efficient car' and 'change your light bulbs,' but won't say 'eat less meat.' They are omitting the single-most powerful, most meaningful action you can take.

Let's say you take a shower every day and that these showers average seven minutes. That's 49 minutes of showering a week. Let's say that's 50 minutes a week, with flow rates of two gallons a minute (which is very strong). At that rate, you'd be using 100 gallons a week for showering. That's 5,200 gallons a year to shower. It takes 5,214 gallons of water to produce one pound of California beef (according to University of California Agricultural Extension).

You'd save as much water by not eating one pound of beef as you would by not showering every day for one year."

– John Robbins, author of *The Food Revolution*

A diet consisting largely of fresh plant matter benefits the planet in many ways. Most significantly, it eliminates the dependence on the wasteful and environmentally damaging meat and dairy industries. And it greatly reduces reliance on processed and corporate foods.

"As human beings, our greatness lies not so much in being able to remake the world as in being able to remake ourselves."

– Mahatma Gandhi

Many people are consuming meat with no idea of the impact the meat industry has on the planet. The methane belched and otherwise emitted from a single cow amounts to about 145 pounds of methane annually. Methane is a greenhouse gas with 23-times the global warming capacity of carbon dioxide. Manure also emits methane.

Tremendous amounts of food are needed to feed the billions of farmed animals being raised throughout the world, including mammals, birds, and fish. More than 60% of the food grown on the planet is grown to feed farmed animals. Additionally, an increasing amount of fish taken from the world's already depleted seas is going to feed farmed animals, and to use as fertilizer to grow grains for feeding farmed animals.

Most commonly, the food grown for farmed animals is grown using nitrogen fertilizer, which is made from natural gas, a fossil fuel. The nitrogen fertilizer was developed using techniques used to develop nitrogen-based bombs used during World War I. The fertilizers are manufactured in factories using large quantities of other fuels, including petroleum drilled from Earth and also electricity made by coal-burning generating plants – which use coal mined from Earth, which causes an extraordinary amount of environmental destruction, such as mountain top removal and the obliteration of forests and river valleys. Nitrous oxide is a greenhouse gas with 296 times the global warming implications of carbon dioxide. It evaporates from fields where the nitrogen fertilizer is applied, and ends up contributing to lung-choking, high-particulate smog.

When most of the farmland on each continent is being used to grow food for farmed animals, which is the situation that we have today, it means that most of the farm equipment is used to grow, harvest, store, and transport food for farmed animals. The equipment used on farms is largely powered by petroleum gasoline and diesel fuel, which emits massive amounts of carbon dioxide into the atmosphere.

Meat, dairy, egg, and seafood products need to be refrigerated, including in temperature controlled trucks, trains, and airplanes. The warehouses where they are stored use more fossil fuels to maintain the storage temperatures. Then the products are shipped inside refrigerated trucks, and taken to stores and restaurants where the products are stored in temperature-controlled rooms and/or put into temperature-controlled display cases. The purchaser must then store the products in a refrigerator or freezer. All of this refrigerating uses fossil fuels, contributing to global warming. More fossil fuels are used to cook the meat, seafood, and eggs, adding more to the global warming gasses.

Additionally, milk is most often pasteurized, which is a heating process involving the use of fossil fuels

> "Our deeds determine us, as much as we determine our deeds."
> – George Eliot

It is estimated that Americans throw away about 25% of the foods they purchase, either through leftovers, or spoiled food. People who eat at home typically waste fewer food products, and people who eat out at restaurants waste more. Most of this wasted food ends up in landfills, where the throwaways are deprived of oxygen. This produces more greenhouse gasses in the form of carbon dioxide and methane. It is better to compost food in home gardens, which improves soil, and reduces dependence on landfills.

An increasing amount of farmland around the planet is being used for raising farmed animals. This has been going on for hundreds of years, and is happening not only on continents, but also on islands.

As you can tell by my name, I am Scottish. My ancestors dealt with the Highland Clearances of 1800s Scotland. This was brought about by Britain's increased demand for meat. To provide land for cattle and sheep, many poor people were kicked off their land, their villages were demolished, and forests were cleared. This is just one small example of the impact cattle ranching has had on poorer people.

As I have traveled around North America, I never fail to be disappointed by the amount of land being used for livestock, and especially by the amount of land and resources used to grow food for farmed animals.

What happened in Scotland years ago has been happening for the past several decades in North, South, and Central America. An increasing amount of land is being cleared to grow food for cattle, and to provide grazing land for cattle. Many thousands of poor people are being forced from their land so that the land can be cleared for the world meat industry. Just as poor people in Scotland were kicked of the land so that the Brits could have more meat, in Central and South

America poor people are being forced from the land to provide space to grow food for farmed animals and land for grazing farmed animals so that meat can be provided for the wealthier people of the planet. All over North America there have been smaller farms taken over by larger farms, and much of this has been to expand the amount of land being used to grow food for farmed animals.

> "According to the United Nations Food and Agriculture Organization, 756 million tons of grain plus most of the world's soybean crop are fed to animals and that amount has increased sharply in recent years as Asian nations have become more prosperous and their populations have started eating more meat."
> – Peter Singer

A few years back NASA conducted a study concluding that the most fertile soil in the United States is now covered by cities. Although cities only take up a little over 3% of the continental land area, that land can produce as much food as the 29% of land used for agriculture. The study concluded that the land being used for agriculture is less fertile and this increases the use of fertilizers and other farming chemicals.

> "If it came from a plant, eat it; if it was made in a plant, don't."
> – Michael Pollan

The fresh food diet is not something that comes in a can, bottle, or plastic bag. It is a diet that consists of edible plant substances that can be grown in your yard, harvested in the wilds, and/or purchased from local organic farmers. The fresh food diet requires more fruiting trees and bushes and other culinary plants to be grown. More plants clean the air, provide oxygen, filter water, create homes for wildlife, and manifest a more healthful environment for all forms of life on the planet.

Additionally, with fewer people consuming meat, land previously used to raise farm animals – and used to grow tremendous amounts of food for those animals – is turned over to the wilds of nature. When a person chooses to follow a sunfood diet, they are also choosing to eliminate their share of the fossil fuels, toxic chemicals, and resources used to maintain the global meat industry.

> "Health depends largely on the foods we eat, and even the commerce of the world is concerned mainly with food supply. By understanding thoroughly, therefore, the meaning of the diet reform movement, we acquire new ideas of living. To become a genuine diet reformer is to recognize that all true and lasting reform begins with oneself. It means further that man will not only become a new creature with a more radiant health, but that he will be better able to promote the higher life of love and brotherhood."
> – Dugald Semple, *The Sunfood Way to Health*

On a sunfood diet your power will awaken from a dormant state induced by unhealthful foods, low-quality life choices, and slothful thinking patterns. Your perceptions will enlighten. What you are capable of accomplishing will become clear to you as you transform into a happier, more healthful and satisfied being in tune with your instinct, intellect, talent, and essence.

A plant-based diet that is free of meat, dairy, eggs, and low-quality foods provides for the restoration of your inner nature, which benefits outer nature.

Not only does following a raw, plant-based diet protect animals from exploitation, it also protects wildlife, wildlands, the oceans, lakes and rivers, and Earth. This is because a raw vegan diet has a much lower impact on Earth than that of the standard American diet (SAD) that consists of meat, dairy, eggs, and highly polluting junk food. It starts with the fact that most food grown on the planet is being fed to farm animals. This may come as a surprise to those who thought that there is a food shortage on the planet. Humans could not possibly consume all of the food that is growing on Earth. There is more than enough food to feed every human on the planet. The largest part of the problem is that most food grown on the planet is used to feed farm animals so that the rich countries can have their meat and dairy products.

> "We are the living graves of murdered beasts, slaughtered to satisfy our appetites. How can we hope in this world to attain the peace we say we are so anxious for?"
>
> – George Bernard Shaw

When we refuse to eat animals, eggs, dairy products, and junk food, and instead subsist on a plant-based diet, we are agreeing to live in tune with nature. We are not participating in the animal-killing industries of factory farms and slaughterhouses. We are not part of the farming industry that grows more than 60 percent of its products to feed animals on meat farms. We are not a part of the fishing industry that kills hundreds of millions of fish and hundreds of thousands of sea mammals and aquatic birds every year. We are not part of the ranching industry that kills many millions of wolves, bear, lions, raccoons, prairie dogs, predator birds, and other wild animals every year. We are not part of an industry that is cutting down the rainforests to provide cattle-grazing land and land to grow food to feed farmed animals. When we follow a sunfood diet we are protecting wildlife, wildlands, and forests, and the oceans, lakes and rivers, and Earth.

> "I am in favor of animal rights as well as human rights. That is the way of a whole human being."
>
> – Abraham Lincoln

"Everyone has control over what they put in their mouth and these choices make a huge difference for our shared environment – our biosphere, as well as our individual environments – our bodies! Choosing organic, vegan raw foods is not only supporting our individual bodies with optimally nutritious foods, but supporting the growth of the whole organic and vegan industry – basically, our health and the health of our planet."

– Rod Rotundi, Leaf Organics, Culver City, CA; LeafOrganics.com

"It should not be believed that all beings exist for the sake of the existence of man. On the contrary, all the other beings too have been intended for their own sakes and not for the sake of something else."

– Maimonides

"A man can live and be healthy without killing animals for food; therefore, if he eats meat, he participates in taking animal life for the sake of his appetite. And to act so is immoral."

– Leo Tolstoy

"Many years ago, I was fishing, and as I was reeling in the poor fish, I realized, 'I am killing him – all for the passing pleasure it brings me.' And something inside me clicked. I realized, as I was watching him fight for breath, that his life was as important to him as mine is to me."

– Paul McCartney

ADAPTT (Animals Deserve Absolute Protection Today and Tomorrow), adaptt.org. Gary Yourofsky gives seminars about the truth of the animal farming industry.
FarmUSA.org
GreenPeople.org/AnimalRights.htm
MercyForAnimals.org
United Poultry Concerns, UPC-Online.org
Shark Savers, SharkSavers.org
WeDontEatAnimals.com

• Livestock by the Billions: A Global Environmental Disaster

"Ask the questions. "Who produced my food?" "What did they use on it?" What's it doing to me, the environment, and the animals?" I want you to think about this. Is it right? Is it right that we should end up with more cancer? Should it be right that we end up with less top soil? It is right that we end up with fewer trees? When are we as the American people going to stand up and say, "Enough is enough!" When in god's world are we going to wake up to the fact that we are destroying the planet?"

– Howard Lyman, MadCowboy.com

"Of all agricultural land in the United States, 87 percent is used to raise animals for food. Twenty thousand pounds of potatoes can be grown on one acre of land, but only 165 pounds of beef can be produced in the same space.

[South and Central American] Rainforests are being destroyed at a rate of 125,000 square miles per year to create space to raise animals for food. Fifty-five square feet of land are consumed for every quarter-pound fast food burger made of rainforest beef."

– PETA, VegNow.Com

"Nationwide, factory-farmed animals produce 130 times more manure than the human population – the equivalent of five tons of manure for every U.S. citizen. U.S. factory farms generate more than 350 million tons of manure each year."

– Farm Sanctuary, VegForLife.Org

"Cattle and sheep grazing is ecologically destructive and an abomination against our national park system in areas as pristine as the Grand Canyon Park.

Grazing causes rapid depletion of wooded areas by clearing, cultivating and eroding the soil. Soil losses are as high as 44 tons per acre annually on steep slopes. Woodlands, waterways and wildlife habitats have been significantly reduced or eradicated entirely due to overgrazing."

– FarmSanctuary.Org

"Most wars are fought over control of natural resources: land, water, oil, and minerals. Yet, animal agriculture is by far the largest user and despoiler of natural resources."

– Citizens for Healthy Options in Children's Education, CHOICE.USA

"Cattle are a chief source of organic pollution; cow dung is poisoning the freshwater lakes, rivers, and streams of the world. Growing herds of cattle are exerting unprecedented pressure on the carrying capacity of natural ecosystems, edging entire species of wildlife to the brink of extinction. Cattle are a growing source of global warming, and their increasing numbers now threaten the very dynamic of the biosphere."

– Jeremy Rifkin, in his book *Beyond Beef: The Rise and Fall of the Cattle Culture*

"Livestock (like automobiles) are a human invention and convenience, not part of pre-human times, and a molecule of CO_2 exhaled by livestock is no more natural than one from an auto tailpipe. Moreover, while over time an equilibrium of CO_2 may exist between the amount respired by animals and the amount photosynthesized by plants, that equilibrium has never been static. Today, tens of billions more livestock are exhaling CO_2 than in preindustrial days, while Earth's photosynthetic capacity (its capacity to keep carbon out of the atmosphere by absorbing it in plant mass) has declined sharply as forest has been cleared. (Meanwhile, of course, we add more carbon to the air by burning fossil fuels, further overwhelming the carbon-absorption system.)"

– Robert Goodland, a former World Bank Group environmental advisor, and Jeff Anhang, an environmental specialist at the World Bank Group's International Finance Corporation. They concluded that, of the world emissions of global greenhouse gasses related to human activity, 51% could be attributed to the meat diet. That is a huge jump from the 18% figure concluded on in 2006. *World Watch* magazine, April 2012

"The less animal-based food you eat, and the more you replace those calories with plant-based food, the better off you are, in terms of your health as well as your contributions to the health of the planet."

– Gidon Eshel, assistant professor of geophysics at the University of Chicago, co-author of a study concluding that becoming a vegan does more to reduce greenhouse gasses than the type of car you drive. (*Earth Interactions* journal, April 2006; It's better to green your diet than your car, *New Scientist Magazine*, Dec. 17, 2005)

"Rainforests cover less than two percent of the Earth's surface, yet they are home to nearly half of our planet's living creatures. Butterflies and birds fill the air, their colors are so intense, no artist could ever match them. Noble jaguars, howler monkeys, vines, fish, gorillas, orchids, lizards, and orangutans flourish there – and nowhere else on Earth.

A four-square mile area of rainforest teems with colorful variety: 750 types of trees, 1,500 different flowers, 125 mammal species, and 400 kinds of birds.

But rainforests are disappearing at the rate of a football field every second. The destruction of the Earth's most ancient complex ecosystem threatens the very survival of the human species.

Over 99 percent of the rainforest species have not yet been studied for possible medical use. A plant that holds the cure for AIDS – or a future epidemic – may be growing somewhere in the rainforest. Or a bulldozer may be crushing the last one right now as you read this.

Rice, potatoes, bananas, chocolate, coffee, oranges, tomatoes, yams, and dozens of other food crops originated in the rainforests. The wild strains still found there provide genetic material necessary to keep world agriculture stocks hardy and healthy. Undiscovered rainforest species could provide new sources of food in the future.

Once the rainforest is gone, the vanished species won't return. And once the proud, ancient indigenous cultures are destroyed, the knowledge they possess – knowledge that could benefit all of humanity – will be lost forever."

– The Rainforest Action Network, RAN.Org

"The livestock population of the United States today consumes enough grain and soybeans to feed over five times the entire human population of the country. We feed these animals over 80 percent of the corn we grow, and over 95 percent of the oats… Less than half the harvested agricultural acreage in the United States is used to grow food for people. Most of it is used to grow livestock feed. This is a drastically inefficient use of our acreage. For every sixteen pounds of grain and soybeans fed to beef cattle, we get back only one pound as meat on our plates. The other fifteen are inaccessible to us. Most of it is turned into manure."

– John Robbins, in his book *Diet for a New America*

"In California, the number of gallons of water needed to produce one edible pound of: wheat: 25 gallons; beef: 5,214 gallons.

Energy expended to produce one pound of grain-fed beef: equivalent to one gallon of gasoline."

– EarthSave.Org

"McDonald's equals slavery and starvation."

– Graffiti on a wall in Quito, Ecuador

"More than half of all the water and 33 percent of all the raw materials used for all purposes in the United States are used in meat production… the average chicken-processing plant may use 100 million gallons of water daily. More than 260 million acres of U.S. forest have been cleared to grow crops to feed to cattle. Cattle-grazing in the western United States has led to soil erosion and desertification."

– *Take a Step Toward Compassionate Living*, by the People for the Ethical Treatment of Animals, PETA-Online.Org; 2004

"More than half of US grain and almost 40% of world grain is being fed to livestock rather than being consumed directly by humans. In the United States, more than 8 billion livestock are maintained, which eat about 7 times as much grain as is consumed directly by the entire US population.

Producing 1 kg of fresh beef requires about 13 kg of grain and 30 kg of forage. This much grain and forage requires a total of 43 000 L of water.

A quarter-pound burger with cheese takes 26 oz of petroleum and leaves a 13-lb carbon footprint. This is equivalent to burning 7 lb of coal.

At a time when 20% of people in the US go to bed hungry each night and almost 50% of the world's population is malnourished, choosing to eat more plant-based foods and less red meat is better for all of us—ourselves, our loved ones, and our planet."

– Dr. Dean Ornish, Holy Cow! What's Good For You Is Good For Our Planet: Comment on "Red Meat Consumption and Mortality," Archives of Internal Medicine, March 12, 2012. Ornish is the founder of the Preventative Medicine Research Institute, PMRI.org

"Livestock grazing on public lands accounts for less than one-tenth of one percent of employment in the eleven western states, including in Colorado (according to a study by Thomas Powers, chairman of the University of Montana's Department of Economics). However, this activity costs taxpayers anywhere from three to five hundred million dollars per year (according to the Cato Institute). More significantly, cows and sheep on public lands pollute streams and rivers, and jeopardize the continued survival of many rare wildlife species (according to the Congressional General Accounting Office)."

– *Colorado Wolf Tracks*; 1996; WildEarthGuardians.org

"Last April (2011), Congress eliminated federal protection for wolves in the Northern Rocky Mountains. Hunting in Idaho and Montana has resulted in 410 wolves killed this winter alone – yet, less than 1,300 wolves live in those two states."

– WildEarthGuardians.org

"The U.S. government spent $22 billion to build 133 water projects in the West. Every year the government spends $7 billion on these water projects. Farmers pay less than $1 billion per year to the government for water."

– *NPR*, 1997

"You can use your food choices, your daily habit of eating, to say yes to life in a very profound way, and to say no to the corporate culture that is destroying the planet, and our communities. You can use your food choices, every meal, every bite, as an opportunity to take a stand for life, to take a stand for compassion."

– John Robbins, *The Food Revolution*; TheFoodRevolution.Org

"When emissions from land use and land use change are included, the livestock sector accounts for nine percent of CO_2 deriving from human-related activities, but produces a much larger share of even more harmful greenhouse gases."

– Food and Agriculture Organisation, Rome, Italy; in a report on worldwide pollution caused by the cattle industry; 2006

"Raising animals for food causes more water pollution than any other industry in the U.S. because animals raised for food produce one hundred thirty times the excrement of the entire human population. It means 87,000 pounds per second. Much of the waste from factory farms and slaughterhouses flows into streams and rivers, contaminating water sources.

Each vegetarian can save one acre of trees per year. More than 260 million acres of U.S. forests have been cleared to grow crops to feed animals raised for meat. And another acre of trees disappears every eight seconds. The tropical rainforests are also being destroyed to create grazing land for cattle."

– *Eating for Peace*, by Buddhist teacher Thich Naht Hanh, on mindful consumption. From the FoodRevolution.Org Web site of John Robbins.

"Raising animals for food consumes more than half of all the water used in the United States. It takes 2,500 gallons of water to produce a pound of meat, but only 25 gallons to produce a pound of wheat. The amount of water used in the production of the meat from an average steer could float a destroyer."

– People for the Ethical Treatment of Animals, VegNow.Com

• War on Wildlife

"But it [cattle ranching] is anything but benign. It is the number one source of water pollution in the West. It's the number one source of soil erosion in the West. It's the number one cause of species endangerment in the West. It's the reason we don't have wolves throughout the West. It's one of the major reasons that more than four-fifths of all native fish west of the Continental Divide are endangered or threatened."

– George Wuerthner of Eugene, Oregon. From *Dispelling the Cowboy Myth*, by Tim Lenerich, Earthsave.org/News/03Summer/Cowboy_Myth.htm; 2004

"Every year, tens of thousands of bison, coyotes, wolves, and other wildlife are maimed, shot, poisoned, and even burned alive because the meat industry claims these animals interfere with raising animals for food. This war on wildlife is carried out with the full support of state and federal agencies, which fund so-called predator control programs."

– FarmSancturary.org

"Animal agriculture directly kills annually nearly 50 billion animals worldwide, after subjecting them to the cruelties of factory farming. It also kills uncounted numbers of wildlife on land and in the seas."

– Citizens for Healthy Options in Children's Education, CHOICE.usa

"In reality, ranchers are the most pervasively destructive force on our public land, with logging as a distant second. Via outlandish subsidies, you, I, and Uncle Sam support the cattle industry with drought and fire relief, fencing, water tanks, windmills, and bargain-basement grazing fees. Our government kills hundreds of thousands of wild creatures each year to protect ranchers' herds against predators such as wolves, mountain lions, and coyotes.

In return we get erosion, endangered species, habitat destruction, flash floods, exotic weeds, desertification, and some of the most degraded landscape on Earth."

– Tim Lenerich, *Dispelling the Cowboy Myth*,

"Nearly 20 million taxpayer dollars fund the trapping, poisoning, and shooting of native predators deemed a threat to agriculture by the USDA Wildlife Services agency, which each year kills approximately 100,000 coyotes, bobcats, foxes, bears, wolves, and other predators. In 2001 the program also killed 1.6 million other 'nuisance' animals.

Almost two-thirds of all large mammal species are threatened or endangered in the lower 48 states. Less than 10 percent of all endangered and threatened species in the U.S. is improving.

About 20 percent of all endangered and threatened species are harmed by grazing."

– A Voice for Animals, VoiceForAnimals.net; 2004

"In response to ranchers' complaints of coyotes attacking cattle in southern Arizona, the federal government took to the air this past January, killing 200 coyotes. The hunt was conducted by Wildlife Services, a division of the U.S. Department of Agriculture, and took place on both public and private land."

– *Earth First! Journal*, May-June 2006; EarthFirstJournal.org

"In 1914, Congress first appropriated money for the U.S. Biological Survey (now known as Animal Damage Control) to exterminate wolves from the face of the continent. Though the agency failed to eradicate the species entirely, by 1945 it had killed every wolf in Colorado."

– *Colorado Wolf Tracks*; 1996; wildearthguardians.org

"The ADC program, created by the Animal Damage Control Act of 1931, is greatly responsible for the virtual extinction of the grizzly and wolf in the lower 48 states as well as for putting the black-footed ferret, jaguar, black-tailed prairie dog, bald eagle, and other wild animals in, or close to, the endangered category. ADC reported it poisoned 1.8 million animals in 1991 and distributed thousands of pounds of restricted-use pesticides to private individuals who poisoned untold numbers more. The U.S. Agency for International Development works with ADC to export ADC pest control practices and chemicals, including those banned in the U.S., to developing countries."

– *Wildlife Damage Review*; 1997; WildEarthGuardians.org

"Trapping and/or hunting are allowed on more than half of the 540 U.S. National Wildlife Refuges.

According to the U.S. Fish & Wildlife Service, of 27 million people who visited refuges, 22 million came for wildlife observation, while only 1.2 million visited to hunt or trap animals."

– A Voice for Animals, VoiceForAnimals.net, 2005

"Next to an all-out nuclear war, today's intensive animal agriculture represents the greatest threat to human welfare in the history of mankind."

– Farm Animal Reform Movement, FarmUSA.org; 2005

"The love for all living creatures is the most noble attribute of man."

– Charles Darwin

• Pollution Caused by Farming Animals

Most pollution on this planet is caused by the meat, dairy, and egg industries – including the meat and dairy packaging, distribution, marketing, cooking, and consumption process. This is because of the misuse and abuse of resources such as fuel, metal, plastics, paper, electricity, and other items used to get meat on the plates of humans who choose to eat meat, dairy, and eggs. Consider the following:

1. The supplies and fuel used to manufacture the equipment that is used to farm the food for billions of farm animals.

2. The supplies and fuel used to run and maintain the equipment that grows the food for billions of farm animals.

3. The supplies and fuel used to transfer the food to feed billions of farm animals.

4. The supplies and fuel used to manufacture the equipment that is used to raise billions of farm animals.

5. The supplies and fuel used to run and maintain the equipment that is used to raise billions of farm animals.

6. The supplies and fuel used to transfer billions of farm animals to the slaughterhouses.

7. The supplies and fuel used to create and maintain the trucks and other equipment used to transport billions of farm animals to slaughterhouses.

8. The supplies and fuel used to manufacture the equipment that runs the slaughterhouses where billions of farm animals are killed.

9. The supplies and fuel used to run and maintain the slaughterhouses.

10. The supplies and fuel used to manufacture the equipment that transfers the dairy products to processing and storage facilities.

11. The supplies and fuel used to run and maintain those processing and storage facilities.

12. The supplies and fuel used to manufacture the equipment that transfers the meat and dairy products to the markets.

13. The supplies and fuel used to run and maintain the equipment that transfers trillions of pounds of meat and dairy products to the markets.

14. The supplies and fuel used to manufacture the equipment that is used in the markets – from the buildings to the shelving to the heating and air conditioning and refrigeration units.

15. The supplies and fuel used to run the markets that sell the meat and dairy products.

16. The supplies and fuel used to manufacture all the equipment used to advertise the meat and dairy products.

17. The supplies and fuel used to advertise the meat and dairy products – which take up millions of pages of newspaper and magazine pages, all sorts of outdoor advertising, and hordes of radio and TV commercial time.

18. The supplies and fuel used to keep and display the meat and dairy products in stores.

19. The supplies and fuel used to manufacture and maintain all the hundreds of millions of refrigerators, stoves, and microwaves used in the stores, restaurants, hotels, homes, cruise ships, schools, hospitals, prisons, military bases, and other places where meat and dairy products are kept and prepared for consumption.

20. The supplies and fuel used to fuel all the hundreds of millions of refrigerators, stoves, and microwaves.

21. The massive amounts of water, soaps, and other cleansers used to clean the farms, slaughterhouses, equipment, markets, and kitchens of all sorts where all of that meat and dairy are produced, killed, sold, prepared, cooked, and eaten.

22. All the pollution left from the manufacture, marketing, packaging, and shipping of the meat and dairy products.

23. All the supplies and fuel used to deal with all of that pollution.

When a person considers the environmental destruction caused by the meat, dairy, and egg industries, they should take into account the litter from fast-food and junk food that is strewn among the roads and highways of the cities, towns, and country. These are the main sources of litter. The other two main sources of litter are products that also lead to health problems: cigarettes and unhealthful drinks. Beer, soda, energy drinks, coffee, and sweetened juice bottles, cans, and cups, along with cigarette butts, are tossed around by the billions – every day. If the North American diet were factored based on the litter found around towns and cities, and along country roads, one might conclude that we are eating the worst foods ever, topped off by beer, booze, cola, coffee, and candy. In reality, that is what a large number of people are putting into their bodies on a daily basis. The environment pays the price for our low-quality food choices and sugar, caffeine, tobacco, and alcohol addictions. And the medical, surgery, and pharmaceutical industries cash in on the ignorance, neglect, addictions, and abuse that nurture polluted land, toxic bodies, illness, and degenerative diseases.

Then there are all the resources used to run the allopathic medical industry, which largely exists to treat the results of unhealthful living. It does this by utilizing toxic drugs and risky, invasive surgery.

The entire obesity industry – from liposuction to stomach stapling and intestinal bypass to "diet" pills and programs – is the result of unhealthful living. The large majority of heart surgery is the result of people eating unhealthful food (especially dairy, meat, eggs, and processed foods), and not exercising.

All of this pollution, the animal farming, and the products associated with it, are not good for human health, or the health of Earth.

Humans do not need to drink soda or eat meat or dairy, fried foods, grilled or barbecued foods, or anything containing artificial dyes, preservatives, flavors, scents, emulsifiers, or sweeteners. The world would be a much healthier place without any of these toxic concoctions.

Again I ask, what industries use up the most amount of petroleum in North America?

> "This is a global business, and it's not only that we need to add to supply, but we need to reduce demand… In the United States alone, we have about two percent of world oil reserves, five percent of the population and yet we use about 25 percent of the world's consumption of oil."
>
> – James J. Mulva, chairman of ConocoPhillips Co., speaking on NBC TV's *Meet the Press*, June 18, 2006. On the same show, Shell Oil Co. President John Hofmeister explained that oil companies are holding "discussions with the White House quite frequently" with the goal of gaining greater access to U.S. federal lands (such as Nature preserves and national parks), as well as local waters to explore and drill for oil. That is truly deplorable.

The large majority of the food we grow on the continent is fed to farm animals. Raising, slaughtering, packaging, marketing, refrigerating, and cooking billions of farm animals every year use up tremendous amounts of fuel.

If you want to help save the world, stop eating meat, dairy, eggs, and processed foods.

> "The typical U.S. diet, about 28 per cent of which comes from animal sources, generates the equivalent of nearly 1.5 tons more carbon dioxide per person per year than a vegan diet with the same number of calories… By comparison, the difference in annual emissions between driving a typical saloon [sedan] car and a hybrid car, which runs off a rechargeable battery and gasoline, is just over one ton."
>
> – According to study done at the University of Chicago; It's better to green your diet than your car, *New Scientist* magazine, Dec. 17, 2005

"Raising animals for food requires more than one-third of all raw materials and fossil fuels used in the United States. Producing a single hamburger patty uses enough fossil fuel to drive a small car 20 miles and enough water for 17 showers."

– PETA, VegNow.Com, 2004

"If anyone wants to save the planet, all they have to do is just stop eating meat. That's the single most important thing you could do. It's staggering when you think about it. Vegetarianism takes care of so many things in one shot: ecology, famine, cruelty."

– Paul McCartney

Following a vegan diet is the single most effective way you can improve the environment and the health of the world.

If you are a meat eater and think that eating meat, dairy, and eggs is your business, and none of mine, think again. Similarly to how Howard Lyman and others have stated it, I repeat the defense to the stance of vegans: If your diet style is relying on the mass breeding of animals, then it is my business, and it is the business of everyone on the planet. It impacts us environmentally, socially, physically, and financially. Your diet style pollutes the air I breathe, the water I drink, and the food I eat. It has led to, and is leading to the extinction of species, and the entire animal farming industry, including the resources needed to support it, is the main cause of global warming.

A vegetarian diet uses substantially fewer resources than a wasteful and unhealthful meat-based diet. A plant-based diet is not only healthier for humans, but also for farm workers, for the land, for plant life, for the water, for the air, for the animals, and for Earth.

• Veal

"Endless multitudes will have their little children taken from them, ripped open and flayed and most cruelly cut in pieces."

– Leonardo da Vinci, who was outspoken against the killing and consumption of animals

"Think of me tonight. For that which you savor. Did it give you something real, or could you taste the pain of my death in its flavor?"

– Wayne K. Tolson

"We manage to swallow flesh only because we do not think of the cruel and sinful thing that we do."

– Rabindranath Tagore

"A dead cow or sheep lying in the pasture is recognized as carrion. The same sort of carcass dressed and hung up on a buther's stall passes as food."

– J.H. Kellogg

"It is only be softening and disguising dead flesh by culinary preparation that it is rendered susceptible of mastication or digestion, and that the sight of its bloody juices and raw horror does not excite intolerable loathing and disgust."

– Percy Bysshe Shelley

"A newborn baby is taken from his mother and placed in a 'crate' so narrow he can't turn around or even lie down comfortably. Instead of nourishing mother's milk, he is fed a substitute liquid that is purposely deficient in iron and fiber – the better to keep his flesh pale. And since he can hardly move in his confined space, his muscles won't develop and he will stay soft and tender. He will endure this for four months… and then he'll be slaughtered and eaten.

Male calves are an unwanted 'by-product' of the dairy industry, as they cannot produce milk. They are trucked to livestock auctions within hours or days of being born and sold for just a few dollars to veal producers. If the calves are too weak or ill to sell after the grueling truck ride, they may be left to die in pens or back alleyways at the auction yards.

At the veal factories, each calf is chained at the neck in a crate only 22 inches wide, so he can't walk or turn around. Because the iron-deficient diet makes him anemic and sickly, his formula routinely contains drugs… that can get passed on to the unsuspecting consumer. The calf suffers from chronic diarrhea, and he is not even allowed to have water to drink – just the liquid diet that produces what is misleadingly labeled 'milk-fed' – and also 'fancy' or 'white' – veal.

Because this is considered a 'common agribusiness practice' it is typically exempt from animal-cruelty laws. As a matter of fact, the production of veal is specifically excluded from anticruelty laws in the majority of U.S. states. In Europe, several nations have banned the inhumane, severe confinement producer for calves that is standard operating procedure in the U.S. But, the meat and dairy industries are a wealthy, powerful lobbying and advertising force… and they have been defeating farm animal protection efforts for decades."

– Farm Sanctuary No Veal Campaign; FarmSantuary.Org

"If you had to kill your own calf before you ate him, most likely you would not be able to do it. To hear the calf scream, to see the blood spill, to see the baby being taken away from his momma, and to see the look of death in the animal's eye would turn your stomach. So you get the man at the packing house to do the killing for you."

– Dick Gregory

Compassion Action Institute, PleaseBeKind.Com
Farm Sanctuary East, POB 150, Watkins Glen, NY 14891; 607-583-2225; FarmSanctuary.Org; FactoryFarming.Com; NoVeal.Org
Farm Sanctuary West, POB 1065, Orland, CA 95963; 530-865-4617; FarmSanctuary.Org; FactoryFarming.Com; NoVeal.Org
Humane Society of the United States, HSUS.Org

• ANIMALS

NOT only is animal life directly impacted by food choices when someone chooses to be vegetarian, vegan, or a meat-eater, how food is grown affects wildlife.

"Ecologists assert that the only large mammals to survive the near future will be those which humans allow to live. Biologists predict the Earth could lose one quarter to one third of all known species within our lifetime."

– EarthFirst.org

Many people don't seem to understand that when choosing to support organic foods also is choosing to support a safter environment for wildlife.

Food is the number one way humanity interacts with both the planet and the life on Earth. Everything from the types of beverages you consume to the sweeteners you use has an impact on the environment and on animals.

Coffee is one example of a food product that can be grown in ways that support wilflife, or grown in ways that damage wildlife. Coffee has traditionally been grown in forests with a tree canopy where wildife fourished. But, to meet world demand for coffee, companies have developed coffed that can be grown in fields, and without the shade of trees. This has resulted in clearcutting of forests to plant fields of coffee. The loss of trees has had a very negative impact on wildlife, and particularly on songbirds.

Some may say that the songbirds aren't that important in the circle of life. But, they are overlooking the fact that birds help to fertilize land all over the planet. Birds consume insects, spread seeds by way of their droppings, and their natural activities help to pollinate a number of plants, from flowers to trees, bushes, and vines. When the population of any type of bird is reduced, so too are the types of plants their life supports.

Certain types of sweeteners play a large role in environmental destruction. The leader is corn syrup, which is made from corn grown on mono-cropping farms of many thousands of acres that are treated with large amounts of farming chemicals. The intensive process of creating corn syrup is resource-heavy, and the product is damaging to human health. Sugar cane and beet sugar also come from monocropped fields – which require the clearing land of all other plants, which means a loss of homes for wildlife and a degradation of soil. Sugar cane and sugar beet farms also use tremendous amounts of chemicals that poison wildlife and pollute rivers, lakes, and the oceans.

Some of the more environmentally safe sweeteners include maple syrup and coconut bud sap sugar, and this is because these require trees, and trees provide homes to wildlife, absorb greenhouse gasses, put forth oxygen, and help maintain healthy soil. Dates are also a good source of sweetner, such as in making date paste or using dates to add sweetness to smoothies and deserts. Dates are harvested from date trees. The more trees we have, the more healthful the planet will be for both wildlife and human life.

Beef is often given as the example as the most environemtnally destructive food choice. Previous to the industrial revolution and refrigeration, humans did not consume much beef. When they did have meat, it was often smaller portions, and also to flavor dishes – such as in stews with vegetables. But when refrigeration became popular, and the development of refrigerated trucks, ships, and airplane storage areas increased the ability to store and transport meat, the consumption of meat increased, as did the use of all of the resources needed to grow food for the farmed animals, to shelter and feed the animals, and to slaughter, process, transport, store, market, and cook the meat.

Only after the development of refrigeration did humans start to open millions of restaurants serving meat morning, noon, and night. The increased meat consumption did no favors for human health. The energy and fuel to refrigerate and cooked all that meat also spews greenhouse gasses into the environment. Many areas of the world now have more air pollution from restaurants than they do from cars and trucks. Not everyone drives, but nearly everyone eats cooked food.

On many levels, sea life is directly impacted by the food choices of humanity. As industrial farming spreads, so does the use of toxic farming chemicals, the destruction of native species, and the diversity of life. Massive mono-cropping farms are becoming more common. To support this type of farming, chemicals are added to the soil, sprays are used to control insects, and other chemicals are used to prevent fungal growth and plant diseases. All of these chemicals end up in the water and land, and eventually in the rivers, lakes, and seas. Farming chemicals are a major cause of species degradation, including in hormonal imbalances, birth defects, and cancers being found in wildlife. Farming chemicals cause algae to grow out-of-control in rivers and lakes, depleting oxygen in the water, which suffocates waterlife and this causes a loss of food for birds, bears, and other wildlife that feed from rivers and lakes. Farming chemicals also gather in the oceans, causing oxygen depletion and killing off great numbers of sea creatures.

Air pollution caused by the farming industry includes the fumes from engines used on farms and also the trucks, trains, boats, and airplanes used to ship the food. When the pollution gets into the atmosphere, it increases acid rain, which damages plants and also ends up in the oceans, increasing the acidity of the water, which damages a wide varity of life in the seas, including the coral reefs that support all sea life. When the smaller forms of life in the seas decrease in population, the larger sea creatures that live off the smaller creatures have less food to eat. The sea mammals, sea birds, bears, eagles, and other animals that feed off of fish also have less food. When the water fowl and migrating birds decrease in population, the plants on the land that usually get fertilized by the bird droppings also don't get their food. When the forests, fields, meadows, and wetlands degrade, all life forms that depend on the forests, fields, meadows, and wetlands suffer. That is the circle of life, and it is suffering globally largely because of the low-quality food choices of humanity.

Whereever there are problems with farming, there are solutions. Some of the solutions include alternative sources of energy, such as wind and solar energy, and also cellulosic ethanol. Other solutions include organic farming, a plant-based diet, and composing of food scraps.

Educate yourself about your food choices, and how your foods impact both the environmet and wildlife. Many studies have concluded that your food choices have a greater impact on the environment than your transportation choices.

Nurture native wildflowers and edible plants, and fruiting bushes and trees on wildlands. This will improve your food choices while supporting wildlife and reducing your carbon footprint. Also, grow some of your own food in a culinary garden using organic methods and composing yout kitchen scraps into the soil.

Avoid supporting international food companies involved in monocropping and non-organic farming practices.

When you follow a plant-based diet, which is the diet on which the human body thrives, you are using less land to support your food choices. Animal agriculture uses more land than any other type of farming. Animal agriculture includes massive monocropping farms to grow the food to feed the animals. It also involves all of the land used to feed and incarcerate billions of farmed animals. A plant-based diet uses 75% fewer land, water, and fuel resources than a diet rich in meat, dairy, and eggs. When more people follow plant-based diets, more land can be left to the wilds, supporting wildlife; less fuel and water has to be used to grow food to feed farmed animals, to transport those animals, to slaughter the animals, to clean up after the slaughter, and to transport and refrigerate the meat, dairy, and eggs, and to cook the food.

A plant based diet that is largely or all raw and organic is the most environmentally-friendly and sustainable of all dietary styles.

Animals and Society, AnimalsAndSociety.org
Care for the Wild International, CareForTheWild.org
The Custeau Society, Cousteau.org
Karen Dawn's Dawn Watch, DawnWatch.com
Endangered Species Coalition, StopExtinction.org
Farm Sanctuary's Factory Farming Page, FactoryFarming.com
Farm Sanctuary, FarmSanctuary.org
GreenPeace, GreenPeace.org/usa
Humane California, HumaneCalifornia.org
In Defense of Animals, IDAUSA.org
The Leatherback Trust, LeatherBack.org
Natureserve, NatureServe.org
New England Anti-Vivisection Society, NEAVS.org
No Puppy Mills, NoPuppyMills.com
Paw Project, PawProject.org
Polar Bear SOS, PolarBearSOS.org
Save the Chimps, SaveTheChimps.org
Sea Shepherd Conservation Society, SeaShepherd.org
Sea Turtle, SeaTurtle.org
Shark Savers, SharkSavers.org
The Songbird Foundation, SongBird.org
Taking Action for Animals, TakingActionForAnimals.org
United Poultry Concerns, UPC-Online.org
Voice for Animals, VoiceForAnimals.net
Wildlife Watch, WildWatch.org

• VIVISECTION

"Atrocities are not less atrocities when they occur in laboratories and are called medical research."
– Geroge Bernard Shaw

"They laugh, like us. They are devoted to their families, like us. They show compassion, like us. They have unique personalities, like us. When they are confined, hurt, or experimented on, they get depressed, they get angry, they cry, and they grieve. Like us."
– ReleaseChimps.Org

"Vivisection is the blackest of all the black crimes that a man is at present committing against God and his fair creation."
– Mahatma Gandhi

"Each year an estimated 28 million animals in the U.S. are used in research, testing, and education, including:

- 70,000 dogs
- 23,00 cats
- 54,000 nonhuman primates
- 266,000 guinea pigs
- 201,000 hamsters
- 280,000 rabbits
- 155,000 farm animals, including cattle, sheep, and pigs
- 165,000 others, such as gerbils, ferrets, and minks
- Approximately 20–25 million rats and mice."

– A Voice for Animals, VoiceForAnimals.Net; 2006

ANIMALS kept in "science labs" are often purposefully injured, such as by burning them with a blow torch, breaking their bones, cutting off their limbs or facial parts, and having drills and surgical tools put into their brains and other parts of their body. Some have their eyes sewn shut. Others have harsh chemicals put into their eyes, on their skin, or into their mouths. Some have electrodes implanted into their skin, muscles, and brain. Some are exposed to extreme noise, nonstop wind, heat, cold, and other experiments. When they are of no more use to the lab workers these horribly abused animals are left to die, or are killed.

Who funds these laboratory experiments? Much of it is paid for by grants from the National Institutes of Health, which is funded by tax dollars. Another tax-supported agency involved with animal experimentation is the U.S. Department of Agriculture. Other labs are supported by businesses, such as those that manufacture various products. Some animal farming businesses use animals to experiment on to develop new ways of slaughtering farm animals.

> "But aren't these experiments necessary to save human lives?
>
> No, absolutely not. There are better ways to study human physiology, disease, and injury than inducing disease and injury in a different species.
>
> Clinical human studies, autopsies, epidemiology, human tissue studies, and imaging technologies are only some of the better ways to study human health and disease."
>
> – New England Anti-Vivisection Society, NEAVS.Org

Many cosmetics companies have been involved in animal experimentation. Federally funded agencies that have been involved in vivisection include the National Institute of Neurological Disorders and Stroke; the National Center for Research Resources; the National Institute of Diabetes & Digestive & Kidney Diseases; and the National Heart, Lung and Blood Institute. Many universities also run labs where animals are tortured. These include Boston University, Harvard University, the University of Massachusetts Medical School, and UCLA.

But that is a very short list. For more information on companies, government agencies, schools and others conducting animal experimentation, contact the organizations listed in this section.

> "In the past three years, approximately $15 million taxpayer dollars went into federally-funded cat experiments in the state of Massachusetts alone."
>
> – New England Anti-Vivisection Society, NEAVS.Org; 2002

> "If you agree with vivisection, go and be vivisected upon yourself."
>
> – Morrissey, during a concert in London, May 2006. He was commenting about a new £20 million animal testing lab at Oxford University. The week before, Oxford University won a legal appeal to keep demonstrators away from the "biomedical" animal torture facility.

American Anti-Vivisection Society, AAVS.Org
AnimalAid.Org.UK
Animal Protection Institute, API4Animals.Org
AnimalsNeedRights.Net
AnimalSuffering.Com
British Anti-Vivisection Society, BAVA.PWP.BlueYonder.CO.UK
British Union for the Abolition of Vivisection, BUAV.Org
CloseHLS.org
Coalition to Abolish Animal Testing, OHSUKillsPrimates.Com
CovanceSucks.Com
Dawn Watch, DawnWatch.Com/Animal_Testing.htm
EmoryLies.Com
FreeAnimals.Org
FreeTheAnimals.Homestead.Com
The Humane Society of the United States, HSUS.Org
HuntingdonSucks.Com
In Defense of Animals, IDAUSA.Org; VivisectionInfo.Org
Irish Anti-Vivisection Society, IrishAntiVivisection.Org
Italian Anti-Vivisection Scientific Committee, AntiVivisezione.IT
Last Chance for Animals, LCAnimal.Org
***Liberation* magazine**, Liberation-Mag.Org.UK
National Anti-Vivisection Society, NAVS.Org
New England Anti-Vivisection Society, NEAVS.Org
New Zealand Anti-Vivisection Society, NZAVS.Org.NZ
Northern Animal Rights Network, NARN-Online.Com
People for the Ethical Treatment of Animals, PETA.Org; StopAnimalTests.Com
Physicians Committee for Responsible Medicine, PCRM.Org
Stop Animal Exploitation Now, All-Creatures.Org/SAEN/
Uncaged.CO.UK
Vivisection-Absurd.Org.UK

• Down Feathers & Feather Hair Extensions

> "Down is the soft breast feathers of birds. Down-filled clothing made and sold by Armani, Ralph Lauren, Benetton, Gap, and other designers is in fashion. The filling for much of this clothing

originates on farms where feathers are ripped from the bodies of live geese, leaving them bleeding and in pain. Other feather fillers – about 98 percent of all feathers according to the Eurupean Down & Feather Association – are byproducts of the foie gras and duck meat industries. The most prized down is hand-stripped from live birds, , because mechanical stripping from slaughtered birds affects prduct quality. Feathers are pulled from the bird's breast, back, under the wings, and neck.

... Birds who are not plucked alive, but whose feathers are used for pillows, comforters, and clothing, suffer no less. If they're raised for foie gras (fatty liver food product), tubes are rammed down their throats several times a day to force-feed them until their livers are ten times the normal size. If they're intended for goose, duck, or chicken meat, they sufer the same as all animals donfined in filthy, disease-ridden industrial buildings and then slaughtered."

– *Feathers ripped from live birds for coats and pillows: birds suffer horribly for these consumer products*, Poultry Press, Winter-Spring 2013; Summerizing Daily Mail report from November 30, 2012; published by United Pultry Concerns, UPC-Online.org

"In 2011, United Poultry Concerns launced a campaign to educate people about the source of rooster feather hair extensions popularized by rock star Steven Tyler on American Idol. Rooster feather hair extenstions are extracted from thousands of roosters who are battery-caged and suffocated to death with carbon dioxide by companies that tear out their tail feathers then trash the dead birds who are brought into the world only so that a few feathers from each bird can be made into cosmetic ornaments and fly fishing lures. Entire breeding flocks of hends and roosters are factory-farmed strictly for these uses."

– United Pultry Concerns, UPC-Online.org

• Chemicals and Drugs in Milk, Meat, and Eggs

Most farm animals are given drugs by mouth or injection from their first day to nearly their last. These drugs may include hormones, antibiotics, milk stimulants, tranquilizers, and chemicals that influence the birth rates. The animals are also sprayed with toxic insecticides, fungicides, miticides, and pesticides.

The insecticides that are used on and around the animals not only kill flies but also kill needed insects such as bees that pollinate plants; preying mantises and ladybugs that help control damaging insects; and other helpful bugs and insects. The chemicals also poison the air, water, and land.

The drugs farm animals are given along with the pesticides, insecticides and other chemicals used on and around them as well as the chemicals used to grow their feed accumulate in the fat cells of the animals. These residues are transferred into the humans that consume the meats, milk products, and eggs.

The fats in farm animals contain residues of all the chemicals used to grow their food. Because the feed given to animals raised in factory farms often contains portions of ground-up farm animals that died prematurely or in accidents, the amount of drug and chemical residue found in meats from these animals contains a larger dose of the residues.

As if giving the naturally vegetarian animals a cannibalistic diet were not bad enough, some farm animals are also fed their own excrement. Some pigs are fed their own urine. Poultry waste and feathers are mixed in with feed that is fed to other farm animals. Other farm animal feed contains the leftovers of slaughterhouses, road kill, and the bodies of animals from county and city animal control shelters. Not only does this magnify the amount of chemical and drug residues in the fat of the animals, it also increases the likelihood that the animals are harboring infectious diseases. The farm animals that die are not tested for diseases. Using ground-up animals to increase the protein content of animal feed increases the likelihood that contagious diseases, such as mad cow, are becoming rampant within farm animals.

Leonardo da Vinci considered the bodies of humans who eat animals to be the tombs of the animals. A modern-day Leonardo might consider the bodies of humans who consume farm animals, eggs, and dairy to be toxic waste dumps of all the farming chemicals and drugs found in the animals.

• MILK

> "Scant evidence supports nutrition guidelines that focus specifically on increasing milk or other dairy product intake for promoting child or adolescent bone mineralization."
>
> – *Pediatrics*, March 2005

> "Our work showed that casein [the chief protein in milk] is the most relevant cancer promoter ever discovered.
>
> Casein causes a broad spectrum of adverse effects.
>
> Among other fundamental effects, it makes the body more acidic, alters the mix of hormones and modifies important enzyme activities, each of which can cause a broad array of more specific effects. One of these effects is its ability to promote cancer growth (by operating on key enzyme systems, by increasing hormone growth factors and by modifying the tissue acidity). Another is its ability to increase blood cholesterol (by modifying enzyme activities)

and to enhance atherogenesis, which is the early stage of cardiovascular disease.

And finally, although these are casein-specific effects, it should be noted that other animal-based proteins are likely to have the same effect as casein.

The biochemical systems which underlie the adverse effects of casein are also common to other animal-based proteins. Also, the amino acid composition of casein, which is the characteristic primarily responsible for its property, is similar to most other animal-based proteins. They all have what we call high 'biological value', in comparison, for example, with plant-based proteins, which is why animal protein promotes cancer growth and plant protein doesn't."

– Dr. T. Colin Campbell, TColinCampbell.org. Interview conducted by Kathy Freston, author of *Veganist.*

"Dairy cows are truly sick, miserable, abused creatures that are fed a high-protein (often animal-based) diet counterproductive to their health. They are then often drugged with bovine growth hormones and antibiotics, and abused to provide more milk than they have been created by nature to give – little or none of which goes to their own young."

– Howard Lyman, *No More Bull;* MadCowboy.Com

"There's no reason to drink cow's milk at any time in your life. It was designed for calves, not humans, and we should all stop drinking it today."

– Dr. Frank A. Oski, former Director of Pediatrics, Johns Hopkins University

"Interestingly, many long-term studies have now examined milk consumption in relation to risk of fractures. With remarkable consistency, these studies do not show reduction in fractures with high dairy product consumption. The hype about milk is basically an effective marketing campaign by the American Dairy industry."

– Walter Willet, M.D., M.P.H., Dr.P.H., Harvard School of Public Health's Nutrition chairman, *Scientific American*, January 2003

"Did you know that 90 percent of hamburger meat in America comes from the dairy industry? When cows no longer give huge amounts of milk after three to seven years, they go to the slaughterhouse. No exceptions. If every given the chance, cows can live to be eighteen to twenty-five. And dairy cows are like all female mammals. In order for a female mammal to give milk, she has to get pregnant. Every year, every cow on every dairy farm is raped. A long steel device is shoved into their vaginas just to inject them with bull semen. Sometimes they use a bare hand. This forces the milk flow. And after she gives birth, babies are stolen. And why do they take away the babies from their mothers? Well, the dairies can't have little babies sucking up all that milk that was meant for them, when the dairy would rather sell it to you instead. Every time you have a glass of cow milk, some calf is not."

– Gary Yourofsky, ADAPTT.org

"Of the beasts from whom cheese is made… The milk will be taken from the tiny children."

– Leonardo da Vinci, writing of how taking milk from a cow is stealing from the calf. da Vinci was a vegetarian and outspoken about his beliefs in protecting the animal kingdom.

I encourage people to eliminate dairy from their diet. But if you consume dairy, please avoid dairy from factory farms, pasteurized dairy, dairy containing additives, homogenized dairy, and all heated dairy. Please research xanthine-oxidase, oxidized cholesterol, and neurotoxic amino acids in dairy.

"Of 14 case studies that have been done on dairy and prostate cancer, 12 have shown a statistically significant relationship – and the other two just aren't strong enough to see anything – and they conclude that all of the predictors of prostate cancer, the consumption of dairy is the best predictor of prostate cancer."

– T. Colin Campbell, author of *The China Study;* TColinCampbell.org

In addition to the cancer-causing casein in milk (including cheese, ice cream, creamer, yogurt, keifer, butter, and whey), consider the sialic acid sugar protein molecule called Neu5Gc (N-glycolylneuraminic acid) in non-human mammal milk. Neu5Gc is also in meat. It is produced by non-human mammals; can't be synthesize by humans - because they lack the enzymes to produce it; binds to cell surfaces; causes an immune response and inflammation; is often found in human cancers, such as of the breast, colon, and prostate; and can make cancer more aggressive. To avoid Neu5Gc, simply don't consume animal milk or mammal meat. Doing both will also decrease your risk of cardiovascular disease, heart attacks, strokes, diabetes, arthritis, macular degeneration, Alzheimer's, kidney disease, osteoporosis, and other degenerative diseases.

"My perspective of veganism was most affected by learning that the veal calf is a by-product of dairying, and that in essence there is a slice of veal in every glass of what I had thought was an innocuous white liquid - milk."

– Rynn Berry

Be aware that the dairy industry is the meat industry, as the dairy cows are eventually slaughtered for their meat. To get milk from a cow, the cow needs to become pregnant. Because they can't produce milk and are therefore not needed on a dairy farm, almost all of the baby male cows are killed within days or weeks of their birth, and are cut up and sold as the meat product called "veal." The dairy industry consists of hundreds of millions of cows the world over, and each of them consumes many times the amount of food needed to feed humans. To feed all of those cows, a tremendous amount of land, water, fossil fuels, and other resources are used. The number one use of farmland on every continent is to grow food to feed to farmed animals. The meat, egg, and dairy requirements for a human body to thrive in health are absolute zero. The only milk a human needs is that of human breast milk during the initial years of life. Beyond that, humans do not need milk.

Raw, organic milk from animals consuming a natural diet contains helpful lactic-acid-generating bacteria; enzymes, and higher levels of omega-3 and omega-6 essential fatty acids. Pasteurization of milk damages these nutrients. In this way, even though I do not consume milk, would not advise anyone to consume it, and believe that the milk is best for the animals' young (to turn a small animal into a large animal), I tell people that, if they are going to consume dairy products, be sure to consume dairy that is raw, unpasteurized, organic, and from animals spending most of their time outdoors grazing in fields. One example is organic raw goats' milk keifer rich in probiotics. Find it through local organic family farmers, or natural foods co-ops. Check the Weston A. Price Foundation's Campaign for Real Milk (RealMilk.com). (I also do not endorse the Weston A. Price Foundation, or their meat-eating ways.)

Also, if you choose to consume dairy, learn about the difference in the milk of A1 breed cows (Friesians and Holsteins) compared to the milk of A2 breed cows (African, Asian, Guerney, and Jersey). Find an organic farmer who is raising A2 breeds. A1 breeds are common in the U.S., Northern Europe, Australia, and New Zealand. For more information, read *Devil in the Milk: Illness, Health and the Politics of A1 and A2 Milk*, by Keith Woodford.

> "Residues of hormones widely used to promote growth in beef cattle, dairy cows, and sheep (especially rBST or rBGH) may increase the risk of breast, prostate, and colorectal cancer. Their use also increases the risk of health problems in animals (especially mastitis), which leads to highter antibiotic use."
>
> – Environmental Working Group, July 2011

Recombinant bovine growth hormone (rBGH) is a genetically modified drug given to cows so they produce more milk. It is also known as bovine somatrotropin (rbST). If you drink milk, please make sure that the cows have not been treated with these terrible drugs.

> "The use of rBGH (rbST) in milk production has been shown to elevate the levels of insulin-like growth factor 1 (IGF-1), a

naturally-occurring hormone that in high levels is linked to several types of cancers, among other things.

rBGH (rbST) use induces an unnatural period of milk production during a cow's 'negative energy phase.' Milk produced during this stage is considered to be low quality due to its increased fat content and its decreased level of proteins.

Milk from rBGH-injected cows contains higher somatic cell counts, which makes the milk turn sour more quickly and is another indicator of poor milk quality."

– Organic Consumers Association

It may surprise those who have lived in a milk-consuming society that people in many parts of the world frown on drinking milk and on eating cheese, and think of consuming animal milk in any form as disgusting.

The main reason people drink milk is for the calcium. At least, that is what they have been brainwashed into believeing by the dairy industry. A vastly better choice for getting minerals in the diet is raw green vegetables, which is what the cows eat. There is no reason to eat the cow to get the minerals that the cow gets from eating greens. Simply, eat a salad. If you want even more minerals, add some seaweed flakes to that salad. Seaweed is rich in a variety of minerals.

Pasteurization of milk is a heating process, which damages the fats and creates a product that leads to degenerative conditions in the human body, such as heart disease. The casein protein in milk can also cause mood swings, depression, and anxiety. Those who experience depression would be wise to avoid milk.

"The source of most commercial milk is the 'modern' Holstein, bred to produce huge quantities of milk--three times as much as the old-fashioned cow. She needs special feed and antibiotics to keep her well. Her milk contains high levels of growth hormone from her pituitary gland, even when she is spared the indignities of genetically engineered Bovine Growth Hormone to push her to the udder limits of milk production.

Real feed for cows is green grass in Spring, Summer and Fall; stored dry hay, silage, hay and root vegetables in Winter. It is not soy meal, cottonseed meal or other commercial feeds, nor is it bakery waste, chicken manure or citrus peel cake, laced with pesticides. Vital nutrients like vitamins A and D, and Price's 'Activator X' (a fat-soluble catalyst that promotes optimum mineral assimilation, now believed to be vitamin K2) are greatest in milk from cows eating green grass, especially rapidly growing green grass in the spring and fall. Vitamins A and D are greatly diminished, and

Activator X disappears, when milk cows are fed commercial feed. Soy meal has the wrong protein profile for the dairy cow, resulting in a short burst of high milk production followed by premature death. Most milk (even most milk labeled "organic") comes from dairy cows that are kept in confinement their entire lives and never see green grass!

Pasteurization destroys enzymes, diminishes vitamin content, denatures fragile milk proteins, destroys vitamins C, B12 and B6, kills beneficial bacteria, promotes pathogens and is associated with allergies, increased tooth decay, colic in infants, growth problems in children, osteoporosis, arthritis, heart disease and cancer. Calves fed pasteurized milk do poorly and many die before maturity. Raw milk sours naturally but pasteurized milk turns putrid; processors must remove slime and pus from pasteurized milk by a process of centrifugal clarification. Inspection of dairy herds for disease is not required for pasteurized milk. Pasteurization was instituted in the 1920s to combat TB, infant diarrhea, undulant fever and other diseases caused by poor animal nutrition and dirty production methods. But times have changed and modern stainless steel tanks, milking machines, refrigerated trucks and inspection methods make pasteurization absolutely unnecessary for public protection. And pasteurization does not always kill the bacteria for Johne's disease suspected of causing Crohn's disease in humans with which most confinement cows are infected. Much commercial milk is now ultra-pasteurized to get rid of heat-resistant bacteria and give it a longer shelf life. Ultra-pasteurization is a violent process that takes milk from a chilled temperature to above the boiling point in less than two seconds. Clean raw milk from certified healthy cows is available commercially in several states and may be bought directly from the farm in many more. (Sources are listed on RealMilk.Com.).

Homogenization is a process that breaks down butterfat globules so they do not rise to the top. Homogenized milk has been linked to heart disease.

Average butterfat content from old-fashioned cows at the turn of the century was over 4% (or more than 50% of calories). Today butterfat comprises less than 3% (or less than 35% of calories). Worse, consumers have been duped into believing that low-fat and skim milk products are good for them. Only by marketing low-fat and skim milk as a health food can the modern dairy industry get rid of its excess poor-quality, low-fat milk from modern high-production herds. Butterfat contains vitamins A and D needed for assimilation of calcium and protein in the water fraction of the milk. Without them protein and calcium are more difficult to utilize and possibly toxic. Butterfat is rich in short- and medium chain fatty acids which protect against disease and stimulate the immune system. It contains glyco-spingolipids which prevent intestinal distress and conjugated linoleic acid which has strong anticancer properties."

– RealMilk.Com

"Cows make milk for their babies, and for their babies alone. Case is closed. Forever. Permanently. No debate. No discussion. They don't make milk for baby elephants, baby orangutans, baby hedge hogs, baby rabbits, baby rats, baby humans, adolescent humans, or adult humans. This body of ours has absolutely no need for cow milk, like it has absolutely no need for giraffe milk, and zebra milk, and rhinorcerous milk, hippopatomus milk, camel milk, deer milk, antelope milk, horse milk, pig milk, dog milk, or cat milk. The only milk that we ever need is our own mother's breast milk when we are born. And that's it. And when we're done weaning, we never need one drop of milk, ever again. No species on this planet needs milk after they are done weaning."

– Gary Yourofsky, ADAPTT.org.

If you consume cheese made of dairy, you may also be eating the stomach lining of a slaughtered calf. On the label, this ingredient is called "rennet." Some cheese companies will list rennet as an ingredient, and some don't – even when there is rennet in the cheese. Some that don't contain rennet will mention on the label that it is "rennet-less cheese," which means they are being sensitive to the vegetarians that are trying to avoid consuming rennet.

"Different meats affect our health and environment differently. Lamb, beef, cheese, and pork generate the most greenhouse gases. They also tend to be higher in fat and have the worst environmental impacts, because producting them uses the most resources – mainly feed, chemical fertilizer, fuel, pesticides, and water. Lamb has the greatest impact. Beef is second. Cheese is third. Beef has more than twice the emissions of pork, nearly four times more than chicken, and more than 13 times as much as vegetable proteins such as beans, lentils, and tofu. But vegetarians who eat dairy aren't off the hook, because pount for pount, cheese generates the third-highest emissions."

– The Environmental Working Group, July 2011

Book: *Whitewash: The Disturbing Truth About Cow's Milk and Your Health*, by Joseph Keon.

Farm to Consumer Legal Defense Fund, FarmToConsumer.org

Dr. John McDougall, DrMcDougall.com

NotMilk.com

Physicians Committee for Responsible Medicine, PCRM.org

• B-12 Vitamin
(Cobalamin, Cyanocobalamin, Methylcobalamin)

B-12 comes from microorganisms and is present in meat, milk, and eggs.

While the claim is often made that vegans and vegetarians don't get enough B-12 in their diet, this depends on what type of veggie diet the vegan or vegetarian is following. While, vegans and vegetarians often test lower for B-12 than do people who consume animal protein, many people who consume meat and dairy have been found with low levels of B-12.

The health of the stomach and intestinal tract play a major role in the presence of B-12 in the body. The quality of the food also is key to getting and maintaining sufficient amounts of B-12. Those who take diabetes medications, painkillers, and some other medications may experience low B-12 absorption.

It may be good to include several sources of B-12 in the diet so that there is no possibility of B-12 deficiency.

Cyanocobalamin is a cheap form of B-12, in which a cyanide molecule is used as a binding agent. Because cyanide isn't exactly something you want in your body, it is advisable to avoid cyanocobalamin. For the body to remove the cyanide from your body, through your liver, the body's natural resources of methyl group molecules are used, which can interfere with the system's ability to metabolise homocysteine. Too much homocysteine can play a role in heart disease.

A better choice for a B-12 supplement is to take methylcobalamin in sublingual form (a tablet that you place under your tongue and let it dissolve there). There are also methylcobalamin skin patch products that deliver B-12 through the skin, such as by placing the patch on the skin behind an ear. The skin patches also usually contain the B vitamin folic acid, which also plays a role in heart health. Methylcobalamine is a coenzyme form of B-12 that is more bioavailable than cyanocobalamin, and is more easily absorbed into the system.

B-12 plays a role in cell replication, in the construction of DNA, and in the formation of red blood cells in the bone marrow. It is the red blood cells that bring oxygen to the body tissues. B-12 is also needed to maintain healthy nerve fiber sheeths, and for converting carbohydrates, fat, and protein into sources of energy.

A diet lacking in B-12 could lead a person to experience hyperhomocystemia, which is a condition defined by an elevated level of homocystine in the blood. Homocystine is an amino acid that is produced normally in the process of breaking down methionine, an amino acid. Too much homocystine can damage the walls of the arteries, cause the accumulation of atherosclerotic plaque, and lead to cardiovascular disease and stroke, and damage the eyes, kidneys, and other organs.

Vitamin B-12 deficiency can also cause weakness, dizziness, fatigue, shortness of breath, depression, paranoia, delusions, intestinal upset, upper respiratory infection, nerve damage, macrocytic anemia, sore tongue, indigestion, diarrhea, slow reflexes, and numbness and tingling in the fingers and toes. A woman with low levels of B-12 is more likely to have a baby with birth defects. Women who are breastfeeding and who have low levels of B-12 may produce nutritionally weak breastmilk, which can stunt brain and nerve cell growth.

Where do vegans get B-12?

- **Algae**: Spirulina, chlorella, wild blue green algae. Not the most reliable sources. Chlorella does contain cobalt, which is at the center of the B-12 molecule, and may be a source of B-12, but it should not be the only thing a person consumes to rely on obtaining adequate amounts of B-12. Wild blue green algae can also help to maintain B-12 levels. Seaweeds may also contain inactive B-12 analogs that can take up the same receptor sites as true B-12, and give a false-positive on the serum B-12 test.
- **Fermented seed or nut cheeses**: When they contain Red Star Vegetarian Support Formula nutritional yeast, which is available in most natural foods stores.
- **Intestinal flora**: The good bacteria in your digestive tract, including the mouth. While the bacteria in the large intestine does manufactur B-12, that ends up leaving the body. The receptor sites are in the small intestine.

  You can increase the amount of intestinal flora in your system by taking a vegan probiotic supplement. They are sold in the refrigerated section in the nutrition section of natural foods stores in either capsule or powder form.
- **Kimchi:** A fermented vegetable salad. Best if made using raw, unheated, organically grown ingredients. It is much more likely to contain B-12 if it is made in a wooden vat rather than a ceramic or steel container, or if a reusable wooden compression weight is used within the non-wooden container. See Sauerkraut, below.
- **Mushrooms**: specifically, cultivated white button and flush mushrooms. In 2009, the *Journal of Agricultural and Food Chemistry* published a study conducted at the Centre for Plant and Food Science, College of Health and Science, University of Western Sydney, concluding that B-12 was found on and in white button and flush mushrooms from a variety of farms. Because B-12 was found to be more present in the peel than other structures of the mushrooms, the study suggested that the B-12 is likely bacteria-derived from bacteria originating in the soil.

- **Noma shoyu:** A raw, fermented, soy sauce-like product made with wheat, soy beans, salt, and a bacterial starter. Only purchase if it says it is raw, and has not been heated. Although the product is made using cooked wheat and soy, the sauce is the product of months of fermentation, which results in a vat of enzymes, amino acids, good bacteria, and other nutrients, usually including B-12. For a variety of reasons, including because of the salt content and the processing, many raw foodists do not consume Noma Shoyu. Those who are avoiding gluten-containing foods may also wish to avoid Noma Shoyu.
- **Nutritional yeast:** Grown on mineral-enriched molasses. Red Star Vegetarian Support Formula nutritional yeast is available in most natural food stores, either in bulk form, or in a container. It is also rich in other B-complex vitamins as well as in amino acids. Nutritional yeast is NOT baker's yeast, which is different. It has been found to be beneficial in helping to reverse B-12 deficiency, but not as helpful as B-12 suppliments. Regularly using nutritional yeast is one way of helping to maintain healthful B-12 levels. Nutritional yeast should be stored in a covered container kept in a cool, dry place (not frozen); and in a place where it isn't exposed to constant light. Cooking it will damage the nutrients. It can be added to salads, hummus, dips, dressings, spreads, and patés, and to nut and seed cheeses.

"A number of reliable vegan food sources for vitamin B12 are known. One brand of nutritional yeast, Red Star T-6635+, has been tested and shown to contain active vitamin B12. This brand of yeast is often labeled as Vegetarian Support Formula with or without T-6635+ in parentheses following this new name. It is a reliable source of vitamin B12. Nutritional yeast, Saccharomyces cerevisiae, is a food yeast, grown on a molasses solution, which comes as yellow flakes or powder. It has a cheesy taste. Nutritional yeast is different from brewer's yeast or torula yeast. those sensitive to other yeasts can often use it."

– Vitamin B-12 in the Vegan Diet, by Reed Mangels, Ph.D., R.D.; Vegetarian Resource Group;

- **Rejuvelac:** While some bacteria in rejuvelac may produce B-12, it should not be considered a reliable source. If it is made using the water from soaking organically grown wheat berries or other seeds to the sprouting stage, rejuvelac may contain more B-12. Rejuvelac is often used in raw vegan cheese recipes, including those that also contain B-12-rich nutritional yeast and/or vegan probiotic powder.
- **Organically grown raw fruits and vegetables**: Soil organisms are on the leaves and skins of these. It can be reasoned that some B-12 is obtained from the bacteria. An organic garden using composted kitchen scraps from organic fruits and vegetables can contain more soil organisms that form B-12 than a garden grown using chemical fertilizers.
- **Probiotic powder**: Vegan probiotic powder is often used in raw foods, such as in cheeses, dressings, spreads, and sauces. It provides healthy

doses of beneficial flora for the intestines, but it should not be considered a way of obtaining adequate amounts of B-12.

- **Recycled B-12**: The body does reclaim and reuse some B-12. The bile extracts B-12 that has been absorbed into the small intestines, and then reabsorbs the vitamin again in the small intestine. Some people's systems are more able to do this than are others, but this should not be considered as a reliable source of adequate amounts of B-12. Those who consume a diet that is free of heated oils, including sautéed foods and fried foods, and those who stay away from gluten, dairy, eggs, meat, bleached grains, processed sugars, and synthetic food chemicals while consuming a diet rich in fresh fruits and vegetables are more likely to have a more healthful alimentary tract that is able to absorb nutrients, including B-12.
- **Sauerkraut:** A fermented cabbage salad that may also contain other vegetables. It should be made using raw, unheated, organically grown ingredients. Sauerkraut sold in your market is likely to have been pasteurized, which kills the enzymes and bacteria. Sauerkraut is relatively easy to make. Some natural foods stores and vegan restaurants now sell raw sauerkraut. It is more likely to contain B-12 if it is made in a wood container, rather than a ceramic, glass, or metal container. A reuseable wooden compression weight used inside a non-wooden container can also increase the presence of B-12.
- **Sea vegetables:** The seaweeds dulse, nori, kelp, and wakame, may contain little or no B-12. The algaes chlorella and spirulina may be a more reliable source of B-12. While they may contain some B-12, they may also contain inactive B-12 analogs, which can use the same receptor sites as B-12, and may lead to a false positive on a B-12 blood test.
- **Sprouts:** Not a reliable source, but some beneficial organisms producing B-12 may be obtained from these, particularly sprouts grown in organic soil, such as sunflower seed sprouts used for salads and also sprouted grasses used for juicing.
- **Wheat, barley, and other grass juices** made from grass grown in organic soil.
- **Vegan B-12 supplements**: For those who have any concern at all that they are not getting enough B-12 through their food choices. Companies that make vegan B-12 supplements include Freeda, Nature's Bounty, Solgar, and Veg Life. As mentioned above, if you purchase B-12 supplements, make sure they are methylcobalamin, and not cyanocobalamin. Get the sublingual methylcobalamin B-12 tablets. There are also injecible B-12 products, and, as mentioned above, the skin patch B-12 delivery products that work by placing the patch on the skin behind an ear.

While a vitamin B-12 rich diet isn't necessarily required every day, or even every week, and stores of B-12 can last months in the body, some people use their stores more quickly than others. While little of it is needed, B-12 is truly an essential nutrient, and people should be sure to get adequate amounts of it in their diet. Taking a quality B-12 supplement of at least 10 micrograms (10 mcg) is a reliable way to guarantee that your system receives adequate amounts of B-12. Many people advise taking a sublingual B-12 supplement, which is one that is held under the tongue until it is dissolved.

Expectant mothers, women who are breastfeeding, and women expecting to become pregnant should be sure to get sufficient amounts of vitamin B-12 (and a wide variety of other nutrients – especially those present in raw fruits and raw vegetables).

> "Some people on raw diets include raw animal products in an effort to get vitamin B-12. With age, the body's ability to absorb the form of vitamin B-12 that is present in animal products diminishes. In animal products, vitamin B-12 is attached to a protein, and as people get older, production of the stomach acid that can split this complex of vitamin B-12 and protein diminishes. The recommendations for vitamin B-12 take into account that up to one in three of all individuals age fifty and older have low stomach-acid secretion. The form of vitamin B-12 that is present in fortified foods and supplements is not attached to protein; therefore, its absorption is not affected by a change in acid production. It is recommended that people over the age of fifty, regardless of their diet choice, rely either on foods fortified with vitamin B-12 or supplements to meet their recommended intakes."
>
> – *Becoming Raw: The Essential Guide to Raw Vegan Diets*, by Brenda Davis, Vesanto Melina, and Rynne Berry.

For more about B-12, read *Becoming Raw: The Essential Guide to Raw Vegan Diets*, by Brenda Davis, Vesanto Melina, and Rynn Berry.

FoodStudies.org
GoVeg.com
Dr. Michael Greger, DrGreger.Org
Dr. Michael Klaper, VegSource.Com/Klaper/
Vegan.com
VeganHealth.org
VeganHealthStudy.Com
Vegan.org
VeganOutreatch.org
VeganSociety.com
VeganSociety.Com/html/Food/Nutrition/B12/
Vegetarian Resource Group, VRG.org
VegInfo.org
VegSource.com

• BIRTHING

SISTERS are taking control of a most amazing life experience. While the medical establishment continues to medicalize and pharmaceuticalize birth to make it into an even bigger money-making venture for doctors, hospitals, drug makers, and medical technology companies, more women are educating themselves and others about natural and home birthing methods.

It is important to make sure the birthing arrangement is clean. My grandmother died from a simple infection after childbirth that in the modern age would have been easy to treat. There are some good things about modern meds. Other than that, I'm an advocate for home births of well-informed expectant mothers assisted by midwives and doulas.

If you are expecting, or expect to be expecting, eat a variety of fresh fruits and vegetables, get adequate amounts of vitamin B-12, and educate yourself about what feels right for you in the way of birthing. Also, be especially sure to maintain a healthy diet when you are breastfeeding.

If you are expecting a baby, or expect to be, clean up your diet. Eat organic foods. Localize your food choices, such as by shopping at farmers' markets and/or by growing some of your own food. Use non-toxic, biodegradable cleaners and toiletries. Use less plastic. Doing so will help to reduce the industrial chemicals that will end up in your baby.

Unfortunately, we are living in a polluted world and many of the industrial pollutants that have been produced in the past 150-or-so years are in our tissues. These chemicals found in our tissues include those that have been banned for decades. They also include heavy metals and chemicals being used today, including preservatives, fire retardants, phthalates, synthetic fragrances, parabens, sulphates, insecticides, fertilizers, and various pharmaceutical drugs. When we follow a clean diet, we reduce our exposure to toxic chemicals, and our bodies are better able to rid toxins from our tissues.

Birth As We Know It, birthasweknowit.com. A documentary and a helpful Web site.
Birth Balance, New York, birthbalance.com
Birth Into Being, Birthintobeing.com. This is a documentary and a helpful Web site.
Bornfree, unassistedchildbirth.com
The Business of Being Born, the businessofbeingborn.com.
Circumcision Resource Center, circumcision.org
Home Midwifery Association, Australia; HomeBirth.org.au
Journey Into Birth, journeyintobirth.com
Mothering Magazine, mothering.com
The Mother Magazine, themothermagazine.co.uk
National Organization of Circumcision Information Resource Centers, nocirc.org
Orgasmic Birth, orgasmicbirth.com. A book and documentary.
Sacred Birthing, sacredbirthing.com.

• CHILDREN

SOME people are treating children these days as some sort of commercialized robotic mechanisms that are to be infused with some variety of synthetic chemical pills and manufactured foods to get them to function at a level acceptable to being a performer in a TV advertisement for perfect children.

Unfortunately, more and more children these days are more likely to be overweight and to eat an unhealthful diet consisting of a variety of unnatural and health-negating ingredients, too may calories, too much sugar, too much salt, a variety of cooked oils, dressings, and sauces, a shortage of omega-3 fatty acids, and that is seriously lacking in the biophotons that exist in raw fruits, raw vegetables, fresh sprouts, germinated seeds, and soaked raw nuts.

While most people today get their food education from commercials, it would be wise to realize that commercialized food is not the best thing to consume.

It would greatly benefit children to keep their diets free from synthetic food chemicals, clarified sugars, gluten, processed salts, bleached grains, MSG, and fried and sautéed oils.

Real food for real children includes some combination of raw fruits, raw vegetables, fresh sprouts, germinated seeds, raw soaked nuts, whole raw gluten-free grains, and water.

Teach children how to make there own simple foods, such as green smoothies, which are better enjoyed slowly, and not guzzled. Access: RawFamily.com. Freeze peeled ripe bananas, and blend or use a food processor to whip them into what tastes like soft serve ice cream. It's one ingredient: frozen peeled bananas.

Teach children to grow some food plants, even if it is in pots, and to grow sprouts.

Have children involved in artistic expression. It will relieve frustrations, help wire the brain in alignment with the talents, and connect them to what they are: a being of expression and energy that can create their reality.

Physical activity and cooperative sport strengthens the bones and muscles, enlivens the organs, balances hormones, and helps to wire the brain and the nerves throughout the body. It improves sleep, evens the temperament, nurtures reasoning, and builds community.

Reading actual books, and not techno screens, does something beneficial for the brain and intellect that scientists still do not fully understand and continue to study. Many people who work in the computer industry understand this and limit the time their own children spend in front of computer screens. Read books to children, and have them read to you, and also get them to read silently.

While many children are not in a household situation that allows them to have a pet, it is good to have children regularly interact with animals, be they other people's pets, or those in an animal shelter or rescue sanctuary.

None of us would exist if it were not for a healthy planet with vibrant forests and wildlands. Have children plant trees, join in with community trash cleanup days, and, where possible, compost food scraps into soil.

Use biodegradable soaps and cleaners. Learn about greening your home, and keep it free of toxic paints and finishes. If you have a microwave oven, get rid of it. Avoid plastic drinking bottles and plastic cups.

Be a good example in word and deed.

> "The psychiatric/pharmaceutical industry spends billions of dollars a year in order to convince the public, legislators and the press that psychiatric disorders such as Bi-Polar Disorder, Depression, Attention Deficit Disorder (ADD/ADHD), Post Traumatic Stress Disorder, etc., are medical diseases on par with verifiable medical conditions such as cancer, diabetes and heart disease. This is simply a way to maintain their hold on an $84 billion dollar-a-year psychiatric drug industry that is based on marketing and not science. Unlike real medical disease, there are no scientific tests to verify the medical existence of any psychiatric disorder. Despite decades of trying to prove mental disorders are biological brain conditions, due to chemical imbalances or genetic factors, psychiatry has failed to prove even one of their hundreds of so-called mental disorders is due to a faulty or 'chemically imbalanced' brain. To counter this obvious flaw in their push to medicalize behaviors, the psychiatric industry will claim that there are certain medical conditions that do not have a verifiable test so this is why there isn't one for 'mental illness.' This is frankly a lame argument; whereas there may be rare medical conditions that do not have a verifiable medical test, there are virtually no psychiatric disorders that can be verified medically as a physical abnormality/disease. Not one."
>
> – Psychiatric Disorders: The Facts Behind the Billion Dollar Marketing Campaign, by the Citizens Commission for Human Rights International; cchrint.org/psychiatric-disorders/.
>
> Because the public has been so mislead by the psychiatric/pharmaceutical industry on the dangers of psychiatric drugs, CCHR has created a one-of-a-kind, easy to search psychiatric drugs side effects database, containing all international studies and drug regulatory warnings that have been issued on both classes of drugs (antidepressants, antipsychotics, anti-anxiety drugs, stimulants, etc) and brand names such as Prozac, Zoloft, Paxil, Risperdal, Seroquel, Ritalin etc. These are provided by CCHR as a free public service to help people make educated decisions based on facts, not marketing campaigns.

FoodStudies.org
Karen Ranzi, Super Healthy Children; SuperHealthyChildren.com. Karen (at) SuperHealthyChidlren.com
Kristen Suzanne's Green Mommy Blog, GreenMommyBlog.com
Raw Power Kids, RawPowerKids.com

• CANCER

If you want to greatly reduce your chances of experiencing cancer, do these things:

- Don't eat meat, or anything containing meat extracts, such as chicken broth, lard, rennet (the stomach lining of a slaughtered animal and used in cheese), gelatin, and other meat "products" and extracts. Fish, birds, frogs, and other small animals are also meat. Don't eat them. The human nutritional need for animal protein is absolute zero.
- Don't eat eggs. Including anything containing eggs, such as mayonnaise, meringue, some mustards, and other foods that may contain egg as an ingredient, such as baked foods, some breads, crackers, cookies, sauces, creams, soups, and even some types of beer. If choosing to consume these items, look for products that say "vegan."
- Don't eat milk, including cheese, creamer, yogurt, cottage cheese, ice cream, butter, whey, and caseine, and foods containing milk or milk extracts.
- Avoid added sugars, including white sugar, brown sugar, agave, corn syrup, rice syrup, and products labeled as "fruit sweetened."
  Yes, agave is a garbage sweetener, and can cause the same health problems as corn syrup.
- Avoid artificial sweetners. These synthetic chemicals can alter brain function; cause brain lesions; damage the lining of nerves; increase the incidence of asthma; interfere with nutrient absorption and transfer; and increase the risk of seizures, tumor growth, cancer, and fertility issues.
- Avoid bleached foods, such as bleached rice and gluten grains.
- Don't eat margarine.
- Follow a plant-based diet rich in raw fruits and raw vegetables.
- Aim for a diet that is organic and non-GMO.
- Follow a low-fat diet, with few or no added oils, including olive oil, canola oil, palm oil, cottonseed oil, corn oil, and other bottled oils marketed or perceived as health foods. If you do choose to eat foods containing oil, choose raw coconut oil and raw hemp seed oil. Read: *The China Study*, and research the points it makes.
- Avoid foods containing synthetic chemicals, including artificial sweeteners, colors, scents, preservatives, flavors, and emulsifiers

- Don't use Teflon kitchen products
- Avoid canned foods, as the cans are lined with extracts of petroleum, known carcinogens
- Exercise daily.
- Follow a regular sleeping pattern.
- Use non-toxic cleansers that are free of synthetic chemicals
- Avoid cosmetic products that contain parabens and synthetic chemicals
- Plant and maintain a food garden, and compost your organic food scraps into soil for the garden
- Support local organic farmers
- Locate a local co-opportunity that sells natural foods.
- Consider getting deliveries of organic fruits and vegetables from a local CSA (Community Supported Agriculture).

"I believe that coronary artery disease is preventable, and that even after it is under way, its progress can be stopped, its insidious effects reversed. I believe, and my work over the past twenty years has demonstrated, that all this can be accomplished without expensive mechanical intervention and with minimal use of drugs. The key lies in nutrition – specifically, in abandoning the toxic American diet and maintaining cholesterol levels well below those historically recommended by health policty experts.

– Dr. Caldwell B. Esselstyn, author of *Prevent and Reverse Heart Disease*; HeartAttackProof.com

• Heart Health

"I believe that coronary artery disease is preventable, and that even after it is under way, its progress can be stopped, its insidious effects reversed. I believe, and my work over the past twenty years has demonstrated, that all this can be accomplished without expensive mechanical intervention and with minimal use of drugs. The key lies in nutrition – specifically, in abandoning the toxic American diet and maintaining cholesterol levels well below those historically recommended by health policty experts.

– Dr. Caldwell B. Esselstyn, author of *Prevent and Reverse Heart Disease*; HeartAttackProof.com

"We spend incredible amounts of money annually to get the best health care we can afford. With all the money we throw at it, we should expect to be some of the healthiest people in the world. Sadly, that is not the case. We keep spending more money, only to find ourselves getting sicker. It feels at times like we are paying to become ill.

Chronic illnesses, and acute illnesses for that matter, are primarily due to biochemical and physiological imbalances. Studies have shown that chronic illnesses are the direct result of our poor lifestyle choices, the most damaging of which is our food choices. We eat too many unnatural, processed foods that are toxic to our bodies, in place of foods that are natural and supply what our bodies' need.

We need a paradigm shift in our approach to healthcare. Our efforts need to start with removing unnatural foods from our diet, and replacing those foods with ones that are 'natural,' as a way of reversing illness and facilitating health. This new approach would be a shift away from the standard approach of using medical and surgical interventions as our primary protocols."

– Dr. Baxter Montgomery of the Houston Cardiac Association, DrBaxterMontgomery.com

WE know very clearly that the average American diet of junk food, processed salts, bleached grains, clarified sugars and oils, fried food, and sautéed food, along with dairy, meat, and eggs damages the heart, creates arthritis, promotes diabetes, increases the incidence of cancers of the colon, prostate, breasts, bladder, and kidneys, and increases the risk of macular degeneration, asthma, stroke, heart attack, kidney stones, attention disorders, and obesity. It is a fact. Meanwhile, if you go into school cafeterias, hospital cafeterias, prison cafeterias, and other institutional eating establishments and popular restaurants and grocery stores, you will see that they are selling the very foods that cause heart disease, cancer, diabetes, and a variety of health problems.

"I don't understand why asking people to eat a well-balanced vegan diet is considered drastic, while it is medically conservative to cut people open."

– Dr. Dean Ornish

Some of the best things you can do for your heart, brain, and health include getting daily exercise, and to follow a plant-based diet that is largely or completely raw and organic, and that is free of processed salts, clarified sugars (including agave), preservatives of any kind, MSG, synthetic chemicals, fried substances, heated oils, and bottled oils. Even better if the diet contains a variety of fruits, fresh greens, and is rich in omega 3s (such as from raw green vegetables, freshly ground flax seeds, fractured or ground raw hemp seeds, unheated walnuts, and germinated chia and buckwheat). It isn't a maybe or a kind-of, it is an absolute.

"By eating these whole foods, and getting away from processed foods, getting away from the dairy, and anything with a mother, anything with a face – meat, fish and chicken – it's incredible how powerful the body can be. If we are going to have a seismic revolution of health in this country, which is really right at our fingertips, then the major behavior that has to change is our food (intake). That is absolutely the key card, it trumps everything."

– Dr. Caldwell B. Esselstyn, author of *Prevent and Reverse Heart Disease.*

For those who advocate taking fish oil for heart health, I strongly advise that you avoid taking fish oil, because:

1) We don't need to kill fish. The fish and sea life populations have suffered greatly because of industrial fishing, and from pollution. Sea life around the planet has been decimated and is at a fraction of what it was just a few decades ago.

We also don't need to be harvesting krill from the seas for it's oil. Krill is a shrimp-like crustacean and is the food for sea life, such as baleen whales, mantas, and whale sharks, which are suffering from what humans have done to the seas.

2) Ingesting fish and extracts of sea creatures increases your exposure to mercury, PCBs, and other environmental toxins from industrial pollution the creatures are exposed to in the increasingly polluted lakes and oceans. Consuming these contaminates leads to an accumulation of them in your cells, which then increases your risk of cancer and other health disorders.

Some may say that the fish oil products they get are from uncontaminated waters free of industrial pollution. Unfortunately, there is no longer such a thing. Industrial pollution flows into lakes and rivers and into the oceans, and it also ends up in the air, which is then absorbed into the rivers, lakes, and oceans around the world. Mercury from coal-fired electric generating plants and cement kilns travels in the atmosphere, and is absorbed into the oceans thousands of miles from where it was released into the air. The main reason polar bears are now so contaminated with industrial pollution, such as fire retardants and heavy metals, is because they are getting these toxins by eating fish. It is impacting polar bears to such an extent that it is affecting their bones, their nerves, and their ability to reproduce.

3) The benefit of taking fish oil is to obtain the omega 3 essential fatty acids. Instead of taking fish oil to get omega 3s, you can take algae supplements (which is where the fish get the omega 3s), and/or also include things like hemp seed powder, germinated chia, germinated buckwheat, soaked flax seeds, and other plant sources rich in essential fatty acids in your diet, including raw fruits and vegetables. All raw fruits and all raw vegetables contain sufficient amounts of omega 3 fatty acids.

The eggs that are advertised as being rich in omega 3s are simply from chickens that have been fed raw flax seeds. Skip the eggs, eat the flax. The beef that is marketed as rich in omega 3s is from cattle that have grazed in meadows, eating raw greens. Skip eating the cow, simply eat fresh green salad as raw greens are rich in omega 3s. For more information, see my book, *Sunfood Diet Infusion: Transforming Health Through Raw Veganism.*

> "Men dig their graves with their own teeth, and die more by those instruments than by all weapons of their enemies."
>
> – Pythagoras

A study conducted at McMaster and McGill universities in Canada, and published on the October 11, 2011 by *PLoS Medicine* journal (published by Public Library of Science) reported that a diet rich in raw fruits and vegetables favorably modified the chromosome 9p21 region genetic variant, which had been identified as a marker for heart disease. The study, titled, The Effect of Chromosome 9p21 Variants on Cardiovascular Disease May Be Modified by Dietary Intake: Evidence from a Case/Control and a Prospective Study, included data of over 27,000 people from a variety of ethnic ancestries, including Chinese, European, Latin American, and Arabian. The study authors concluded that the people with the genetic variant could, if they followed a diet rich in raw fruits and vegetables, reduce their risk of heart disease to the level experienced by those who do not have the genetic variant. The authors of the study concluded that, "The risk of myocardial infarction and cardiovascular disease conferred by chromosome 9p21 SNPs appears to be modified by a prudent diet high in raw vegetables and fruits."

> "We know that 9p21 genetic variants increase the risk of heart disease for those that carry it. But it was a surprise to find that a healthy diet could significantly weaken its effect."
>
> – Dr. Jamie Engert

> "We observed that the effect of a high risk genotype can be mitigated by consuming a diet high in fruits and vegetables. Our results support the public health recommendation to consume more than five servings of fruits or vegetables as a way to promote good health."
>
> – Sonia Anand

Scientists have known that certain chemicals that form in cooked food, including acrylamides, glycotoxins, polycyclic aromatic hydrocarbons, and heterocyclic amines, can damage DNA and trigger the growth of cancer cells. But, the McMaster and McGill study identified how a diet rich in raw plant matter favorably alters human genes to prevent disease. This was no surprise to me. I have learned that dietary choices certainly can alter genes and make genes express favorable or unfavorable health events.

"Since we know that these foods are injuring people, why would we ever want to have them on the menus of our schoolchildren? Why wait until people do have heart disease? We know, for instance, that if we do autopsies on our guys who died in Korea and Vietnam, roughly eighty percent of young GIs will already have gross evidence of coronary heart disease that you can see without a microscope. If we are ever going to make a breakthrough in this epidemic of cardiac disease, we really have to start when it's young."

– Dr. Caldwell B. Esselstyn, author of *Prevent and Reverse Heart Disease.*

"When it comes to heart healthy eating, fresh fruit and vegetables are essential. A natural plant based diet can not only help prevent heart disease and other chronic illnesses, but help to reverse it, even in its most advanced forms."

– Dr. Baxter Montgomery

Books of Interest:

- *Becoming Raw: The Essential Guide to Raw Vegan Diets*, by Brenda Davis, RD, Vesanto Melina, MS, RD, and Rynn Berry
- *The Engine 2 Diet: The Texas Firefighter's 28-Day Save-Your-Life Plan that Lowers Cholesterol and Burns Away Pounds*, by Rip Esselstyn. This is the son of Dr. Caldwell Esselstyn of the Cleveland Clinic. Rip is a firefighter who persuaded his Austin, Texas firehouse workers to go vegan.
- *The McDougall Program for a Health Heart: A Life-Saving Approach to Preventing and Treating Heart Disease*, by John McDougall, MD, and Mary McDougall
- *Prevent and Reverse Heart Disease: The Revolutionary, Scientifically Proven Nutrition-Based Cure*, by Caldwell B. Esselstyn, Jr., MD
- *The Spectrum: A Scientifically Proven Program to Feel Better, Live Longer, Lose Weight, and Gain Health*, by Dr. Dean Ornish

Dr. Mary Clifton, Traverse City, MI; drmarymd.com

Dr. Joel Fuhrman, DrFuhrman.com

Dr. John McDougall, DrMcDougall.com

Preventative Medicine Research Institute, Sausalito, CA, USA; pmri.org. Dr. Dean Ornish has proved that heart disease and narrowing of the arteries can be reversed through a vegan or near vegan diet combined with exercise, stress reduction, and lifestyle-changes.

Dr. Baxter Montgomery, Houston Cardiac Association, 10480 Main St., Houston, TX; DrBaxterMontgomery.com

True North Health, 1551 Pacific Ave., Santa Rosa, CA 95404 USA; healthpromoting.com. Staffed by vegan and vegetarian doctors. The food is all vegan. The facilities include yoga classes. Howard Lyman of Mad Cowboy fame has stayed here. He was a Montana cattle rancher who went vegan, greatly improving his health. He wrote the books *Mad Cowboy* and *No More Bull.*

• Diabetes

Books of interest:

Becoming Raw: The Essential Guide to Raw Vegan Diets, by Brenda Davis, RD, Vesanto Melina, MS, RD, and Rynn Berry

Defeating Diabetes, by Tom Barnard, MD and Brenda Davis, RD

Dr. Neal Barnard's Program for Reversing Diabetes: A Scientifically Proven System for Reversing Diabetes without Drugs, by Neal D. Barnard

There is a Cure for Diabetes: The Tree of Life 21-Day + Program, by Gabriel Cousens

Documentary of interest:

Raw for Thirty, access: RawFor30Days.com. This involved taking a group of people diagnosed with diabetes and placing them on a raw foods diet.

ONE of the most amazing things about a well-balanced raw foods diet is that it can greatly improve the health of those who have suffered from blood sugar issues, including diabetes. The Boutenko family of RawFamily.com originally became interested in raw foods to improve the diabetic condition of their son, Sergei, who now writes raw food recipe books and tours the world teaching seminars about raw foods, wild food foraging, and chef skills.

On January 26, 2011, the United States Centers for Disease Control released updated facts about diabetes:

- Diabetes affects 25.8 million people in the U.S.
- 8.3% of the U.S. population has diabetes
- 18.8 million people with diabetes are diagnosed
- An estimated 7.0 million people with diabetes have not been diagnosed
- Among U.S. residents aged 65 years and older, 10.9 million, or 26.9% had diabetes in 2010
- About 215,000 people younger than 20 years had diabetes (type 1 or type 2) in the U.S. in 2010
- About 1.9 million people aged 20 years or older were newly diagnosed with diabetes in 2010 in the U.S.
- In 2005-2008, based on fasting glucose or hemoglobin A1C levels, 35% of U.S. adults ages 20 years or older had prediabetes (50% of adults aged 65 years or older). Applying this percentage to the entire U.S. population in 2010 yields an estimated 79 million American adults aged 20 years or older with prediabetes.
- Diabetes is the leading cause of kidney failure, nontraumatic lower-limb amputations, and new cases of blindness among adults in the U.S.
- Diabetes is a major cause of heart disease and stroke
- Diabetes is the seventh leading cause of death in the U.S.

Preventative Medicine Research Institute, Sausalito, CA, USA; pmri.org. Dr. Dean Ornish has proved that heart disease and narrowing of the arteries can be reversed through a vegan or near vegan diet combined with exercise, stress reduction, and lifestyle-changes.

Tree of Life Rejuvenation Center, POB 778 Patagonia, AZ 85624, USA; treeoflife.nu. Dr. Gabriel Cousens' retreat and education center teaching raw foods and holistic health practices.

True North Health, 1551 Pacific Ave., Santa Rosa, CA 95404, USA; healthpromoting.com. Staffed by vegan and vegetarian doctors.

• ARTIFICIAL SWEETENERS AND MSG: THE EXCITOTOXINS

Book of interest:

Excitotoxins: The Taste that Kills, by Russell Blaylock, MD

Documentary of interest: *Sweet Misery*
The documentary can be watched for free by accessing: topdocumentaryfilms.com

PLEASE avoid artificial sweeteners, including those listed on ingredient labels as Aspartame, Aspartate, Nutrisweet, Equal, Splenda, and Amino Sweet. Other sweeteners include Neotame and Sweetos. These chemicals are classified as neurotoxins and have been proven to cause or contribute to brain lesions, brain tumors, brain lymphoma, memory loss, seizures, depression, and lupus, and to interfere with vision, protein synthesis, brain function, nerve synapse function, and the function of neurotransmitters. Aspartame alters brain chemistry. Chemicals released into the body when a person consumes Aspartame include methyl ester, phenylalanine, and aspartic acid, and each of these can work to trigger or cause a variety of health problems.

The FDA, which approved Aspartame after a lot of political maneuvering by the Reagan administration, published a list of 92 side effects of Aspartame. The FDA employees who were in office before Regan took office wouldn't approve Aspartame, but the FDA employees appointed by Reagan quickly approved Aspartame for use in foods, drinks, snacks, and candies.

Some of these chemical sweeteners are used in animal feed. Sweetos has specifically been marketed to farmers and farmed animal feed companies. It covers the smell and taste of rancid feed that animals wouldn't normally consume. If you are a consumer of animal products (eggs, meat, milk [cheese, casein, yogurt, ice cream, creamer, whey, etc.]), you may also be consuming residues of Sweetos – and a variety of other chemicals used on farms.

Other artificial food chemicals that are excitotoxins include MSG, and any ingredient that is MSG-related, such as those listed on ingredient labels as casein hydrolysate, hydrolyzed vegetable protein, vegetable protein, broth stock, yeast extract, whey protein, carrageenan, textured protein, protein extract, autolyzed yeast, l-cystine, and even vaguely as "spices" and "natural flavoring." These are contained in processed foods, and may also be in some foods sold at "healthfood" or "natural foods" stores. Anything that is hydrolyzed can contain glutamate. So, avoid any foods with labels listing anything as hydrolyzed. (Access MSGMyth.com or NoMSG.com)

Excitotoxins interfere with intellectual and physical development, degrade concentration, alter immunity, and wreak havoc on hormonal balances, including the production and reception of testosterone and estrogen. Excitotoxins can impact puberty, tissue growth, and aging, and interfere with the ability to fight off and heal from diseases.

If a product label says it is "sugar-free," it likely contains artificial sweeteners. If a product says "MSG-Free," it may still contain MSG, but under misleading names that sound nice, but are simply disguises for unnatural and health-damaging ingredients.

Synthetic sweeteners and artificial food flavorings are contained in many products, including sodas, candy, cookies, chips, sweet snacks, gum, some brands of bottled and canned drinks, sports drinks, energy drinks, coffee additives, canned foods, dressings, soups, and mixes, some brands of children's vitamins, and some brands of baby foods. They may also be in meat, especially processed meats, and in fake meats sold as "vegetarian." Many restaurants include artificial sweeteners and food flavorings in their dishes.

To avoid excitotoxins, don't eat processed foods. Learn to make foods using whole ingredients. Grow some of your food, shop at organic farmers' markets and organic food co-ops. If you eat at restaurants, be aware of what may be in your food. Find your local organic raw vegan or raw vegan fusion (may serve some cooked vegan foods) restaurant. Learn to make salad dressings from scratch.

• Food Waste = Energy Waste, and Pollution of Land, Water, and Air

The standard American diet (SAD diet) is the most energy-intensive diet in history. And a large amount of America's food is wasted, both because of overeating, and because of food that is thrown away because it is unwanted, expired, or spoiled.

Not only do Americans eat more food than other people on the planet, they also throw away more of it. Every bit of wasted food was grown, processed, transported, and prepared with the use of various types of energy-using equipment, including farm equipment, vehicles, storage facilities, and often refrigerators and/or ovens (including microwave ovens), stoves, or dehydrators.

> "Nearly 20 percent of all edible meat ends up in landfills. That makes chemical fertilizer, pesticides, and water used to produce the wasted meat unnecessary, and the resulting emissions and environmental damage entirely avoidable."
>
> – Environmental Working Group, July 2011

According to a 2010 study by the University of Texas' Center for International Energy and Environmental Policy, food waste in America is the energy equivalent of 350 million barrels of petroleum. That is enough energy to power the country for a week at levels current to the use at the time the study was being conducted.

And that wasted energy use is only related to the food that is thrown away. According to study, which used 1990s statistics provided by the Department of Agriculture, Americans throw away about 27 percent of their food. Because Americans are heavier than they were in the 1990s, and the population has increased, the amount of energy being wasted has increased.

A 2005 study conducted by the National Institutes of Health concluded that Americans throw away about 40 percent of their food. The study also concluded that, in 2005 Americans were eating about thirty-percent more calories than they were in 1970.

When it is taken into consideration that most Americans are eating at least a third more calories than they need to live healthfully, and that more Americans are overweight than of a healthful weight, it is clear that Americans are wasting vast amounts of resources on a lifestyle of gluttony. Unfortunately, many countries have been following in the culinary footsteps of the U.S., which means that more and more countries are wasting vast resources on wasted food.

The growing, production, transport, processing, packaging, storage, marketing, and preparation of food results in more greenhouse gasses than all sources of transportation combined – including the pollution put out by all cars, trucks, ships, planes, and trains. In other words, more than anything else, the food choices of humanity are resulting in the environmentally ruinous climate change. And, more than any other country's populace, this applies to the large majority of Americans.

This topic is covered well in the book *American Wasteland*, by Jonathon Bloom.

Because most people do not compost their food into their nearby soil, most of the billions of tons of food that is tossed into the garbage every year in America also results in a large percentage of the garbage being hauled to landfills and trash dumps using trucks that use petroleum as fuel. Some municipalities, such as in Hawaii, incinerate their waste, which uses a large amount of fossil fuels and causes pollution of the air, water, and soil.

Even when the food waste ends up in landfills, it causes air pollution because decomposing food results in methane gasses, which are more damaging to the environment than carbon dioxide exhaust from petroleum-burning engines. Landfills result in about one-third of methane gasses caused by human society. This all factors more environmental damage into the food waste quagmire that also is related to billions of dollars being spent on food that ends up as trash.

U.S. households, restaurants, stores, cafeterias, prisons, hospitals, hotels, catering companies, food trucks, and cruise ships are all throwing away food scraps, expired or spoiled food, and unwanted food, and every day it adds up to a pile of food that, according to University of Texas researchers, can fill the 90,000-seat Rose Bowl stadium in Pasadena, California.

While it is good to reduce your food waste, and to eat a sensible diet that in tune with health, largely or all raw, and consists mostly or all of plant matter, it is also good to compost food scraps so that the nutrients they contain return to the soil.

• Composting

In past centuries people grew or wildharvested most or all of their food. Then they put their food scraps back into the soil. This returned nutrients to Earth and built up their soil base so that their culinary gardens grew amazingly well.

These days most people are disconnected from growing food. They purchase their food from stores, then go about the toxemian practice of throwing their food scraps into the trash, which gets taken to a landfill – where it is mixed with all sorts of toxic substances. Then, if people want to grow a garden they often use synthetic chemical fertilizers to feed the plants. This practice is a double-edged sword. Not only are they depleting the soil by *not* returning the plant and food scraps to the soil, which feeds the beneficial bacteria and fungi, they also are poisoning the land and their bodies with chemical fertilizers made from fossil fuel substances that are known to cause cancer, birth defects, learning disorders, and other health problems. Large amounts of fertilizers end up in underground aquifers, and in rivers, lakes, and oceans, where they cause damage to the environment and waterlife.

Plants that are grown in weak soil are not as hardy as they would be if they had been grown in nutrient-rich soil containing healthful amounts of bacteria and fungi. Plants grown in weak soil also are more susceptible to infestation. To deal with that issue people use pesticides and insecticides that are designed to kill living things. Pesticides, fungicides, and insecticides are toxic to humans, pets, and wildlife, and damage beneficial soil organisms.

Ideally, in addition to households, all restaurants and food stores would return vegetable food scraps to the land, and not send them to trash dumps. In 1997, the city of New York estimated that compostable food scraps made up 16% of the city's trash. On a national level, about 13% of U.S. trash consists of compostable food scraps.

There are many ways of composting food scraps. These include under-the-sink worm composting containers, outdoor compost bins, and compost pits dug into the ground.

Lately, there have been many people in cities getting into composting their food scraps by using ventilated worm bins, or "worm condos." These are containers containing hundreds of worms and that are kept under the kitchen sink, in a cabinet, or in an out-of-the way area of the home. This is known as "vermicomposting," and the worms that are used eat about half their body weight every day. As the worms consume the food scraps, which are often mixed with shredded newspaper lightly misted with water, the "worm casting" are what make up the compost, which can then be used in potted plants, in gardens, or spread among landscaping.

One family I know that uses an indoor worm composting system uses the worm castings to grow their wheatgrass for juicing, and their sunflower and bean sprouts that they use in salads. After they have harvested the wheatgrass and sprouts, they put the soil back into the worm bin along with more kitchen scraps.

When composting indoors, it is especially important to keep bread, dairy (milk products), oil (including lard and vegetable oils), and meat (including fish and fowl) out of the compost bin. Strictly include veggie waste scraps consisting of vegetables, fruits, berries, seeds, and nuts, and shredded, uncoated paper, such as newspaper (no wax- or plastic-coated papers).

Some cities have community gardens that accept food scraps for their compost bins. Check with your city to find out if they offer this option.

Where I live, we burry our kitchen scraps about once a week by simply digging a hole, tossing in the scraps, and covering them with dirt. Once the container we use for the scraps is emptied, it is rinsed out, and we start all over again.

I have found that I need to burry the scraps beneath at least a foot of soil to keep the raccoons and possums from digging them up.

Composting our kitchen scraps has greatly improved the condition of the soil. The ground was once hard, sandy, and difficult to dig. It is now moist and rich and holds onto moisture. It has become easy to dig holes two or three feet deep. When I first began composting here, there were no worms to be found. Worms are now everywhere in the soil. Composting the kitchen scraps this way also has fed the good bacteria and fungi in the soil, which is excellent for growing edible plants.

The soil has also improved in areas where we haven't buried compost; this is because the beneficial bacteria and fungi feeding on the compost have spread into nearby soil.

This soil rich in worms has also attracted more birds to nest in surrounding trees as they feed the worms to their young.

Sometimes random plants sprout from the composting pits, such as melon, tomato, and bean vines, which I've transplanted to places where they can grow – which results in more homegrown organic food.

When soil rich in bacteria and fungi is added to potted plants, the plants grow better as it is the microorganisms in the soil that help the plant roots to absorb nutrients.

> "We abuse land because we regard it as a commodity belonging to us. When we see land as a community to which we belong, we may begin to use it with love and respect."
> – Aldo Leopold, *A Sand County Almanac*

Although I already had an understanding of the importance of fungi in garden soil, I didn't really understand how composting was improving the soil until I heard what Paul Stamets had to say about composting.

According to Stamets, the guy who knows a lot about the fungus among us (check him out on YouTube.com), "Fungi are the mycomagicians of nature, in that they create soil (out of rock). And so engaging these fungi – if everyone individually began to compost, began to grow their own food, began to localize their use of resources and reinvest literally in their backyards as standard practice throughout the world, then I think that would create a big difference. People may not realize we are more closely related to fungi than we are to any other kingdom. We separated from fungi about 650 million years ago. We exhale carbon dioxide; so do fungi. We inhale oxygen, so do fungi."

Knowing that plants absorb carbon dioxide that we exhale, it only seems reasonable to assume that the carbon dioxide that the fungi in the soil exhales is helping to feed the roots of the plants. So... adding the nutrient-rich kitchen scraps to our garden soil will help spur the growth of fungi, which, as Stamets points out, "digest nutrients through fine, web-like cells called mycelium."

It is known that fungi help to decontaminate soil. So, nurturing the soil with kitchen scraps improves the fungi growth, which benefits your soil in a variety of ways.

According to Stamets, fungi can help detoxify soil that has been treated with farming chemicals: "We can use these fungi for breaking down hydrocarbon-based contaminates like oil, which most pesticides are based upon. We can break down PCBs, PCPs, dioxin, and lots of other recalcitrant toxins that kill life. These fungi can not only neutralize them, but also make them into fertilizer that breeds life. Fungi are the gateway species that leads to ecosystems re-flourishing."

Those who live in regions where it snows, and/or where the ground freezes during the winter months, will need their outside winter composting system to consist of a bin, or to have a compost pile that is covered by a weighted tarp. Throughout the winter, the compostable kitchen scraps can be tossed into the bin, or under the tarp. As the cold temperature months pass, the warmer temperatures of the spring months will speed up the microbial activity, causing the scraps to decompose. This is especially true with a compost pile covered by a tarp, which will trap the solar heat. As the compost pile warms, the worms will also become active in consuming the kitchen scraps.

Many coffee cafes will give you their used coffee grounds, which make an excellent coverage for compost piles. This also provides a way to prevent coffee grinds from going to landfills and garbage dumps.

In addition to improved soil conditions, another benefit of composting has been that we produce very little trash. We recycle nearly everything possible (glass, plastic metal, and paper) and have greatly reduced purchasing items that contain packaging. We produce about three bags of trash per year, and much of that consists of biodegradable materials that we can't put in our compost. Some of the trash also consists of junk mail that is on coated paper that can't be composted or recycled (and, yes, we have tried everything we know of to try to stop junk mail from arriving… but nothing seems to stop it).

Things that are good to include in your outdoor compost:

- Leftover and/or expired and/or rotting and/or scraps and peels of fruits, vegetables, berries, nuts (no produce labels or stickers)
- Egg and nut shells
- Coffee grounds
- Tea bags
- Weeds, leaves, and bark
- Grass and plant trimmings
- Wood chips, sawdust
- Wood ashes (no plastics, or ash from wood containing toxic chemicals or heavy metals)
- Old bread, rolls, muffins, cookies, and crackers (no icing)
- Tissues and paper towels
- Shredded paper and uncoated paper (no plastic or wax coated paper)
- 100% natural fibers (cotton, hemp, bamboo) cut into pieces
- Nut butters are okay, but no dumping of vegetable oils (no: olive oil, corn oil, canola oil, flax oil, etc., but foods containing them are okay.)

Things to keep out of your compost:

- Pet waste
- Meat, poultry, and fish
- Bones, animal fat, and oil (lard, expired oils: corn, canola, olive, etc.)
- Dairy products (milk, cheese, yogurt, keifer, and creamer)

A separate burying pit of at least three feet deep can be maintained to burry these items. A weighted, secure lid should be kept over the pit to avoid attracting wildlife, such as raccoon, bear, and possum. It is good to cover these items in the pit with ash, landscape clippings, soil, and/or coffee grinds to keep them from becoming an insect breeding ground.

These should be taken to a recycle center

- Plastic
- Glass
- Metal

These should be kept out of the compost:

- Branches (over 1/2" diameter)
- Crab or Bermuda grass

• Diseased plants
• Weeds that have gone to seed
• Non-native, invasive plants that will germinate or take root in the compost

Things to be disposed of by taking them to a toxic waste disposal station:

• Chemical pesticides, insecticides, and fertilizers (don't even purchase them!)
• Paints, varnishes, finishes
• Engine oils
• Chemical cleaners (use biodegradable cleaners)
• Light bulbs, especially compact fluorescent bulbs
• Batteries
• Electronics

BioCycle, biocycle.com
Eco•Cycle, EcoCycle.org/compost
Find a Composter, findacomposter.com
How To Compost, HowToCompost.org
US Composting Council, CompostingCouncil.org

• Slow Food

"Find the shortest, simplest way between the earth, the hands, and the mouth."

– Lanza Del Vasto

WHEN McDonald's planned to open a McDonald's near the Piazza di Spagna in Rome in 1986, a man named Carlo Petrini organized a protest. As their weapons the protesters used bowls of penne. Petrini wrote a manifesto against the fast-food culture and he founded the Slow Food Movement. The movement promotes traditional and regional foods as well as agricultural biodiversity, home culinary gardens, small farms, and sit-down dinners.

The Slow Food Movement has been key to reviving the "victory gardens" people planted in their yards, on their rooftops, and in their neighborhoods during WWII. But, this time people are planting home and neighborhood culinary gardens to provide personal independence from corporate agriculture, from the industrial food chain, and from mass marketed foods, and to save money, water, energy, and other resources.

The spread of home culinary gardening is reviving a connection to nature people lost by becoming too attached to commercialism, restaurants, and store-bought and industrialized foods.

Many affiliate groups have been started around the world.

Eat the Weeds, eattheweeds.com
Food Not Lawns, FoodNotLawns.com
Food Routes, FoodRoutes.org
Goode Green, goodegreennyc.com. Green rooftop design and installation.
KitchenGardeners.org
Local Harvest, LocalHarvest.org
Slow Food Nation, SlowFoodNation.org
Slow Food USA, SlowFoodUSA.org

Urban Organic Gardener, UrbanOrganicGardener.com. Mike Lieberman's blog
Yards to Gardens, y2g.org

• Low Fat Raw Veganism (LFRV)

Low Fat Raw Veganism These are people who follow a raw vegan diet that is more in tune with what Douglas Graham writes about in his book, *The 80/10/10 Diet*. These people are basically sunfoodists, but they follow a diet that is high in raw carbs (fruit), and low in fat (nuts, seeds, avocadoes, etc.). They mostly consume fruit (including vine fruits, such as cucumbers, zucchini, and tomatoes), and a smaller part of their diet consists of green leafy vegetables, nuts, and seeds. They also tend to avoid spicy foods, garlic, onions, peppers, salt, condiments, refined oils (olive oil, flax oil, hemp oil, etc.), and all synthetic food additives. They may consume some dehydrated foods, such as dried fruit and unsalted raw seed or veggie pulp crackers.

The majority of my meals tend to be aligned with the LFRV style of eating, but I don't consider myself to be a LFRV.

The people who closely follow a LFRV style of eating mostly or totally avoid what they call "gourmet raw," which is the food served in many of the raw restaurants, such as raw vegan cheesecake (made largely of creamed nuts), dehydrated seed breads (containing salt and oil), and salads with nut, avocado, or oil-based dressings. Many consider the occasional binge on gourmet raw to be fine.

Some people follow a mostly LFRV diet, but don't stick to it so strictly. They may eat some raw gourmet and heated vegan foods.

Two of the most active educators in the low fat raw vegan lifestyle are Harley Johnstone and Freelee Love in Australia. They hold retreats and also run the popular social networking site 30BananasADay.com.

Another well-known LFRV is Michael Arnstein, who has ran and won marathons. He refers to himself as a *fruitarian* and has an inspirational Web site: thefruitarian.com. In July 2011, he won the Vermont 100 mile race in 15 hours, 26 minutes.

Whether or not one follows LFRV, including a variety of raw, unheated, organically grown fruits in the diet is an excellent way of obtaining top quality nutrients, such as antioxidants, biophotons, enzymes, amino acids, minerals, vitamins, and other beneficial substances.

Some people question the energy used to import the tropical fruits often eaten by LFRVs, and say that this is unsustainable. While it is true that the carbon footprint of a diet consisting of a large amount of fruits can be a bit much, it is more sustainable than the typical meat-eating diet, which uses up enormous supplies of water, land, and fuel, and also food to feed the farmed animals, then to transfer them, slaughter them, and then to package the meat, which then has to be transferred to markets, bought, and cooked. The amount of water used to clean up after all of the meat eating is tremendous. Also not to be overlooked is that methane emitted from cows is more damaging to the environment than the burning of fossil fuels, which are also used to cook the meat, and to heat the water used in cleaning the slaughterhouses, the ovens and stoves, and the pots and pans. In other words, if anyone who is following the common SAD (standard American diet: meat, dairy, processed and junk foods containing fried oils, bleached grains, processed salts and sugars, and synthetic chemical additives) is critical of the environmental implications of importing fruit, they are certainly not dealing with the reality of their own diet.

Some people are putting up greenhouses and growing fruiting trees, berry bushes, and fruiting vines inside these. Some people travel and work as volunteers on organic fruit farms, such as through an organization called Worldwide Opportunities on Organic Farms (Access: WWOOF.org). Some people follow lifestyles in which they can travel with the seasons, going to the tropical regions during colder months, and moving north or south into the summer seasons of the hemispheres.

You may be interested in what Kristina Carrillo-Bucaram did in Texas. She connected with local organic farmers and founded the Rawfully Organic Co-op, which quickly grew into what is now a successful member co-op through which a growing variety of people are getting locally-grown organic fruits and vegetables. (Access: RawfullyOrganic.com)

American Community Gardening Association: CommunityGarden.org

AppleLuscious Organic Orchards, AppleLuscious.com

Michael Arnstein, TheFruitarian.com.

Bautista Dates, Mecca, CA; 7HotDates.com; KissMe (at) 7HotDates.com. The Bautista family has a mail-order date company so they can sell the dates they grow directly to the public.

Beyond Pesticides, BeyondPesticides.org

Bioneers, Bioneers.org

California Rare Fruit Growers, CRFG.org. Paul Thomson and John Riley founded this association in 1968. There are now chapters with thousands of members in many countries

California Rare Fruit Growers, CRFG.org/nurlist.html. Site listing nurseries selling both rare and common fruiting trees and bushes.

California Tropical Fruit Trees, TropicalFruitTrees.com. Vista, CA. California Tropical Fruit Trees sells a variety of both rare and common fruiting trees and berry bushes.

Chris Kendall, TheRawAdvantage.com; Nutritionist, yoga practitioner, professional skateboarder.

City Farm Organic Produce Markets, 1 City Farm Pl., East Perth, Australia; cityfarm.org.au. Saturday 9-noon. Organic produce and nursery.

Community Garden, CommunityGarden.org

DurianRider's Blog, DurianRider.org. Blog of Harley "Durianrider" Johnstone.

Eat Fruit Feel Good, eatfruitfeelgood.com

Eat the Weeds, eattheweeds.com

811 Directory, el-camacho.com/811friendly. Information about the lfrv lifestyle, includes listings of stores, places to travel, roommates, farms, etc.

Edible Forest Gardens, edibleforestgardens.com

Fallen Fruit, fallenfruit.org. Fruit share site. This began in Los Angeles with property owners who had fruit trees willing to allow other people to harvest the fruit and share it with others.

Farmers' Market Finder: AMS.USDA.Gov/FarmersMarket

Food Not Lawns: FoodNotLawns.com. Promotes the growing of organic food gardens instead of manicured lawns.

Food Routes, FoodRoutes.org

TheFruitarian.com. This is Michael Arnstein's Web site.

Fruitarian Nirvana, fruitariannirvana.ning.com. A social networking site for those interested in LFRV.

Fruit Co-op, califruit.webs.com. Good source for dates and raw almonds.

Fruit for Our Children, New Zealand, fruitforourchildren.com.

The Fruit Shack, 55 Dunn Bay Rd., Dunsborough, Australia; fruitandvegshack.com.au.

Brian Greco, thefruitandvegetablecuisine.com. Brian wrote a recipe book for low fat raw vegans.

Green Guerillas, New York, NY; GreenGuerillas.org.

Guerilla Gardening, guerrillagardening.org.

Home Orchard Society, HomeOrchardSociety.org

Jourdan's Beautiful Food, Florida; jourdansbeautifulfood.com. Tropical fruit.

KitchenGardeners.org

Local Harvest, LocalHarvest.org

Local Harvest, Santa Cruz; CALocalHarvest.org. Searchable database of farmers' markets, small farms, and related groups and businesses.

Neighborhood Fruit, neighborhoodfruit.com. Fruit- and vegetable-sharing site.

North American Fruit Explorers, NAFEX.org

Organic Food & Farmers' Markets, Australia; organicfoodmarkets.com.au. Site lists organic farmers' markets in Sydney area.

Permaculture, Permaculture.net

Pesticide Action Network, San Francisco, CA; PANNA.org

Pick Your Own, PickYourOwn.org. Lists farms where you can harvest your own produce. Blake2007 (at) PickYourOwn.org

Rare Fruit Society of South Australia, rarefruit-sa.org.au.

RawfullyOrganic.com. An organic food co-op in Texas founded by Kristina Carrillo-Bucaram, KristinaBucaram.com; Kristina (at) RawFullyOrganic.com; FullyRaw.com.

RawNaturalLiving.com. Matthew Warner is the author of *Fruitarians are the Future.*

30 Bananas A Day, 30BananasADay.com

Tropical Fruit World, TropicalFruitWorld.com.au. Gold Coast, store with variety of fruit.

Veggie Trader, veggietrader.com. People sharing homegrown and wild produce.

Willing Workers on Organic Farms, OrganicVolunteers.org

Worldwide Opportunities on Organic Farms, WWOOF.org

Urban Organic Gardener, UrbanOrganicGardener.com. Mike Lieberman's blog

Yards to Gardens, y2g.org

• Raw Vegan Fusion

WHILE many people who are into raw vegan food aim for consuming a nearly 100% raw diet, many people who are otherwise raw also eat some foods that have been heated.

Rather than high temperature cooked foods, such as fried, sautéed, grilled, or baked foods, these heated foods that people who are otherwise raw foodists may consume are likely to be along the lines of simmered vegan soups that don't have any oil or salt added until the soup is in the serving bowl, and steamed vegetables, quinoa, and lentils.

One goal is to avoid cooking starchy foods to above 247 degrees Fahrenheit, which is when acrylamides form. Also, avoid cooking that would make foods brown, which is when glycotoxins form (such as toast). Acrylamides and glycotoxins are chemicals that trigger the immune system and have been shown to increase the risk of cancer, kidney disease, and other health issues.

Water boils at about 212 degrees Fahrenheit at sea level, and at lower temperatures at higher elevations, such as in the mountains. So steaming and summering foods are ways of avoiding heating foods to the point where harsh chemicals will form in the foods.

While heating food does damage or destroy some nutrients, including biophotons, some vitamins, some antioxidants, some amino acids, and also essential fatty acids, a few foods contain beneficial substances that may become more bioavailable when the foods are lightly heated. These include carrots, broccoli, and tomatoes. And there are also some foods that become more digestible when low temperature steamed or simmered. These include beans, bamboo shoots, and yams.

For more information on heated foods in an otherwise raw vegan diet, read the book *Becoming Raw: The Essential Guide to Raw Vegan Diets*, by Brenda Davis, Vesanto Melina, and Rynn Berry. I also go into more detail about glycotoxins and acrylamides in my book, *Sunfood Diet Infustion: Transforming Health through Raw Food Veganism.*

The heated foods that otherwise raw foodists may also include truly fermented whole grain sourdough bread – which is to say, not your typical sourdough bread sold at the grocery store.

There are some well-known otherwise raw vegan restaurants that have some heated foods on the menu. These include the California restaurant chain Cafe Gratitude, and Rod Rotundi's Leaf Organics restaurant in Culver City, California. Also, Cherie Soria of the Living Light Culinary Institute, which is the main raw vegan chef school, knows about preparing some foods at low temperatures, and avoiding putting oil or salt in the foods until after they are ready to serve – as a way of avoiding damaging the essential fatty acids and salts.

Here is what Rod Rotundi says about raw vegan fusion:

> "Since I have been a raw foods chef and restaurateur for nearly 10 years, some of you are probably surprised to see that I am

offering some cooked vegan foods in addition to my extensive array of raw dishes. Allow me to explain…

While I do believe that raw foods are optimally healthy foods for most people in most situations, I also realize that we don't always eat only for "optimizing health". In fact, there are many other reasons to eat! One of the most obvious ones is pleasure- and it's not a sin! Taking pleasure from our culinary experiences is in my opinion a natural and normal way to eat. In fact, if the food we eat isn't delicious and pleasant tasting then we probably won't continue eating it for very long.

Now I know that some in the raw foods community think that every bite we take should be done with optimal health in mind. And indeed, there is certainly much merit in this approach. However, I believe that the ultimate objective is not optimal health but optimal happiness.

And let me tell you, I love food. I take great pleasure in tasting and eating different foods. Food offers us culture, community and comfort in addition to sustenance. When I was restricting myself to solely raw foods, I was doing it because I wanted to, because it felt right to me and I was enjoying it. After many years eating this way, I found myself wanting to broaden my culinary boundaries to include some cooked vegan foods- especially foods from around the world. And so I have. And I feel good with it.

So while I still eat a predominantly raw foods diet, I also enjoy some cooked foods. And I find that including probiotic foods together with cooked vegan foods helps with the digestion. I have included some of my favorite world cuisines in my new menu; Ethiopian, Indian and Mexican, and combined them with our raw creations and pro-biotic sauerkrauts to create my Vegan Fusion dishes."

– Rod Rotundi, owner of Leaf Organics restaurant, Culver City California; http://www.leaforganics.com; author of *Raw Food for Real People*.

• Fruiting Trees and Bushes

Fruits and berries are some of the most nutritious foods you can eat. One way to guarantee that you have access to fresh fruits and berries is to plant some of your own fruiting trees and bushes. If you don't have your own land, consider planting them on a cooperative neighbor's property, or on nearby wildland. I know people who hike into a canyon near their home where they have been planting fruit trees and berry bushes. Little-by-little they are creating an amazing fruit forest. They are also saving money, getting exercise, improving their nutrition, and disconnecting from the corporate food chain.

California Rare Fruit Growers, CRFG.org. Paul Thomson and John Riley founded this association in 1968. There are now chapters with thousands of members in many countries

California Rare Fruit Growers' San Diego chapter, CRFGSanDiego.org

California Rare Fruit Growers, CRFG.org/nurlist.html. Site listing nurseries selling both rare and common fruiting trees and bushes.

California Tropical Fruit Trees, TropicalFruitTrees.com. Vista, CA. California Tropical Fruit Trees sells a variety of both rare and common fruiting trees and berry bushes.

Common Vision, CommonVision.org. California-based organization plants fruiting trees at schools and other community facilities, and also helps reforest areas that were formerly forested.

Northern Nut Growers Association, NutGrowing.org

• Trees and Forests

> "The planting of trees is the planting of ideas. By starting with the simple step of digging a hole and planting a tree, we plant hope for ourselves and for future generations."
> – Wangari Maathai

> "The American reading his Sunday paper in a state of lazy collapse is perhaps the most perfect symbol of the triumph of quantity over quality.... Whole forests are being ground into pulp daily to minister to our triviality."
> – Irving Babbitt

TREES and forests are one of the many keys to life on this planet. Without them, we could not survive.

The average human living in North America uses paper and wood products that amount to hundreds of trees during their lifetime. To replenish the trees we use is a noble venture.

> "To me a lush carpet of pine needles or spongy grass is more welcome than the most luxurious Persian rug."
> – Hellen Keller

Please be involved with planting and protecting trees and forests. Support organizations that work to do the same.

Learn the types of trees that are native to where you live. There are over 970 species of trees that are classified as endangered. It is likely that some of them are native to your area. Find out which ones they may be, and then plant some of them.

> "Trees shade our ground, create topsoil, clean the air and help the land attract, hold and filter water. The trees and their roots purify the water as the rains fall. Clean streams keep millions of aquatic and other species alive."
> – Tim Hermach; *Forest Voice*, Spring 2006; ForestCouncil.org

> "We have nothing to fear and a great deal to learn from trees, that vigorous and pacific tribe which without stint produces

strengthening essences for us, soothing balms, and in whose gracious company we spend so many cool, silent and intimate hours."

– Marcel Proust

"Destruction of forests is a leading cause of global environmental breakdown, including global warming."

– AncientTrees.org, 2006

"A society is defined not only by what it creates, but by what it refuses to destroy."

– John Sawhill

"We must protect the forests for our children, grandchildren and children yet to be born. We must protect the forests for those who can't speak for themselves such as the birds, animals, fish and trees."

– Qwatsinas, Nuxalk Nation

American Chestnut Foundation, ACF.org
Alliance for Community Trees, ACTrees.org
American Forests, AmericanForests.org
Ancient Trees, AncientTrees.org
Budongo Forest: Budongo.org. African site.
Campaign for Old Growth, ancienttrees.org
California Rare Fruit Growers, CRFG.org
California Tropical Fruit Trees, TropicalFruitTrees.com. Vista, CA. California Tropical Fruit Trees sells a variety of both rare and common fruiting trees and berry bushes.
Common Vision, CommonVision.org. California-based organization plants fruiting trees at schools and other community facilities, and also helps reforest areas that were formerly forested.
Earth First!, EarthFirst.org
Forest Advocate, ForestAdvocate.org
Forest Council, ForestCouncil.org
Forest Ethics, ForestEthics.org
Forests Forever, ForestsForever.org
Forest Protection Portal, Forests.org
Friends of The Trees, friendsofthetrees.net
Friends of the Urban Forest, FUF.net
Global ReLeaf, GlobalReLeaf.org
Gifford Pinchot Task Force, GPTaskForce.org
Living Tree Paper Company, LivingTreePaper.com
Australia's Men of the Trees, menofthetrees.com.au
North American Native Plant Society, NANPS.org
Native Forests, NativeForest.org
Natural Resources Defense Council, NRDC.org
Northern Nut Growers Association, NutGrowing.org
Protect Our Woodland, ProtectOurWoodland.co.uk
Rainforest Action Network, RAN.org
World Rainforest Information Portal, RainForestWeb.org
Sanctuary Forest, SanctuaryForest.org
Save the Memorial Oaks Grove, SaveOaks.com

Save the Redwoods League, SaveTheRedwoods.org
Sequoia Forest Keeper, SequoiaForestKeeper.org
TasForests, TasForests.green.net.au. Tasmania, Australia.
Tree Muskateers, TreeMusketeers.org
Tree People, TreePeople.org
Tree For Life, TreesForLife.org
Trees for the Future, TreesFTF.org
Trees Foundation, TreesFoundation.org
We Save Trees, WeSaveTrees.org
North Coast Earth First is working to protect the last remaining stands of ancient redwood forests on the planet. Lumber companies controlled by billionaire investors, pension funds, and endowments own much of these forests and want to cut them down for profit. Help protect the redwoods! Send donations to:
North Coast Earth Firs, POB 4646, Arcata, CA 95518-4646; northcoastearthfirst.org

• BAMBOO

THERE are over 1,000 varieties of bamboo. It is a fast-growing plant that can be used for food, flooring, shelter, clothing, soil detoxification, flood control, oxygen, and cleaning the air of pollution.

American Bamboo Society, AmericanBamboo.org
Bamboo Central, BambooCentral.org
Bamboo Man, BambooMan.com.au
Bamboo 2000, Bamboo2000.com
Environmental Bamboo Foundation, BambooCentral.org
International Network for Bamboo and Rattan, INBAR.int
Panda Bamboo, PandaBamboo.com
Smith & Fong Plyboo, Plyboo.com

• HEMP

HEMP is perhaps the most useful single plant on the planet. It can be used for food, fuel (both ethanol made from the cellulose for gasoline engines and oil pressed from the seeds for diesel engines), fabric, flooring, insulation, plastic, nylon, fiberglass, plywood, resin, bricks, filters, ink, paint, soap, paper, medicine, furniture, and hundreds of other products.

Even though you can't get high from hemp, and it is a plant that absorbs pollution; improves air and water quality; protects wildlife habitat; localizes economies; and provides a more sustainable culture, as if this writing, hemp remains illegal to grow in the U.S., and all hemp material must be imported. Right now, if any farmer planted hemp in the U.S., they could be charged with a felony, be imprisoned, and have their land and belongings confiscated by the federal government.

Solar and wind energy are part of the solution to breaking away from fossil fuels. But hemp can also play an important role in reducing and eliminating fossil fuel use.

Unlike solar power and wind turbines, hemp absorbs greenhouse gasses while producing oxygen.

Unlike the creation of solar energy farms where thousands of solar panels are placed on large plots of land in regions where the cloudless days are common, such as in the Nevada desert, hemp requires a small investment for farmers, can be grown in every region of the continent, and improves soil conditions. While solare energy energy farms and solar electric generating plants are owned by corporations and stockholders, family farmers can be growing hemp, and employing local people in every region.

Unlike petroleum, coal, natural gas, and tar sands that need to be drilled and pumped or mined from the ground, hemp can be grown without destroying, drilling, or mining deep into the land.

Hemp can be used to make plastic that is safer for the environment than the plastics made from petroleum.

Growing hemp for both ethanol and diesel fuel would mean that American countries become more energy independent. We would reduce drilling and digging into Earth to obtain billions of gallons of petroleum. Our air would be cleaner. The number of ships traveling around the planet to transport petroleum would be greatly reduced. Millions of acres of hemp would be absorbing more pollution than the same number of acre of trees.

When you consider that the pollution put out by the world's shipping barges amounts to the pollution put out by most countries, you can get an idea of how much petroleum is being burned by the ships, and how much they contribute to global warming, the acidification of the oceans, the melting of the ice caps, and the death of wildlife.

When hemp is used to make ethanol, the fiber is left over. That can be used as insulation in homes, helping us to save money on heating costs while also reducing the amount of fuel we use to heat our homes and buildings. The fiber can also be used to make fiberboard to build those structures.

Meanwhile, as the U.S. continues its hemp farming prohibition, other countries are allowing and encouraging their farmers to grow hemp. They are also being innovative in creating products from hemp. But, if U.S. companies need raw hemp material, they have to import it.

With a legalized industrial hemp farming we could also stop cutting down our forests for paper and plywood. Hemp paper is stronger, lasts longer, and is more recyclable than wood pulp paper. Hemp has longer and stronger fibers than wood. Fiberboard made with hemp is four times stronger than fiberboard made using tree wood, and is less susceptible to rot and infestation.

Hemp paper was used in the first printing presses, bringing humanity out of ignorance and into mass education.

Now that the machinery exists to more easily process hemp into paper, cardboard, fiberboard, and plywood, it no longer makes economic or environmental sense to keep destroying our forests to create those products when we can be using hemp.

Hemp is believed to be the first crop that was used to create fabric. Evidence of this has been found in China where hemp fabric and rope has been unearthed in settlements believed to be over 10,000 years old. The use of hemp fabric brought about the end of using animal skins as clothing.

Hemp was used in the first fabric sails that allowed humans to travel the seas. And the ropes that were used on the ships were also made of hemp fiber. The lamps on board were fueled with hemp seed oil. Hemp oil, resin, and fiber were used to waterproof the hulls and decks.

After the invention of the cotton gin, cotton became king of the south on the backs of slave labor. At the same time, the hemp farms of the north began to close down, or to transition into other crop farms, or animal farms.

When you consider that cotton uses enormous amounts of water, and that cotton farming uses more pesticides than any other crop, and that an acre of hemp provides more fabric-making material than an acre of cotton, you can get the idea of what hemp can do to benefit farmers, local economies, and the environment.

Hemp is a crop that grows easily without the pesticides and fertilizers used on cotton. Unlike cotton, hemp can be grown in every region of the U.S. Hemp uses much less water than cotton. Hemp can be made into a variety of fabrics that easily can be stronger, softer, and warmer than cotton. Hemp can also be made into more varieties of fabric than cotton can provide, and not just the rough, potato-sack material that people visualize when they think of hemp. Henp can also be combined with bamboo to create an amazingly soft and sturdy fabric that is both softer and sturdier than cotton.

The hemp market already exists. You can walk into any natural foods store, and an increasing number of mainstream grocery stores, and find products made from hemp.

Hemp contains more omega 3 fatty acids and tastes better than than flax. Hemp seeds and its oil can be used in a variety of foods.

There are a number of industries that already use hemp fiber in the U.S. These include companies that make rugs, clothing, curtains, and the sound insulation boards of trucks and automobiles. Many vehicles also contain carpeting and seating fabric that is made partially of hemp.

Today's farmers are struggling. And the high price of fuel is creating more of a strain on farmers. Why not allow them to grow hemp farmers' fuel co-ops that would press the seeds into oil, which could then be used to run the diesel engines in the farm machinery that largely run on diesel fuel? The hemp plants could also be used to make ethanol, which could be sold to regional gas stations. We shouldn't be importing billions of gallons of petroleum from other countries to then refine and use as fuel for farm equipment when we could be allowing farmers to grow their own fuel, and for lower cost.

Throughout history, hemp has been used to transform human culture. It is time for a hemp renaissance. Not only does it need to happen in the U.S., but also it needs to happen around the world. It will localize our economies, improve our condition, and make us less dependant on imported goods and services. It will help us break our ties to the corporate giants that rely on our money for their tremendous profits.

> "And I will raise up for them a plant of renown, and they shall be no more consumed with hunger in the land, neither bear the reproach of the heathen anymore."
>
> – Ezekiel 34:29; Geneva Study Bible (A. D. 1599)

Documentary: *The Hemp Solution*, TheHempSolution.com.au

Book: *Marijuana & Hemp: History, Uses, Laws, and Controversy*, by John McCabe

Canadian Hemp Trade Alliance, HempTrade.ca
Hemp Industries Association, TheHIA.org
Hemp Nation, HempNation.com
Hemp Oil Canada, HempOilCan.com
The Hemp Solution, TheHempSolution.com.au
Hemp Stores, HempStores.com
Hemptydoo, Shop 140 Belmont Forum, 227 Belmont Ave., Cloverdale 6105, Australia; hemptydoo.com.au. Hemp clothing, accessories, beauty products, and foods.
Margaret River Hemp Co., 133 Bussel Hwy., Margaret River – and – 85 Market St., Fremantle, Australia; hempco.net.au. Clothing and accessories.
North American Industrial Hemp Council, NAIHC.org
Nutiva Hemp Foods, Nutiva.com
Seattle Hempfest, HempFest.org
Vote Hemp, VoteHemp.com

• Solar Energy and Wind Turbines

If you are looking for where the energy will come from to power households and businesses of the future, look up – to the rooftops and the sun, and to the wind. And not to mining, drilling, fracking, or pumping, and not to the lie of clean coal or the disaster that is nuclear energy. And not to desert or wild lands, or the oceans or lakes – which should be protected from development.

One of the more promising technologies to be developed is solar molten solar electic generating plants (Google that!), which use mirrors and steam to create electricity. Those, and siilar solar electric generating plants, which can be built on sprawling rooftops, can help fuel many households.

> "California has the commercial and residential rooftop potential for more than 70,000 megawats of photovoltaic (PV) generation. This does not include the capacity for PV generation over the massive parking lots that clutter California cities. Currently, California electricity consumption peaks at 65,000 megawats on the hottest summer days."
>
> – David Myers, Got A Light? Earth Island Journal, Autumn 2010

American Solar Energy Society, ASES.Org
eSolar, eSolar.com
Green Energy News, NRGLink.Com
Green Home Building, GreenHomeBuilding.Com
Hat Creek Publishing, HatCreekPublishing.Com
Home Power Magazine, HomePower.Com
International Solar Energy Society, ISES.Org
Red Solar, CubaSolar.Cu. Site is in Spanish. The Cuban government has been very active in converting schools to solar energy.
Solar Energy Society of Canada, SolarEnergySociety.Ca
Solar Living Institute, POB 836, 13771 S. Hwy. 101, Hopland, CA 95449; 707-744-2017; SolarLiving.Org
Sol West, SolWest.Org
Urban Green Energy, UrbanGreenEnergy.com. Manufactures home wind turbines.

• GREEN YOUR HOME

LEARN about nontoxic paints and finishes; composting; solar power; solar hybrid lighting; tankless hot water systems; graywater systems; landscaped roofs; biodegradable soaps; safe cosmetics; recycled and rescued wood furniture; natural insulation; recycling; native plants; low-impact housing; organic culinary gardening; recycled paper products; nonpetroleum candles; open brick paving; and ways you can live a more environmentally sustainable life.

Alcohol Can Be A Gas, PermaCulture.com
Building Green, BuildingGreen.com
Earth 911, Earth911.org
Earth Garden Magazine, POB 2, Trentham, VIC 3458, Australia; earthgarden.com.au. Magazine for sustainable living
Goode Green, goodegreennyc.com. Green rooftop design and installation.
The Green Life, theGreenLifeCo.com
Green Roofs, GreenRoofs.com
Permaculture Activist, PermaCultureActivist.net
Regreen, RegreenProgram.org
We Can Live Green, WeCanLiveGreen.com

• Biodegradable Soaps and Detergents

DID you know that the most common cleaning substances contain chemicals that can poison you? The colorings, astringents, scents, and other substances found in soaps and detergents are often made out of carcinogenic and hormonal disrupting chemicals that can cause birth defects, learning disabilities, and other health problems. Disinfectants may contain phenol and cresol, which can cause fainting, diarrhea, and dizziness and well as damage to the kidneys and liver.

Additionally, wood and floor polishes may contain nitrobenzene, which is a carcinogen that can also cause birth defects. Metal polishes may contain petroleum distillates that interfere with vision and cause damage to the kidney and nerves.

Safer choices for cleaning include vinegar and baking soda. Non-chlorine bleaches and hydrogen peroxide can be used as disinfectants.

Avoid soaps and detergents made out of petrochemicals. Either make your own cleaner, or purchase those that are more environmentally safe.

Look for cleaners that are made of plant substances, and that are produced by companies that do not test their products on animals. Many of these may be found in your local natural foods market.

• Cosmetics

> "I apply the same principals to skin care as I apply to food. Both are entering my body, whether through my skin or through my mouth. Therefore, both need to be as close to nature as possible, completely pure, and entirely free of chemicals and synthetics. Unlike the food industry, there are no legal standards for personal care products sold in the United States, meaning that we need to be savvy when shopping for healthy skin care."
>
> - Jill Bickford, Living Earth Beauty. Find out 5 Ways to Start Making Healthy Skin Care Choices at blog.livingearthbeauty.com/go/healthyskin

> "It is amazing how there is such a lack of regulation when it comes to cosmetics. Many ingredients in cosmetics contain toxic substances that are on the Environmental Protection Agency's lists of hazardous wastes and hazardous substances. Since there was the long-ago myth that the skin is an impermeable barrier, cosmetics laws became a low priority – much to the chagrin of the American people."
>
> – Elizabeth Howard, RawRawGirls.Com, a living foods catering and cosmetics company in Oregon.

DID you know that many of the skin, hair, and oral care products sold in stores today contain toxins that can cause cancer and that also poison our lakes, rivers and oceans; and can cause birth deformities, miscarriages, sterility, and learning disabilities in both humans and wildlife?

Many skin, hair, and oral care products contain petroleum-derived parabens. These are known carcinogens and are used as preservatives in the products. Parabens are known to mimic estrogen and disrupt testosterone levels. Many of the same chemicals used on insecticides are often used in body scents and other cosmetics. Other chemicals used on the most popular cosmetic products include coal tar coloring, labeled as D&C and FD&C colors (dyes made from coal tar may also be in soda, candy, icing, and other foods); formaldehyde, a known carcinogen; lead, phthalates; and nonylphenols, chemicals that disrupt hormonal balance and that are contained in many shampoos, shaving creams, and hair dyes.

Perfumes and colognes are some of the most toxic substances people put onto their skin. They often contain chemicals that are derived from petroleum and coal and that can interfere with respiratory function, hormonal balance, and the function of the brain and neurons. Additionally, many of the chemicals in perfumes and colognes are known to cause asthma, birth deformities, and cancer. When the chemicals are put onto the skin they are absorbed into the body where they collect in fat cells and in the blood.

Perfumes and colognes contain so many toxins that municipalities advise people to avoid disposing the products by pouring them into the sink or toilet, but to take them to the nearest hazardous-waste collection center. Do you really think you should be putting these substances on your skin?

Many people think that the Food and Drug Administration is a gatekeeper that protects consumers from exposure to toxins by not allowing companies to use them. The truth is that the FDA does not get involved until a problem arises. And even then they may have to be dragged into it through lawsuits and consumer outrage.

Companies that make body care products may conduct some testing, including horrible and torturous tests conducted on incarcerated animals, but the companies are known to use some of the most toxic chemicals in their products. Some of the very same chemicals have been identified by the U.S. Environmental Protection Agency as hazardous to the health of humans and wildlife.

Why are companies permitted to use such toxic chemicals in their personal care products, and advertise them using “super models”? Good question. I don’t have the answer other than that the industry trade group for the hair, skin, nail, and oral care product companies, the Cosmetic, Toiletry and Fragrance Association, may like the way things are done.

There is no government agency testing the combination of chemicals used as ingredients in body care products. Nobody knows what happens when you mix some of the chemicals with others because testing has never been done.

Meanwhile, those who use the products are absorbing the synthetic chemicals into their tissues, and the chemicals often end up lingering in the fat cells of the body, where they can cause or contribute to an assortment of ailments.

Remember that what you put on your skin, hair, nails, and use to care for your teeth ends up in your body, and in your environment.

If you are vegan, you want to read labels of cosmetics to make sure they don't contain beeswax or other bee products, as well as animal products. Also, many of the most popular cosmetic products contain ingredients derived from processing the remains of animals from slaughterhouses as well as roadkill and dead animals from animal shelters sold to rendering plants. (See Howard Lyman's *Mad Cowboy*.)

Some companies that sell themselves as "natural" hair and skin care product companies do use animal by-products and other ingredients that are not so good for you, for wildlife, or for the planet.

Check out the cosmetics at your local natural foods store. Look for those that state on the label that they consist of organic ingredients, do not contain animal by-products, synthetic chemicals, or ingredients that were tested on animals.

Better yet, learn to make your own cosmetics. You may invent new types of cosmetics using the substances of nature. Some of the ingredients can be found in your kitchen, your garden, nearby wildlands, and the local farmers' market, or the produce section of your natural foods store.

> "Contrary to popular belief, the U.S. government doesn't regulate cosmetics and body care products for safety, long-term health impacts or environmental damage. Many synthetic chemicals and petroleum-based ingredients found in non-organic certified brands are harmful to people and the environment.
>
> Consumers can avoid toxic ingredients by using USDA certified Organic Body Care and Cosmetics. The trouble is, while the USDA allows cosmetics and body care products meeting National Organic Program food and agricultural standards to be certified organic, it doesn't police the rampant labeling fraud in the industry, where many brands make organic claims on their front label, but in fact are neither organic nor certified."
>
> **Top 10 Reasons to Use Organic Body Care and Cosmetics. Non-Organic Body Care and Cosmetics...**

> 10. Fuel Oil (petroleum) Addiction; 9. Spawn Super Weeds; 8. Unleash Biocides; 7. Contaminate Water; 6. Make Us Fat; 5. Speed Up Puberty; 4. Increase Infertility; 3. Cause Birth Defects; 2. Give Us Cancer; 1. Aren't Regulated
>
> – The Organic Consumers Association

The Organic Consumers Association has put together a "coming clean campaign" that is working to bring organic integrity to the cosmetic market. Watch the seven-minute short documentary, *The Story of Cosmetics*, which approaches the questions, "What are all those chemicals in your shampoo? Your lipstick? Your aftershave? And what do they have to do with asthma, breast cancer and learning disabilities?" It was produced by the Campaign for Safe Cosmetics, Annie Leonard's Story of Stuff Project, and Free Range Studios. (Access: OrganicConsumers.org or FreeDocumentaries.org)

• Toilet Paper

Toilet paper was first created in China in the 1300s. It has since become one of the most environmentally destructive materials in the common home. According to the Natural Resources Defense Council, toilet paper uses about ten percent of all paper in the U.S., and is responsible for about 15 percent of deforestation in North America, including from old-growth forests and from toxic-farming chemical-treated monocropped tree plantations. While many companies in a variety of countries manufacture toilet paper, the largest are the Kimberly-Clark company located in Texas, and the Yuan Xiang Paper company in China. These are among the companies manufacturing and shipping toilet paper products to markets all over the world.

According to the Earth Island Journal article, Not a Square to Spare, by Noelle Robbins, one in every seven trees cut down by the forest industry goes right down the toilet in the form of toilet tissue. Increasing the negative impact on the environment is that toilet paper is made using toxic pulp-processing chemicals, dried with high-octane machinery, and is then treated with perfumes and wrapped in plastic.

When you purchase toilet paper or tissue, please purchase those brands that use 100% recycled paper and that are unscented. Also, choose to support VoteHemp.com, which lobbies to get industrial hemp farming legalized in the U.S. (hemp can be used to make paper products – and can help us preserve and replenish forests).

• Light Bulbs

MOST lights on the planet rely on electricity produced by coal-burning power plants. The mining of coal destroys mountains, valleys, rivers, and lakes, and leaves gaping holes in Earth. Burning coal spews soot, greenhouse gasses, radioactive fly ash, and mercury into the atmosphere. The burning of coal for electricity is the chief cause of mercury poisoning in fish.

About half of the electricity in the U.S. and a third of its carbon dioxide pollution is produced by coal-burning power plants. Please reduce your use of electricity created by coal-burning power plants.

Using a compact fluorescent light instead of the typical 100-watt incandescent light bulb eliminates the burning of about 100 pounds of coal. Use LED lights, which use even less electricity than, and don't contain the mercury found in compact fluorescent bulbs.

In addition to solar and wind energy, check into the emerging technology of solar hybrid lighting.

Always turn off lights not in use.

Wildlife, including migrating birds and nocturnal animals, need darkness at night. Please eliminate or greatly reduce exterior lighting.

> "Two-thirds of Americans live in places that no longer afford a sight of the Milky Way. Light pollution increases at rates that experts say will cancel out every dark sky in the contiguous United States within 15 years – until there will be no more Milky Way for us. The alien light burns out the people it touches. Light pollution in excess – and it always appears in excess – correlates with higher rates of cancer. It poisons sleep, sucking melatonin from the brain. It is unnatural and invasive, and accepted as the norm."
>
> – Christopher Ketcham, Night Vision; *Earth Island Journal*, Autumn 2010

International Dark Sky Association, DarkSky.org

• AIR CONDITIONING

INSULATE with natural, biodegradable insulation. If you use an electric or gas heater, insulating is one of the main ways you can reduce your use of fossil fuels, especially if you live in a cooler climate where you use heat, or a climate where you use air conditioning.

If you use air conditioning: Install a Cool-n-Save kit to reduce costs, electricity, and pollution by 25% or more.

Install solar panels to cut your use of fossil fuels. Home wind turbines may be a solution for creating your own electricity. But the technology for small wind turbines isn't quite there yet – unless you live in a particularly windy area, or a place with a constant breeze.

Consider landscaping your roof with native plants. This will insulate your home while reducing the heat pond of your roof and will be providing safe habitat for native insects and birds.

Cool-N-Save, CoolNSave.com
Earth Pledge, earthpledge.org/gr
Goode Green, goodegreennyc.com. Green rooftop design and installation.
Green Grid Roofs, greengridroofs.com
Green Roofs, greenroofs.org
Roof Meadow, roofmeadow.com

Rooftop Farms, rooftopfarms.org
Swift Wind Turbine, SwiftWindTurbine.com

• School Campus Sustainability

MANY organizations are helping to transform school campuses into sustainable villages, to get their energy from renewable resources, to recycle, to reduce their use of plastics, to compost food scraps, to use biodegradable cleaning agents, to provide bike-friendly campuses, and to have local, organic foods available for students and staff, including by having students grow culinary gardens on campus.

> "The global food system, from seed to plate to landfill, is responsible for as much as one-third of all greenhouse-gas emissions, largely because it is the single greatest force behind deforestation and soil degradation, both of which release carbon dioxide into the atmosphere. Indeed, livestock production alone is responsible for 18 percent of the world's emissions, more than those produced by all transportation – every SUV, steamer ship and jet plane combined."
>
> – Anna Lappe, author of the books *Diet for a Hot Planet,* and *Hopes Edge.*

California Student Sustainability Coalition, sustainabilitycoalition.org
Campus Climate Challenge, climatechallenge.org
The Edible Schoolyard, edibleschoolyard.org
Real Food Challenge, realfoodchallenge.org

• Reducing Trash

> "We need to think about creating things rather than buying them, and say, taking a walk with friends rather than shopping. We are not going to shop our way out of resource depletion."
>
> – Deborah Koons Garcia, director of the documentaries *The Future of Food* and *In Good Heart: Soil and the Mystery of Fertility*

EVERY product you use has something to do with natural resources and the stream of trash being produced on the planet. Everything from the substances used to produce the product to how the product is manufactured, packaged, shipped, and used impacts the planet.

Even products as simple as a staple use resources. Staples are made of steel, which is mined from Earth. The number of staples used every year in the U.S. amounts to over 200 tons of steel, and the great majority of them end up in trash dumps. When you have the choice, use a reusable paperclip instead of a single-use staple.

There is more trash collected in the month of December than during any other part of the year. This is simply because of massive amounts of people involved in abundant holiday shopping and extravagant holiday meals. If you are a person who celebrates the traditional end-of-year holidays, consider ways that you can make your celebrations less toxemian and more sustainable.

Basel Action Network, Ban.org
Eco Cycle, EcoCycle.org
Free Cycle, FreeCycle.org
Freegans, Freegans.info
Free Geek, FreeGeek.org
Global Recycling Network, GRN.com
Life Box Company, LifeBoxCompany.com. Has created boxes that contain seeds within the cardboard. When the box is done being used, you plant it, and it will grow into a garden.
Planet Green Recycle, PlanetGreenRecycle.com
Recycle Bank, RecycleBank.com
Zero Waste America, ZeroWasteAmerica.org

• Shopping Bags

CHOOSE cloth, not paper or plastic. Bring a cloth shopping bag with you when you shop.

Hundreds of millions of plastic bags are used every day. The U.S. population used 380 billion plastic bags in 2007. Nearly 2.5 billion of those were used in Los Angeles County. It is likely that over a trillion were used worldwide. These choke landfills, end up as littler, clog waterways, shut down drainage systems, provide breeding areas for mosquitoes, and billions of bags end up in lakes and oceans, leaching chemicals into the water. Plastic bags cause the death of birds, fish, turtles, and other wildlife when bags choke or strangle them, or end up in their digestive tract and cause them to starve.

Paper bags are not the solution to avoiding the use of plastic bags. Hundreds of thousands of trees that are home to wildlife and that also clean the air, filter water, build soil, and put forth oxygen are cut down every year to produce paper bags, literally trashing forests: the lungs of Earth, and the starting base of many rivers.

Ireland was the first country to require stores to charge for plastic bags. Since the law went into effect in 2002, the use of plastic shopping bags has dropped by 90 percent. An increasing number of cities have been banning single-use plastic grocery bags, including San Francisco, Los Angles, and Mexico City. Some smaller cities are also banning single-use plastic bags, including Santa Monica, California, and Modbury, England.

Please avoid using paper and plastic bags by using non-synthetic, biodegradable cloth shopping bags. Biodegradable fabrics include cotton, hemp, bamboo, and sisal.

Get your local stores to stop using plastic and paper bags. Encourage laws that require a fee for paper and plastic bag use.

Green Jute, 15930 Cypress Trace Ct., Chesterfield, MO 63017, USA; greenjute.com; marjula (at) greenjute.com. Marjula Pothuri.

• Kitchen Food Stock

THERE are a number of companies that specialize in quality, organic foods common in raw food kitchens.

There are a lot of choices to be made with how and what to use when making food.

Some people avoid certain ingredients, such as gluten, while others don't seem to have an issue with it.

Some people will use agave as a sweetener, but others avoid it. I almost totally avoid it, and don't buy it.

Some people that are otherwise raw will use maple syrup, while others consider maple syrup to be a cooked food, and they avoid it. (Maple syrup is maple tree trunk sap that is a watery substance and that has been slowly simmered into syrup.)

Some people will eat raw chocolate, and some people avoid it. Some don't use chocolate because it makes their heart race, or because they aren't sure of it, such as if it came from a modern slave farm in Africa. Some consider it a neurotoxin. Some may use raw carob instead.

Some people use lemon instead of vinegar in their dressings. Some people don't use vinegar for anything.

Some people use Nama Shoyu, while others avoid it because it contains gluten. At Matt and Janabai Amsden's Euphoria Loves Rawvolution restaurant in Santa Monica (EuphoriaCompany.com), they use Coconut Secret, a 100% organic, raw coconut aminos, and no longer use Tamari or Nama Shoyu.

The best foods you can have in the kitchen are those you grow organically yourself with soil enriched by kitchen compost, and those you get from local organic farmers. Research organic home gardening.

If you have a food co-op nearby, it is good to join so that you can get discounts on organic foods. Co-ops typically purchase in bulk, and share the discount with members. If there isn't a co-op near you, consider starting one.

It is also good to have a variety of organic sprouting seeds. Sprouts are rich in a variety of nutrients, and a low-cost way to keep greens in your daily diet. Typically, in my kitchen, there are seven jars of sprouts going at the same time – using one jar of sprouts every day, and starting a new one. See the Sprouting section of this book for more information about sprouting.

Blessed Herbs, Oakham, MA, USA, BlessedHerbs.com. For organic herbs.

Bautista Family Organic Date Ranch, POB 726, Mecca, CA 92254-0726; 760-396-2337

Fat Uncle Farms, California; funclefarms.blogspot.com. Raw almonds.

Fronteir Natural Products Co-op, Iowa; FrontierCoop.com. Sells sprouting supplies.
Handy Pantry, Utah; HandyPantry.com. Sprouting supplies.
Heirloom Organics, Sprouting-Seeds.com.
Mountain Rose Herbs, Eugene, OR; MountainRoseHerbs.com. Sells herbs and sprouting supplies.
Mumm's Sprouting Seeds, Saskatchewan, Canada; Sprouting.com.
Ocean Harvest Sea Vegetable Company, Mendocino, CA; OHSV.net. Wild, raw Mendocino seaweeds. Terry Nieves.
Selina Naturally, Arden, NC, USA; CelticSeaSalt.com. Markets high-quality salts.
Sprout House, New York; SproutHouse.com.
Sprout People, San Francisco, CA; SproutPeople.com. Sells organic sprouting seeds.

• CHOCOLATE

IN much of the chocolate sold through the world, there is a dark secret called *modern day slavery*. Children as young as 8 are sold into labor, including to work on chocolate farms. Many are used to spread toxic farming chemicals and to perform labor that is taxing and dangerous even for adults. If the slaves don't work hard enough, they are mistreated, beaten, maimed, or even killed. If you consume chocolate, be aware of from where the chocolate is sourced. Also, you may be interested in a documentary titled *The Dark Side of Chocolate*. The documentary exposes slavery and child labor among the cocoa farms of Africa's Ivory Coast.

Many people who are into raw food are also into raw chocolate and consider it to be a tremendous superfood. However, chocolate can make the heart race, interfere with sleep, contribute to stress, tax the adrenal glands, and many consider it an addictive neurotixin (Google: chocolate neurotoxin). Some of those who sell it make outlandish claims about the health benefits of raw chocolate. Most people who ever lived on the planet never had access to chocolate. It certainly isn't a necessity, and is not essential for vibrant health. I went through a raw chocolate phase, but didn't like the way it made me feel. I tend to avoid it. If I am going to eat something along that line, I prefer carob – which is calming rather than stimulating. Many raw chocolate products also contain agave, which I also try to avoid, as that processed sugar also is not something I consider to be a healthfood – but is one step away from corn syrup.

The Dark Side of Chocolate, TheDarkSideOfChocolate.org
International Cocao Initiative, Cocoainitiative.org

• FOOD STORAGE

IN uncertain economic times and in emergencies, having a variety of foods available in a food storage cabinet, closet, cellar, fridge, and/or freezer can be a huge help.

Purchasing foods in bulk can be a lot less expensive than purchasing small amounts of the same items.

Growing foods, learning to wildharvest and nurture food plants on open land, and knowing about sprouting and keeping a variety of sprouting seeds are all ways of eating inexpensively, organically, and nutritionally, including in good times and not so good.

If you keep food storage, remember to rotate it, consuming the oldest things first, and writing the dates on containers so that you know how old they are, and when to use them before they get too old. Learn to determine when foods have passed their state of being edible, such as by looking at them, smelling them, and at the first taste of them.

There are many ways of protecting the nutrients in your fruits and vegetables that will make them keep longer.

Storing certain fruits and vegetables in airtight containers is not an option as they are alive and need oxygen. Even storing things in a plastic bag can smother them and/or alter their flavor.

Many people have had problems with fruit flies. Simple solutions include storing things in paper or cloth bags.

A box with a screen on top, or a cabinet that has been fitted with screens or fabric stretched across the door frame, where windows would normally be, is another way of allowing fruits and vegetables stored at room temperature to continue to be exposed to air, but not get exposed to pests.

Seeds, nuts, legumes, grains, dried herbs, and dehydrated foods can be stored in jars with a tight cover and kept in a cool, dry, dark place.

Seeds that are good to keep on hand and use regularly include those used for germinating, such as buckwheat, quinoa, chia, and lentils, and those used for sprouting, such as mung bean, sunflower, and alfalfa, and those used dry, such as hemp and millet.

If you grind seeds, grains, or beans, it is good to only grind what you need for the meal you are making so that you protect the nutrients. Some people will soak seeds, grains, and beans for a few hours, then allow them dry for a day, or in a dehydrator, before grinding, and this increases nutrients. A coffee grinder or small grain mill is a helpful tool.

If you are one who isn't totally raw, and you consume simmered soups, remember that you can increase the nutrients in beans by soaking them for a day in water, and even allowing them to germinate for a day after that in a loosely covered container at room temperature (being sure to rinse them at least two times per day), then simmering them at the lowest temperature. Soaking beans before simmering will also decrease the amount of time needed to soften them by simmering – thus, you get more nutrients and save fuel. (Be sure to keep the heat at the lowest temp needed for simmering, and far below the temperature that causes the creation of acrylamides: keep the temperature below 247 degrees

Fahrenheit.) If you use salt, don't add any salt to beans until after they are in the serving bowl.

Seed and bean sprouts and germinates need air. Best to sprout or germinate seeds in containers that allow for airflow, such as a screened wide-mouth jar, or a bowl covered with a cloth. To slow the germinating and sprouting process, keep them in the fridge. To increase the nutrients in sprouts, expose them to sunlight before consuming.

Powders that can be stored for months in jars placed in a cool, dry, dark place include hemp powder (although it is best to freshly grind the seeds), maca powder, mesquite powder, lucuma powder, seaweed powders, green powders, and dehydrated coconut bud sap sugar (if you choose to use a sweetener).

While eating fresh fruits and vegetables is best, dehydrating certain fruits and vegetables is one way to build your long-term food storage, and to prevent fruits and vegetables from going bad if you have too many of them. Also, learn how to make dehydrated vegetable and seed crackers, which, when dehydrated well, can be stored for a few months in tight containers. Tomatoes, corn freshly cut from the cob, grapes, berries, figs, apples, pears, bananas, and even kale are examples of foods that can be dehydrated for long-term storage.

Certain fruits and vegetables can also be frozen. This should be done in the smallest containers possible so that there is little air in the container. If you are going to freeze bananas, they need to be peeled before they are frozen, and stone fruit will need to be cut in half and the pit removed before freezing. A friend showed me that whole strawberries freeze perfectly well in paper bags. I imagine that other fruits and vegetables can also be frozen in paper rather than in plastic. The less plastic we use, the better.

I'm not into canned foods, so those who aren't totally raw are on their own to learn how to can foods in glass jars for long-term storage. There are certain safety measures that should be followed to protect against pathogens. Canning your own home-grown produce is one way to be self-reliant, and to rely less on stores and restaurants for food.

If you want to be more self sufficient, and to be able to use electric kitchen tools without being plugged into the grid that gets its electricity from coal-fired and nuclear power elecricity generators, get a solar electric generating panel and/or rig up a stationary bike so that it can generate electricity. Another option is to get a diesel-powered generator that can also run on vegetable oil.

Storing fruits and vegetables: Getting more life from your greens

By Runi Burton of Australia's LiveFoodEducation.com:

Knowing how to store your food is a very important factor in maximising its nutritional value. Any type of storage results in some deterioration. Produce bought from the store has already begun to lose vitamins, with nutrient losses increasing each day. Wilted produce contains far fewer nutrients than its fresh counterpart, especially Vitamin C content which is partial to rapid decay. While a certain amount of nutrient loss is inevitable, we can minimize it by purchasing the freshest possible produce and storing it under the following optimal conditions:

- Dry and place all leafy greens in airtight containers in the fridge to prevent loss of moisture and vitamins.
- Store cucumbers and eggplant in paper bags in the fridge crisper.
- Refrigerate carrots in bags or containers that allow for air circulation and to protect them against heat and light.
- Place tomatoes in a basket that allows the air to circulate. If you place them in the fridge they will lose their flavour.
- Don't refrigerate any produce that continues to ripen after picking, for example bananas, avocados and stone fruit. These should be stored in a brown paper bag at room temperature until ripe.
- Store citrus fruits at room temperature for several days, alternatively store them in the fridge for up to two months.
- Apples should be refrigerated and it is best to store them away from any vegetables to prevent the vegetables from spoiling.
- Store your vegetables whole. Sliced vegetables exposes the flesh to air and light, which breaks down nutrients.
- Store root vegetables in a dark, cool place.

• COTTON

RANKING just below animal farming as a water intensive industry, including all of the water needed to support the meat industry and to grow food for billions of farmed animals, is cotton farming. Cotton is the most water intensive crop.

The non-organic cotton industry does a lot of damage to the world's water systems. According to the Pesticide Action Network, cotton farming uses 25 percent of the world's insecticides and 10 percent of the world's pesticides. These chemicals poison the land, are troubling for farmers, cause birth deformities and learning disabilities, poison and kill wildlife, contribute to global warming, and pollute streams, rivers, lakes, oceans, and underground water aquifers.

One of the worst environmental disasters was chiefly caused by the cotton industry. In the 1900s, the Soviet Union built canals to take water from the Aral Sea to turn the surrounding desert lands into farmland. The main crop grown on the farmland was cotton. The Aral Sea was once the world's 4th largest inland body of water. As of this writing in

2010, the Aral Sea is now less than 20% the size it was in 1950. Where there was once over 35 feet, or more, of water, there is now desertland. Ships are rusting away on this desert land. Winds often kick up the dust and create huge dust storms. Former fishing village are abandoned, their docks and structured rotting. Fish and other wildlife have died.

The Aral Sea disaster is only one of many tragedies caused by the cotton industry.

When you purchase new cotton fabric, choose organic cotton. Also, consider fabrics that are more sustainable, such as those made of bamboo and hemp. For clothing, consider second-hand shops, and clothing made from reclaimed fabrics.

Co-op America, coopamerica.org/pubs/greenpages
Organic Trade Association, OTA.com
Pesticide Action Network, PANNA.org
Sustainable Cotton, SustainableCotton.org
Vote Hemp, VoteHemp.com

• Blue Jeans

Building Green TV, buildinggreentv.com/keywords/blue-jean-insulation
Cotton From Blue To Green, cottonfrombluetogreen.org/
Green Talk, green-talk.com/2009/01/02/recycle-your-old-blue-jeans/
Planet Green, planetgreen.discovery.com/fashion-beauty/donate-blue-jeans.html

• Bees

A MAJOR threat to honeybees is the various toxic chemicals being used as pesticides. Bees are especially sensitive to these chemical poisons that are used on farms, around homes, on golf courses, and on the property of campuses and other public and private land. Pesticides are chemicals designed to poison living things. When pesticides are spread across farm fields, bees are particularly susceptible to poisoning because bees harvest from the flowers at the tops of plants, where the pesticides settle. When the bees unknowingly carry the poisons back to the hives, more bees, and their larvae, are poisoned, and many die.

When you support organic agriculture, and nongenetically engineered agriculture, you are protecting the bee populations of the world.

Nonstop urban sprawl and industrial agriculture has also damaged bee terrain. Huge amounts of land have been covered by buildings, homes, sidewalks, roads, freeways, and parking lots. This construction along with agriculture has wiped out many of the flowering plants the bees depend on. The situation now exists where the over 4,000 different species of bees (not honeybees) in America are in danger. Similar situations exist for the worldwide bee species that are estimated to be over 30,000. It is important to have a diverse population of bees because some bees will only pollinate certain plants.

Because the wild bee population has been on a dramatic decrease, farmers are depending more on beekeepers to pollinate their plants. Formerly beekeepers used to pay farmers to be able to place their hives in their fields, but now farmers are paying the beekeepers.

The bees kept by the beekeepers are not enough to make up for the loss in the native bee populations. In the 1940s there were an estimated 5 million bee colonies being kept by American beekeepers. By 2004, that figure had decreased by half.

Honeybees aren't the only type of bee needed. Some native bees harvest from plants that honeybees do not. Because of the reduction in wild bee populations farmers increasingly rely on bees brought in from other parts of the world. This bee importing increases the risk of transferring infectious diseases among bee populations. At least one native American bee species, *Bombus occidentalis*, has been devastated by an infection disease brought to North American soil by bees imported from Belgium.

In an attempt to bring back and preserve native bee populations, some farmers plant parts of their fields with native flowering plants.

Because bees are so sensitive to pesticides, nobody knows how long some of the fields sprayed with pesticides will be poisonous to bees. Increased urban and government sprawl will continue to reduce bee habitat.

You can help the bee populations in your region by planting native wildflowers, bushes, and trees, by protecting fields of native weeds, by stopping urban sprawl, and by never using pesticides or other toxic gardening chemicals.

Backyard Hive, BackyardHive.com
Bee Culture Magazine, BeeCulture.com
Bees Wax Co, BeesWaxco.com/HowBeesMakeHoney.htm
Phillip Chandloer, biobees.com. He is the author of *Barefoot Beekeeper.*
Scientific Bee Keeping, ScientificBeeKeeping.com
Vanishing Bees, VanishingBees.com
Wild Flowers, Wild-Flowers.com

• WATER

WE all need clean water to grow our food, feed our bodies, and refresh us.

Many of the world's water sources are so polluted that the life within them is altered.

Streams, rivers, lakes, underground water aquifers, and other sources of water are being depleted by supplying water to golf courses, to farms growing food for the world's billions of farmed animals, for lawns, and for greatly unsustainable industrial practices.

> "Water, like religion and ideology, has the power to move millions of people. Since the very birth of human civilization, people have moved to settle close to it. People move when there is too little of it. People move when there is too much of it. People journey down it. People write, sing and dance about it. People fight over it. And all people, everywhere and every day, need it."
>
> – Mikhail Gorbachev

Please protect water by using only biodegradable, plant-based cleaning products. Also, to protect water, reduce your use of plastics and fossil fuels, follow a plant based diet, grow some of your own food using organic gardening techniques, compost your food scraps into soil to support new plant life, support local organic farmers, and use non-toxic paints and finishes.

> "There is but one ocean though its coves have many names; a single sea of atmosphere with no coves at all; the miracle of soil, alive and giving life, lying thin on the only Earth, for which there is no spare."
>
> – David Brower, first executive director of the Sierra Club; founder of Friends of the Earth; founder of Earth Island Institute; father of the modern environmental movement

Avoid using personal care products that contain these substances that are poisonous to you and to wildlife:

Parabens
Monoethanolamine, diethanolamine, and triethanolamine (MEA, DEA, and TEA)
Formaldehyde
Socium sulfate, amonyl lauryl sulfate, and laureth sulfate
Petroleum jelly
PVA/VA copolymer
Stearolkonium chloride
Synthetic or other coal-tar colors/dyes
Phthalates and synthetic fragrances
Chemical antibacterials
Glyco ether
Phenylenediamine (PPD)

> "On average, only 10% of plastic water bottles are recycled while a whopping 90% are thrown away. In the Unites States alone, Americans consume more than 30 billion - BILLION! - bottles of plastic water bottles per year, spending upwards of $11 billion dollars. Imagine what we could do with $11 billion dollars a year! Just by not buying plastic water bottles! We could fund low-income students to get a college education, we could help build proper homes for people who live in garbage dumps and we could plant trees. We could start a nonprofit that educated Legislation and the US Board of Education why organic, sustainable food is so important and impel these forces to commit to introducing a new,

public food system nationwide! If you would like to learn more, please join the NO MORE PLASTIC BOTTLES, NO MORE PLASTIC BAGS AND NO MORE PAPER CUPS campaign (On FaceBook)."

– Masumi on cafegratitude.com/our-blog/no-more-plastic-bottles.html

American Rivers, AmericanRivers.org
Corporate Accountability Int., StopCorporateAbuse.org
Environmental Justice Coalition for Water, EJCW.org
Find A Spring, FindASpring.com. An interactive site listing places to obtain free natural spring water from the source.
The Greywater Guerillas, SFUAS.org
International Rivers, InternationalRivers.org
Natural Resources Defense Council, NRDC.org
Rainwater Harvesting, RainWaterHarvesting.org
Reef Check, ReefCheck.org
Sierra Club, SierraClub.org/committees/cac/water
Water Keeper Alliance, WaterKeeper.org
World Water Council, WorldWaterCouncil.org

• WATERLIFE

"All of life is interrelated. We are all caught in an inescapable network of mutuality, tied to a single garment of destiny. Whatever affects one directly affects all indirectly."

– Martin Luther King Jr.

EVERY sea mammal and every type of fish, crustacean, and mollusk is on the critical list. So are the seabirds and the bears that depend on fish for their survival. The microscopic animals of the seas are in also trouble. This is because air and industrial pollution is changing the acidity level of the oceans and poisoning sea life; because synthetic farming chemicals and waste from farmed animals are causing massive algae blooms that block light and choke off waterlife; because of fishing, recreational, cruise line, industrial, and military watercraft; and because plastic trash is both killing marine life and gathering in and leaching chemicals into the rivers, lakes, and oceans. To put it mildly, what is going on in the oceans threatens every form of sea life, every form of life dependent on ocean life, and every human on every area of the planet.

Since the middle of the 1800s, the amount of carbon dioxide (CO_2) in the atmosphere has increased in relation to the use of fossil fuels (coal, petroleum, and natural gas). The burning of fossil fuels releases carbon dioxide into the atmosphere. Plants naturally absorb carbon dioxide. But the amount of carbon dioxide being produced by humans is far beyond the amount that could be absorbed by the plants on Earth. The oceans, lakes, and rivers also absorb carbon dioxide. But the world's bodies of water are absorbing far more carbon dioxide than they would in a balanced atmosphere.

The industrial pollution and carbon dioxide from the use of fossil fuels have greatly increased the acidity of the oceans. The oceans of the world are experiencing the worst acid trips ever. Because pollution can hang in the atmosphere for decades, the oceans keep absorbing more of it, and humans keep creating more of it, there are no signs that the acid trip of the seas is going to come down soon.

The increasingly acidic situation of the oceans doesn't damage the marine life only at the surface, but impacts marine life miles below water. Every part of the ocean, from the surface that is increasingly polluted with floating bits of plastic and oil slicks, to the water that is increasing in acidity and in toxic chemicals, to the bottoms of the oceans, which are becoming coated with sediment pollution and pools of chemicals, and to every living thing in and around the oceans, from the coral reefs to fish and sea mammala and sea birds, and also the land animals reliant on the ocean life, is being impacted by how people live, the products they use, and what they do with water, soil, and garbage.

Consider that you play a role in the health of the oceans. Even if you live more than a thousand miles from an ocean, what you do impacts the water that flows into rivers and lakes, and eventually into oceans. The electricity you use may originate from coal-burning electricisy generating plants, which spew pollution into the air. That pollution contains mercury, which ends up in the oceans, poisoning fish and sea mammals, and the birds and animals that feed off of that sea life. Becaue of mercury pollution, every large fish and every mammal that eats the fish contains mercury – which is highly toxic and leads to birth deformities, miscarriages, cancers, learning disorders, and a variety of health problems in humans.

> "History will not only judge us by our mistakes, but by what we do to fix them."
>
> – Jacques Yves Cousteau

The oceans start where you live. It doesn't matter if you live on top of a mountain, or in the meadowlands in the center of a continent. What you do impacts the distant oceans.

The way you live, including the foods you choose to eat, the variety of cleansers you use, the types of medications you take, the type of transportation you use, and the sources of energy you use, impacts the aquafers, rivers, lakes, and oceans around the planet.

Whenever you eat, consider what types of labor, energy, chemicals, packaging, and other resources and products were used to grow and bring that food to your plate.

When you use electricity, consider what types of resources are being used to create the energy.

When you use cleaning products, consider what sorts of chemicals they contain.

When you breathe, consider that the oxygen you depend on is being produced by trees and plants in forests and meadows, and by sea and water plants, thousands of miles away.

When you see water, realize that you and all life on the planet consist mainly of water. If the water bodies of Earth are not healthy, neither is humanity. If life in and around the water bodies of Earth dies, so will humanity.

Books:
The Great Lakes Water Wars, by Peter Annin
Sea of Slaughter, by Farley Mowat
When the Rivers Run Dry: Water – The Defining Crisis of the Twenty-first Century, by Fred Pearce

Documentaries:
Flow, FlowTheFilm.com
Tapped, TappedTheMovie.com

Please watch this free 22-minute documentary produced by the Natural Resources Defense Council: Acid Test: The Global Challenge of Ocean Acidification; nrdc.org/oceans/acidification/aboutthefilm.asp

The documentary is about the rising acidity of the oceans. Everyone should understand the dire consequences of this problem. If you don't understand what burning fossil fuels is doing to the oceans and all life in and around the oceans, this documentary will explain some of it to you. In 2009, scientists estimated that 22 million tons of carbon dioxide is being absorbed into the oceans every day. In the ocean, carbon dioxide turns into acid, and this interfered with all forms of life in and around the oceans. Because of rising acidity, tiny sea creatures are dying, including those that make up coral reefs. One in every four sea creatures lives in, on, or around coral reefs. When the small life forms in the seas die, it impacts food sources of all fish, sea mammals, sea birds, bears, eagles, and other wildlife. If the microscopic sea life dies, we all die. The microscopic sea life is dying. Currently, only 25% of the sea coral in the oceans is left. The rest has died off in the past 100 years. The smallest forms of sea life, including pteropods and krill, are not as abundant as they once were just a few decades ago, and many of them show forms of damage from acidic water that is the result pollutions. These small forms of sea life are food for larger forms of sea life, including whales.

Scientists from many institutions from throughout the world have estimated that the current loss in sea life will lead to a collapse of ocean life before the year 2050.

Other documentaries about sea life:

The End of the Line, EndOfTheLine.com/Film
Pirate of the Sea, PirateForTheSea.com
The Cove, TheCoveMovie.com

To protect the rivers, lakes, and oceans, and all life that depend on them:

1) Drastically reduce your use of fossil fuels, including petroleum, coal, and natural gas.
2) Choose to eat organically grown foods. Work to distance yourself from depending on foods that have been grown using synthetic chemical fertilizers, pesticides, herbicides, insecticides, miticides, and fungicides. Support local organic farmers. Grow some of your own food using organic gardening methods.
3) Eat low on the food chain: Don't eat fish or meat. Follow a plant-based diet that is largely raw.
4) Compost your kitchen scraps. Don't send them to landfills, trash dumps, or incinerators. Get local restaurants, cafes, and food production facilities to do the same.
5) Use household products, including cleaning products that are plant-based and biodegradable. Don't use chlorine bleach, or cleaning products containing petroleum or coal extracts.
6) Reduce your use of plastic. Look for biodegradable plastics that consist of 100% plant substances, such as corn, sugar cane, and soy.
7) When you shop: Use a nonsynthetic cloth bag, not paper or plastic. Make and/or purchase nonsynthetic cloth bags and give them out to your friends, family, neighbors, fellow students, co-workers, and others.
8) Get your local stores and businesses to reduce and eliminate their use of plastics that end up as trash.
9) Plant and protect trees, restore and protect forests, and protect coastal wildlife habitat. Support organizations that do the same.
10) Legalize industrial hemp farming. Hemp and bamboo can provide the materials we commonly depend on trees to provide, including paper and lumber. Unlike trees, hemp and bamboo can also be made into fabric, food, and engine fuel. An acre of either hemp or bamboo absorbs more air pollution than trees, which helps to reverse global warming. Unlike cotton, which is the most fertilized and water-hungry crop, hemp and bamboo grow easily without fertilizer while providing material that creates fabric that is stronger, softer, and lasts longer than cotton. Visit: VoteHemp.com.
11) Reduce pollution. Reduce your use of products that pollute. Recycle.
12) Pedal instead of driving. Support and promote bike culture.
13) Shop less. Stop trying to replicate corporate imagery in your life. Avoid mimicking commercialized celebrity culture.

These organizations work to protect marine and forest life:

Algalita, Algalita.org
Ancient Trees, AncientTrees.org
Blue Voice, BlueVoice.org
Common Vision, CommonVision.org
EarthEcho.org
Earth First, EarthFirst.org

Earth Island, EarthIsland.org
Earth Garden Magazine, POB 2, Trentham, VIC 3458, Australia; earthgarden.com.au. Magazine for sustainable living
Environmental Justice Coalition for Water, EJCW.org
Fishing Hurts, FishingHurts.com
Forest Advocates, ForestAdvocate.org
Forest Council, ForestCouncil.org
Forest Ethics, ForestEthics.org
Forests Forever, ForestsForever.org
Forest Protection Portal, Forests.org
Global Water Policy Project, GlobalWaterPolicy.org
Great Lakes Water Wars, GreatLakesWaterWars.com
GreenPeace, GreenPeace.org
The Greywater Guerillas, SFUAS.org
Harp Seals, HarpSeals.org
International Rivers, InternationalRivers.org
Leatherback Trust, LeatherBack.org
Native Forest, NativeForest.or
Natural Resources Defense Council, NRDC.org
Ocean Alliance, OceanAlliance.org
The Ocean Project, TheOceanProject.org
Oceanic Preservation Society, OPSociety.org
Ocean Protection Coalition, oceanprotection.org
Oil Sands Truth, OilSandsTruth.org
Protect Our Woodland, ProtectOurWoodland.co.uk
Rainforest Action Network, RAN.org
Rainforest Web, RainForestWeb.org
Rainwater Harvesting, RainWaterHarvesting.org
Rainforest Action Network, RAN.org
Reef Resiliance, ReefResilience.org
Rising Tide Australia, RisingTide.org.au
Rising Tide North America, RisingTideNorthAmerica.org
Rising Tide UK, RisingTide.org.uk
Sanctuary Forest, SanctuaryForest.org
Save Japan Dolphins, SaveJapanDolphins.org
Save Oaks, SaveOaks.com
Save the Manatee, SaveTheManatee.org
Save the Redwoods League, SaveTheRedwoods.org
Sea Otters, SeaOtters.org
Sea Turtle, SeaTurtle.org
Sea Shepherd, SeaShepherd.org
Sequoia Forest Keeper, SequoiaForestKeeper.org
Shark Savers, SharkSavers.org
Surfers for Cetaceans, S4CGlobal.org
Tas Forests, TasForests.green.net.au
Tree Muskateers, TreeMusketeers.org
Tree People, TreePeople.org
Trees for Life, TreesForLife.org
Trees for the Future, TreesFTF.org
Trees Foundation, TreesFoundation.org
Water Keeper Alliance, WaterKeeper.org
We Save Trees, WeSaveTrees.org

The Wilderness Society, Wilderness.org
Wildlands CPR, WildlandsCPR.org
World Watch, WorldWatch.org
World Water Council, WorldWaterCouncil.org

"Water is the driving force of all nature."
– Leonardo da Vinci

"It is imperative to maintain portions of the wilderness untouched so that a tree will rot where it falls, a waterfall will pour its curve without generating electricity, a trumpeter swan may float on uncontaminated water – and moderns may at least see what their ancestors knew in their nerves and blood."
– Bernand De Voto, *Fortune*, June 1947

• Environmental Protection

"The future of the Earth is in the balance. It's up to us – who else? There is no one big fix. It involves everything we do, permanently, forever."
– David Attenborough

"There are more factors than climate change that threaten our existence on Earth. Scientists warn that it is only one of nine 'planetary life-support systems' vital for human survival. The other boundaries are: global freshwater use, chemical pollution, ocean acidification, land use change, loss of biodiversity, and the increasing extinction rate, ozone aerosol levels in the atmosphere, and the nitrogen and phosphorus cycles that regulate soil fertility. We've already crossed three of these critical boundaries – climate, the nitrogen cycle, and biodiversity loss. We are close to breaching the boundaries of the rest."
– Seth Sandronsky, *Earth Island Journal* review of the book, *The Ecological Rift: Capitalism's War on the Earth*, by John Bellamy Foster, Brett Clark, and Richard York; Autumn, 2011

A Delicate Balance is an interesting documentary from Aaron Schreibner, POB 183, Kama, NSW, 2533, Australia; info (at) PhoenixPhilms.com. adelicatebalance.com.au

"We abuse land because we regard it as a commodity belonging to us. When we see land as a community to which we belong, we may begin to use it with love and respect."
– Also Leopald

"The moment one gives close attention to anything, even a blade of grass, it becomes a mysterious, awesome, indescribably magnificent world in itself."
– Henry Miller

PLEASE, become involved with at least one of the following organizations and support their projects to protect the environment.

If possible, also donate funds to them.

Byron Environment Center, POB 782, Byron Bay, NSW 2481, Australia; byronenvironmentcentre.asn.au
Earth Day, EarthDay.net
Earth First, EarthFirst.org
Earth Garden Magazine, POB 2, Trentham, VIC 3458, Australia; earthgarden.com.au.
Earth Island Institute, EarthIsland.org
Global Green, GlobalGreen.org
Green Power, China; GreenPower.org.hk/gp/e_main.asp
Greens, Greens.org.au. Australian environmentalists
Kyoto USA, KyotoUSA.org
Natural Resources Defense Council. NRDC.org
The Nature Conservancy, nature.org
Oil Sants Truth, OilSandsTruth.org
Rising Tide Australia, RisingTide.org.au
Rising Tide North America, RisingTideNorthAmerica.org
Rising Tide UK, risingtide.org.uk
We Can Solve It, WeCanSolveIt.org
The Wilderness Society, Wilderness.org
Wildlands CPR, WildlandsCPR.org
Wildlands Project, Wild-Earth.org
World Watch, WorldWatch.org

"What you people call your natural resources, we call our relatives."
– Oren Lyons Faith keeper of the Onondaga

• CLIMATE CHANGE

"Corporations have given us the climate chaos that we are seeing threatening life at all kinds of levels."
– Vandana Shiva, author of *Soil Not Oil*

Campaign Against Climate Change, CampaignCC.org
Center for Alternative Technology, cat.org.uk
The City Repair Project, CityRepair.org
Climate Challenge, ClimateChallenge.org
Culture Change, CultureChange.org
Climate Change News, ClimateChangeNews.org
Climate Crisis, ClimateCrisis.net
Community Solution, CommunitySolution.org
Cool Mayors, CoolMayors.org
Environmental Media Association, EMA-Online.org
Fight Global Warming, FightGlobalWarming.com
Global Green, GlobalGreen.org
Greenpeace, GreenPeace.org
Mayors for Climate Protection, CoolMayors.org
Oil Sands Truth, OilSandsTruth.org
Redefining Progress, RProgress.org
Union of Concerned Scientists, UCSUSA.org
We Cam Solve It, WeCanSolveIt.org
World Watch Institute, WorldWatch.org

• Bike Culture

SUPPORT bike culture. Get a bike. Don't drive when you can ride a bike or walk instead.

"Get a bicycle. You will not regret it."
– Mark Twain

"Every time I see an adult on a bicycle, I no longer despair for the future of the human race."
– H. G. Wells

"A human body and a bicycle are the perfect synthesis of body and machine."
– Richard Ballantine

"It is curious that with the advent of the automobile and the airplane, the bicycle is still with us. Perhaps people like the world they can see from a bike, or the air they breathe when they're out on a bike. Or they like the bicycle's simplicity and the precision with which it is made. Or because they like the feeling of being able to hurtle through air one minute, and saunter through a park the next, without leaving behind clouds of choking exhaust, without leaving behind so much as a footstep.
– Gurdon S. Leete

"The bicycle is the most civilized conveyance known to man. Other forms of transport grow daily more nightmarish. Only the bicycle remains pure in heart."
– Iris Murdoch

"The bicycle is just as good company as most husbands and, when it gets old and shabby, a woman can dispose of it and get a new one without shocking the entire community."
– Ann Strong

"Let me tell you what I think of bicycling. I think it has done more to emancipate woman than anything else in the world. It gives women a feeling of freedom and self-reliance. I stand and rejoice every time I see a woman ride by on a wheel. The picture of free, untrammeled womanhood."
– Susan B. Anthony

"It is by riding a bicycle that you learn the contours of a country best, since you have to sweat up the hills and coast down them. Thus you remember them as they actually are, while in a motor car only a high hill impresses you, and you have no such accurate remembrance of country you have driven through as you gain by riding a bicycle."
– Ernest Hemmingway

"The bicycle had, and still has, a humane, almost classical moderation in the kind of pleasure it offers. It is the kind of machine that a Hellenistic Greek might have invented and ridden. It does no violence to our normal reactions: It does not pretend to free us from our normal environment."

– J.B. Jackson

"Nothing compares to the simple pleasure of a bike ride."

– John F. Kennedy

IF you ride a bike, please **have lights and reflectors on your bike**, including a rear red light, and a front white light. In addition to lights, install side, front, and rear reflectors. And, **wear a helmet**! Also, simple **biker gloves** will protect the hands. Obey traffic laws. Don't wear headphones that block sounds that you need to hear for safety while riding. Put a bell on your handle bars. Ringing the handle bar bell an easy way to let people know you are approaching. **Ride safe**.

"Think of bicycles as rideable art that can just about save the world."

– Grant Peterson

Books:
Cycling for Profit: How to make a living with your bike, by Jim Gregory
Pedaling Revolution: How cyclists are changing American cities, by Jeff Mapes

Bamboo Bike Maker, bamboobikemaker.com
Bamboosero, bamboosero.com. Bamboo bikes made in Africa.
Bicycle Civil Liberties Union, BCLU.org
Bicycle Paper, BicyclePaper.com. Seattle, Washington
Bicycle Safe, BicycleSafe.com
Bicycle Transportation Alliance, BTA4Bikes.org
Bicycling Info, BicyclingInfo.org/pp/exemplary.htm
Bicycology, Bicycology.org.uk
Bike Blips, Bikeblips.dailyreader.com
Bike Boom: BikeBoom.com
Bike Cart, bikecart.pedalpeople.com
Bike 4 Peace, Bike4Peace.org
BikeRoWave, BikeRoWave.org
Bike School, BikeSchool.com
Bikes at Work, 129 Washington Ave., Ames, IA 50010; bikesatwork.com. Sells bike trailers that can be used for hauling or transporting. They also provide information on starting a bike-based business: bikesatwork.com/cycling-for-profit
Bikes Not Bombs, BikesNotBombs.org
Bike Oven, 3706 N. Figueroa St., Los Angeles, CA 90065; bikeoven.com. A bike co-op workshop and repair shop.
Bike Trailer Shop, biketrailershop.com
Bike Trax, Biketrax.co.uk
Bike Trip, BikeTrip.org
Boneshaker Magazine, BoneShakerMag.com
Busch + Muller, bumm.de. Bike lights.
Car Free, CarFree.com/link/fpor.html

Christiania Bikes, christianiabikes.com
Climate Cycle, Chicago, IL; ClimateCycle.org
CrimAnimalz, CrimAnimalz.com
Critical Mass, Critical-Mass.info
Culture Change, CultureChange.org
Cycling News, CyclingNews.com. Australian racing bike news
Cyclists Inciting Change Thru Life Exchange, CICLE.org
David Hembrow English delivery bike baskets, Hembrow.eu/delivery
The Dog Trike, oaktreevet.co.uk/trike/trike.htm
European Cyclists Federation, ecf.com
Flying Pigeon LA, 3714 N. Figueroa St., Los Angeles, CA 90042; flyingpigeon-la.com
Free Wheelin Farm, Santa Cruz, CA; freewheelinfarm.com/home.html. An organic farm run by bicyclists who even deliver produce to local restaurants by bike.
Henry Work Cycles, workcycles.com/workbike
International Federatioin of Bike Messenger Associations. messengers.org.
International Human Powered Vehicle Association, ihpva.org
Kinetics, kinetics.org.uk. Folding bikes.
League of American Bicyclists, BikeLeague.org
Midnight Ridazz, MidnightRidazz.com
Organic Engines, organicengines.com/
Pedal People, Northampton, MA, pedalpeople.com. A human-powered delivering and hauling service.
Rickshaw Forum, rickshawforum.com
Ride A Cycle, RideACycle.org
San Diego County Bicycling Coalition, San Diego, California; SDCBC.org
Shifting Gears, ShiftingGearsCycling.com. Santa Monica, CA
Stolen Bike Registry, stolenbicycleregistry.com
Ten Links, TenLinks.com/cycling/portals.htm
Velo News, VeloNews.com. Boulder, Colorado
VeloVision Magazine, VeloVision.co.uk
Workbike, zerocouriers.com/workbike. Great source of information about bike-based business, bike trailers, and bike messenger services.
Workbike mailing list, ihpva.org/mailman/listinfo/workbike
Wrench Science, WrenchScience.com. For bicycle parts

• CONVERTING CARS

IN 2007, the U.S. used about 7.6 billion barrels of petroleum, the petroleum industry experienced record profits, and the U.S. government gave $18 billion worth of tax credits to petroleum companies.

If you choose to drive a car or truck, please convert it to run on ethanol or used veggie oil from restaurants. Establish biofuel stations.

Learn about the damage being done to rainforests to supply the world with biofuels. The expanding palm oil industry is doing much harm to the rainforests of Borneo and leading the orangutan to extinction in the wild. Much of the forests are being burned down. The palm oil produced from the growing oil palm plantations is being sold into the world biofuel market.

Become aware of the obscene damage being done to Canada's forests to extract tar sands. First, roads are being built into pristine forests. Then, thousands of acres of trees are cut down. Open pit and strip mining then takes place, leaving behind trashed landscapes, destroyed wildlife habitat, and poisoned rivers, bogs, ponds, lakes, and aquifers. Seventy-five percent of the oil from Alberta's tar sands mining is used by the United States, including for airplanes, fleet trucks, and other vehicles.

Even though it can be used to produce oil for diesel engines and ethanol for gas engines, hemp is a plant that remains illegal in the U.S. Hemp provides more oil per acre than corn, soy, or oil palm. And it does so with less water, and it does so without the use of pesticides, insecticides, fungicides, miticides, or fertilizers. Work to legalize industrial hemp. Access VoteHemp.com.

> "In the old-growth forest of Canada's Alberta Province, a sprawling network of bogs, lakes, and rivers provides a pristine breeding ground for millions of North America's songbirds and waterfowl. Lynx and caribou roam undisturbed among the forest's dense stands of aspen and poplar. But in recent years, soaring demand for oil has driven energy companies to strip bars thousands of acres of this thriving wildlife habitat to produce fuel from buried tar sands – an immensely polluting and energy-intensive process even by oil industry standards.
>
> … Driven by skyrocketing U.S. demand, the tar sands rush has spawned a rapidly expanding web of pipelines, roads, and wells that threatens to destroy and fragment more than 55,000 square miles of boreal forest habitat – and area the size of Florida.
>
> … The staggering environmental impact of this dirty fuel boom extends well beyond the boreal forest. The massive amount of energy needed to extract, upgrade, and refine tar sands oil generates three times the amount of global warming pollution as conventional oil production. In fact, global warming pollution related to tar sands development is projected to quadruple from 25 megatons in 2003 to as much as 126 megatons in 2015, the equivalent of putting 15 million new cars on the road. Even now, tar sands extraction is largely responsible for Alberta's rising levels of air pollution and is Canada's fastest growing source of global warming pollution. Most Americans are unaware that fully 8 percent of our oil supply already comes from Alberta's tar sands – at an unacceptable cost to our continent's boreal forests."
>
> – The Natural Resources Defense Council, nrdc.org; SaveBiogems.or/birds

Berkeley Biodiesel Collective, BerkeleyBiodiesel.org
Biodiesel America, BioDieselAmerica.org

Biodiesel Community, BioDieselCommunity.org
Biodiesel Co-op, BioDiesel-CoOp.org
Biodiesel Now, BiodieselNow.com. Site contains a link to locations where biofuel is available.
Biodiesel, BioDiesel.org
Biodiesel Solutions, BioDieselSolutions.com
Biofuel Oasis, BioFuelOasis.com
Climate Crisis, ClimateCrisis.net
Coalition for Clean Air, CoalitionForCleanAir.org
End of Suburbia, EndOfSuburbia.com
Golden Fuel Systems, GoldenFuelSystems.com
Grease Care, GreaseCar.com
Hemp Car, HempCar.org
Journey To Forever, JourneyToForever.org
Live Green Go Yellow, LiveGreenGoYellow.com
Lovecraft Biofuels, LoveCraftBioFuels.com
Make Biodiesel, MakeBioDiesel.com
Mayors for Climate Change, 436 14th St., Ste. 1520, Oakland, CA 94612; CoolMayors.org
Oil Sands Truth, OilSandsTruth.org
Piedmont Biofuels, Pittsboro, NC; Biofuels.coop.
Path to Freedom, PathToFreedom.com
Stop Global Warming, StopGlobalWarming.org
Sustainable Options, SustainableOptions.com
Sustainable Transport Club, SustainableTransportClub.com
Tellurian Biodiesel, tellurianbiodiesel.com/lasf
Terra Pass, TerraPass.com
Veggie Power, VeggiePower.co.uk
Vote Hemp, VoteHemp.com
Yokayo Biofuels, YBiofuels.org

• Nuclear Energy = War Industry

"Environmentalists have long been fond of saying that the sun is the only safe nuclear reactor, situated as it is some ninety-three million miles away."

– Stephanie Mills, ed., *In Praise of Nature*, 1990

"In 1942 Enrico Fermi led a team of scientists at the University of Chicago in creating the world's first man made nuclear reactor, Chicago Pile 1, and first self-sustaining nuclear chain reaction, nuclear fission. This experiment took place on a squash court underneath the bleachers of the original Alonzo Stagg Field Stadium at the University of Chicago. Heralded as one of the world's foremost scientific achievements, this scientific breakthrough lead to the manhattan project and the unleashing of a Nuclear age of weaponry married to the production of nuclear energy that has defined man's most threatening and destructive scientific discovery to date."

– Dr. Helen Caldicott, NuclearFreePlanet.org

THERE is no such thing as a nuclear power plant that does not leak. They all leak some level of radiation. There is also no international monitoring organizatioin that monitors how much radiation is leaking from the various nuclear power plants that are now built in many different countries.

There is an inextricable link between the nuclear power industry and the nuclear bomb industry.

Don't believe the propaganda put out by the nuclear power industry claiming that nuclear energy is clean energy that is environmentally safe.

There are many extremely problematic sides to the nuclear power industry. But you won't hear about them from the propaganda spewed by the Nuclear Energy Institute. The institute has set up the "Clean and Safe Energy Coalition," which spends multiple millions of dollars on publicity campaigns meant to make nuclear energy look safe and wonderful.

To create nuclear energy uranium has to be mined, which leaves behind highly toxic and radioactive waste on the destroyed land that causes birth defects, cancers, and miscarriages in humans and wildlife. The nuclear power plants create massive amounts of radioactive waste, which remains toxic for many thousands of years. The power plants are not safe in the long term, and they pose an ongoing target for disaster.

Nuclear energy is not cheap, is not green, is not environmentally safe, is not sustainable, and is not good.

The U.S. government has given hundreds of billions of dollars to the nuclear power industry, and the industry wants more. In fact, the nuclear industry could not exist in the U.S. without billion dollar subsidies in loan guarantees, production tax credits, construction insurance, and direct cash infusion into the accounts of companies involved in building and running nuclear plants.

Billionaire investor Warren Buffet's company, MidAmerican Nuclear Energy Company, abandoned plans to build a nuclear power plant in Idaho after the company analysts concluded that the plant would never stop operating in the red.

The 104 operating nuclear power plants in the U.S. supply 19 percent of the nation's electricity. They are decades old, and the older they get the more dangers they pose. The technology used to build them is outdated, the structures are weakening, and the companies that run them are trying to get as much out of them as possible before the plants have to be decommissioned.

In 2006, one of the cooling towers at the Vermont Yankee Nuclear Plant simply crumbled to the ground. In 2002, Ohio's David-Besse

Nuclear Plant was shut down when a basketball-sized corrosion hole was found in the steel cap of the reactor.

The book, *We Almost Lost Detroit*, tells the story of a partial fuel meltdown at a nuclear power plant in 1975.

All of the nuclear power plants are continuing to create nuclear waste that will remain "hot" for over 10,000 years – yes, that's *ten thousand* years. At any time during at least 10,000 years, if any of the fuel rods are exposed to air for more than several hours, they spontaneously combust, spreading extremely toxic radioactive isotopes throughout a region of the planet. That would bring death, cancer, birth deformities, and miscarriages to humans and wildlife. What are we leaving for our future generations? Or, have we already caused their demise?

The government has been trying to build a nuclear waste storage facility in Yucca Mountain, Nevada. 2008 estimates, before cost overruns, to research, build, and run the facility for 100 years range in the area of 100 billion dollars. There is no agreement of how much waste would need to be stored there, or what the size of the facility should be – which indicates that they do not know how much it would cost.

Currently all of the nuclear waste at each nuclear power plant is stored on-site at the nuclear power plants, in "spent fuel pools." If any of these were to malfunction, it would be more disastrous than the meltdown of a nuclear reactor. The Nuclear Regulatory Commission's "Report on Spent Fuel Pool Accident Risk" (NUREG-1738) states that a fire in a spent fuel tank could cause 25,000 fatalities within 500 miles of the fire. What could cause such a fire? Some of the causes could be a plane crash, missile strike, or natural disaster. Does this pose a threat to you? Find out where the nuclear plants are near where you live, locate them on a map, and draw a 500-mile circle around each one.

In 2001, four duck hunters nearly caused a nuclear catastrophe at a nuclear power plant in Maine. The hunters were not aware that lead pellets from their guns were hitting one of the cooling pools where the spent nuclear rods are stored.

The construction of the plants takes tremendous resources, including concrete, steel, fuel, land, and water. Any plant that is built and begins operating remains as an environmental hotspot and potential disaster site that could require the permanent evacuation of surrounding communities.

There is a direct correlation between the nuclear energy industry and the nuclear bomb industry. Spent nuclear fuel rods have been, and are being, used to make weapons-grade plutonium and enriched uranium. The U.S., Japan, Russia, France, and other countries that have nuclear power plants have used their nuclear waste to build atomic arsenals.

Many of the bombs dropped in Iraq contained depleted uranium, a product of nuclear energy plants. The bomb residues have caused rates of cancer, miscarriages, and birth deformities to skyrocket among the people exposed to the residues.

Learn more about the dangers of nuclear energy. Start by considering what happened with the 1975 reactor fire at Browns Ferry, Alabama; and the 1979 meltdown at Three Mile Island in Western Pennsylvania. Consider the horrors of the 1986 Chernobyl disaster that required the immediate abandonment of hundreds of towns and villages that now sit rotting.

There are nuclear power plants near many large cities, such as New York City. Imagine if a Chernobyl disaster happened near New York City, and the entire zone had to be immediately and permanently evacuated and abandoned. To where would more than 20 million New York-area residents permanently move?

Say NO to nukes.

> "Once-through cooling technology is used exclusively in 48 nuclear reactors with 11 additional reactors employing the technology in conjunction with cooling towers and canals. These reactors, situated on coastal waters, major rivers, and lakes can draw in as much as a billion gallons of water per reactor unit a day, nearly a million gallons a minute, in order to dissipate the extraordinary amounts of waste heat generated in the fission process.
>
> The initial devastation of marine life and ecosystems stems from the powerful intake of water into the nuclear reactor. Marine life, ranging from endangered sea turtles and manatees down to delicate fish larvae and microscopic planktonic organisms vital to the ocean ecosystem, is sucked irresistibly into the reactor cooling system, a process known as entrainment."
>
> – Nuclear Information and Resource Service, NIRS.org

> "The average two-reactor nuclear power plant is estimated to cost $10 billion to $18 billion to build. That's before cost overruns, and no U.S. nuclear power plant has ever been delivered on time or on budget… The sputtering decline of nuclear power has been one of the greatest industrial failures of modern times. In 1985 *Forbes* called the nuke industry 'the largest managerial disaster in history.'"
>
> – Christian Parenti, "What Nuclear Renaissance," *The Nation*; May 12, 2008; TheNation.com

The Committtee to Bridge the Gap, CommitteeToBridgeTheGap.org
Mothers for Peace, MothersForPeace.org
Natural Resources Defense Council, NRDC.org
New England Coalition on Nuclear Pollution, NECNP.org
Nuclear Information and Resource Center, NIRS.org
Nuke Watch, NukeWatch.com

Physicians for Social Responsibility, PSR.org
Public Citizen's Critical Mass Energy Program, Citizen.org
Redwood Alliance, RedwoodAlliance.org
Shundahai Network, Shundahai.org
Sierra Club, SierraClub.org/nuclearwaste
Union of Concerned Scientists, UCSUSA.org
Waging Peace, WagingPeace.org

• PEACE

> "War against a foreign country only happens when the moneyed classes think they are going to profit from it."
> – George Orwell

> "If you wish to experience peace, provide peace for another."
> – Tenzin Gyatso

DURING 2010 the U.S. was spending approximately $500 million per day on the wars in Iraq and Afghanistan, which had been carrying on for several years. The wars also have largely been conducted to secure interest in "natural resources," such as minerals and petroleum. At the same time, various branches of federal, state, and local governments were cutting funding to such things as environmental protection, school funding, welfare, unemployment compensation, healthcare, alternative energy development, and the construction of inner-city rail transportation systems.

With $500 million per day spent over several years, the U.S. could have transformed the U.S. to be more sustainable, environmentally friendly, and less dependable on fossil fuels. Instead, that money was being poured into endless war, including supporting and expanding military bases where tens of thousands of U.S. government employees lived and worked to assist the "war effort" (petroleum and mineral protection access effort).

An immediate cost of war is not just the day-to-day operations of the war, but what the wars leave behind, as in demolished lives, damaged people, and a ruined environment. In modern-day-warfare, the costs of wars include radiation left over from bombs made of depleted uranium from nuclear energy facilities, and that radiation remains in the environment – causing cancers, birth defects, and miscarriages in people and wildlife for many years to come.

> "Man is the only animal that deals in that atrocity of atrocities, war. He is the only one that gathers his brethren about him and goes forth in cold blood and calm pulse to exterminate his kind. He is the only animal that for sordid wages will march out – and help to slaughter strangers of his own species who have done him no harm and with whom he has no quarrel. And in the intervals between

campaigns he washes the blood off his hands and works for 'the universal brotherhood of man.'"

– Mark Twain

"To please their kings, they've all gone out to war, and not a one of them knows what they're fighting for."

– Irving Berlin

"A cost of war is not just guns and ammunition and tanks and airplanes. A cost of war is taking care of veterans and also taking care of the deceased service members widows, widowers, and orphans."

– Senator Bill Nelson, D-Florida, 2011

"Can anything be stupider than that a man has the right to kill me because he lives on the other side of a river and his ruler has a quarrel with mine, though I have not quarreled with him?"

– Blaise Pascal

"If we have no peace, it is because we have forgotten that we belong to each other."

– Mother Teresa

"If we all do one random act of kindness daily, we just might set the world in the right direction."

– Martin Kornfeld

Brave New Foundation, BraveNewFoundation.org
Central Committee for Conscientious Objectors, Objector.org
Code Pink, CodePink4Peace.org
Cursor, Cursor.org
Iraq Veterans Against the War, IVAW.org
The National Network Opposing Militarization of Youth, NNOMY.org
National Youth and Student Peace Coalition, NYSPC.org
Veterans for Peace, VeteransForPeace.org
Voices for Creative Nonviolence, vcnv.org
Voters for Peace, VotersForPeace.org
War Resisters, WarResisters.org

"Never do anything against conscience, even if the state demands it."

– Albert Einstein

"What can you do to promote world peace? Go home and love your family."

– Mother Theresa

• Drug War: End It!

Book:
Marijuana & Hemp: History, Uses, Laws, and Controversy, by John McCabe

Ducumentary:
War on Drugs: The Prison Industrial Complex, see this documentary for free on the website: FreeDocumentaries.org

The American Civil Liberties Union, ACLU.org
Australian Cannabis Law Reform Movement, NimbinAustralia.com.Cyber-Pod.com/ACLRM
ChangeTheClimate.org
Common Sense for Drug Policy, CSDP.org
The Drug Reform Coordination Network, DRCNet.org; StopTheDrugWar.org
DrugScope.org.uk
Drug Truth Network, DrugTruth.net
DrugWarDistortions.org
DrugWarFacts.org
Educators for Sensible Drug Policy, EFSP.org
End Prohibition, Canada; EndProhibition.ca
Families Against Mandatory Minimums, FAMM.org
Human Rights and the Drug War, HR95.org
Judges Against the Drug War, JudgesAgainstTheDrugWar.org
Law Enforcement Against Prohibition, LEAP.CC
The Media Awareness Project, MAPInc.org
National Organization for the Reform of Marijuana Laws, NORML.org
The November Coalition, November.org/razorwire
Students for Sensible Drug Policy, SSDP.org
Veterans for More Effective Drug Strategies, VetsForMeds.org

• Raw Magazines

Comunidad Cruda, a community in Balta produces a magazine
Funky Raw Magazine, funkyraw.com; magazine (at) funkyraw.com
Pear Magazine Online, PearMagazine.com
Raw Foods News Magazine, RawFoodsNewsMagazine.com. Judy Pokras
Super Raw Life Magazine, Utah, U.S.A.; SuperRawLife.com
Vegan Views, Longridge, Bankend Rd, Dumfries, DG1 4TP. UK; veganviews.org.uk. Random quarterly magazine produced in England.
Vegan Voice, Australia; Veganic.net. Stopped publication 2011.
Vegetarian Journal, Baltimore, MD. VRG.Org/Journal. Published by the Vegetarian Resource Group, this magazine covers a variety of issues of interest to those who are following a plant-based diet. Some articles specifically cover topics of interest to raw foodists.
VegNews Magazone, San Francisco, CA; VegNews.com. Not a raw magazine, but it includes information about raw food. This magazine wouldn't mention John McCabe's book, *Sunfood Living: Resource Guide for Global Health*, because, as the editor said, "it mentions honey." She said the magazine is against the enslavement of bees. How much food does she eat that is the result of bees from managed hives pollinating the flowers? Perhaps she should consider that most of the food she eats originates of farms using managed hives, or, as she put it, "enslaved bees." Some of the restaurants advertising in the magazine are not vegan, and the magazine also was found to be using photographs of real meat and presenting the photos as if they were of a vegetarian meal. Yet, they won't mention McCabe's books simply because his books mention honey.
Veggie Vision Internet TV, c/o MAD Promotions, Independent House, Radford Business Centre, Radford Way, Billericay, Essex CM12 0BZ; VeggieVision.co.uk. An England-based vegetarian Web-based mag that includes some raw food information.
Vibrance Magazine (formerly: Living Nutrition Magazine); vibrancemagazine.net; livingnutrition.com. Email: Letters (a) PurelyDelicious.net. Anna Sinclair Tipps, publisher, Anna (at) purelydelicious.net

• Publications for Awareness

"Basically, we should stop doing those things that are destructive to the environment, other creatures, and ourselves, and figure out new ways of existing."

– Moby

"It is horrifying that we have to fight our own government to save the environment."

– Ansel Adams

100 Fires, 100Fires.com.

Clamor **Magazine**, POB 1225, Bowling Green, OH 43402; ClamorMagazine.org

Earth First! Journal, POB 3023, Tucson, AZ 85702; EarthFirstJournal.org

Earth Garden Magazine, POB 2, Trentham, VIC 3458, Australia; earthgarden.com.au. Magazine for sustainable living

Earth Island Journal, 300 Broadway, Ste. 28, San Francisco, CA 94133; EarthIsland.org

Earth Light **magazine,** 111 Fairmount Ave., Oakland, CA 94611, USA; EarthLight.org

Eco Logic Books, Eco-LogicBooks.com. England

E the Environmental Magazine, 28 Knight St., Norwalk, CT 06851; POB 5098, Westport, CT 06881; EMagazine.com

Funky Raw Magazine, London, England. funkyraw.com.

Get Fresh, Unit 4, Aylsham Business Park, Shepheards Close, Aylsham, Norwich, Norfolk, NR11 6SZ, UK; Fresh-Network.com. Available in PDF or print version.

Green Teacher **magazine,** Canada: Green Teacher, 95 Robert St., Toronto, ON M5S 2K5; United States: Green Teacher, POB 452, Niagara Falls, NY 14304-0452; GreenTeacher.com

Hope Dance, POB 15609, San Luis Obispo, CA 93406; HopeDance.org

Impact Press, ImpactPress.com

Lantern Books, LanternBooks.com

Mother Earth News, MotherEarthNews.com

Mother Jones **magazine**, POB 334, Mt. Morris, IL 61054; MotherJones.com

Natural Home Magazine, NaturalHomeMagazine.com

Orion, The Orion Society and Myrin Institute, 187 Main St., Great Barrington, MA 01230; OrionSociety.org

Permaculture Activist, POB 5516, Bloomington, IN 47407; PermacultureActivist.net

Permaculture **magazine: Solutions for Sustainable Living**, PermaCulture.co.uk

Pear Magazine **Online**, PearMagazine.com

Revolution Books, SeattleRevolutionBooks.BlogSpot.com

The Sun, POB 469061, Escondido, CA 92046; TheSunMagazine.org

Terrain, Northern California's Environmental Quarterly, 2530 San Pablo Ave., Berkeley, CA 94702; EcologyCenter.org

Threshold, Student Environmental Action Coalition, POB 31909, Philadelphia, PA 19104; SEAC.org

The Trumpeter: **Journal of Ecosophy**, C/O Athabasca University, 1 University Dr., Athabasca, AB T9S 3A3, Canada; TheTrumpeter.athabascau.ca

Utne **reader**, 1624 Harmon Pl., Minneapolis, MN 55403; Utne.com

Vegan Voice **magazine**, POB 30 Mimbin, NSW, 2480, Australia; Veganic.net

Vibrance: Living Nutrition **magazine,** LivingNutrition.com

Whole Life Times Magazine, Los Angeles, CA; WholeLifeMagazine.com. Monthly free publication in California that is also available online.

Wild Earth, POB 455, Richmond, VT 05477; Wild-Earth.org

Z **magazine**, 18 Millfield St., Woods Hole, MA 02543; ZMag.org.

• Activist Directories

"If you are neutral in situations of injustice, you have chosen the side of the oppressor."

– Desmond Tutu

"You must be the change you wish to see in the world."

– Mahatma Gandhi

"People get offended by animal rights campaigns. It's ludicrous. It's not as bad as mass animal death in a factory."

– Richard Gere

"We must educate the public. The average person has no idea of what's going on in factory farms, in laboratories, circuses, roadside zoos, or rodeos."

– Bob Barker

"Revolution is not something fixed in ideology, nor is it something fashioned to a particular decade. It is a perpetual process embedded in the human spirit."

– Abbie Hoffman

"The penalty good people pay for not being interested in politics is to be governed by people worse than themselves."

– Plato

"I am only one, but I am still one. I cannot do everything, but I can do something."

– Helen Keller

"We must use time creatively, and forever realize that the time is always ripe to do right."

– Martin Luther King, Jr.

"Politics is democracy's way of handling public business. We won't get the type of country in the kind of world we want unless people take part in the public's business."

– David Brower, first executive director of the Sierra Club; founder of Friends of the Earth; founder of Earth Island Institute; father of the modern environmental movement

"Activism is getting off your ass and working to try to better something that really bothers you. Something that you know is undoubtedly unfair, corrupt, unjustifiable, or simply wrong. It's being a strong voice for a cause and taking action into your own hands – not assuming that others will do it for you. It's being a missionary – spreading your message no matter how others might judge you or how uncomfortable and alienated you may feel doing it. It's being righteous."

– Jenny Brown, co-founder of Woodstock Farm Animal Sanctuary, WoodstockSantuary.Org; WoodstockFAS.Org; as quoted in *Herbavore* magazine, Fall 2006

"It is one of the most beautiful compensations of this life that no one can sincerely try to help another without helping himself."

– Ralph Waldo Emerson

"Nothing that I can do will change the structure of the universe. But maybe, by raising my voice I can help the greatest of all causes - goodwill among men and peace on earth."

– Albert Einstein

"Corporations are not concerned with the common good. They exploit, pollute, impoverish, repress, kill, and lie to make money. They throw poor people out of homes, let the uninsured die, wage useless wars for profit, poison and pollute the ecosystem, slash social assistance programs, gut public education, trash the global economy, plunder the U.S. Treasury and crush all popular movements that seek justice for working men and women. They worship money and power."

– Chris Hedges

"This country, with its institutions, belongs to the people who inhabit it. Whenever they shall grow weary of the existing government, they can exercise their constitutional right of amending it, or their revolutionary right to dismember or overthrow it."

– Abraham Lincoln, First Inaugural Address

Adbusters, 1243 W. 7th Ave., Vancouver, BC, V6H 1B7, Canada; AdBusters.Org

Albion Monitor, AlbionMonitor.Com. Alternative newspaper on the Internet.

Animal Rights Action Network, Kildare, Ireland; ARAN.Ie

Animal Rights Canada, AnimalRightsCanada.Com

Animals Australia, North Melbourne, Victoria, Australia; AnimalsAustralia.Org

The Artivist Collective, Artivist.Org. International activist film festival held every year in Los Angeles.

Center for the New American Dream, NewDream.Org

Civic Media Center, CivicMediaCenter.Org

Compact, SFCompact.BlogSpot.Com. Perhaps best described as an anti-shopping group.

DawnWatch, dawnwatch.com. Karen Dawn became involved in the animal rights movement after reading Peter Singer's book *Animal Liberation.*

Deep Ecology Index, Home.C2I.Net/DEI. DEI is an index of deep ecology resources.

Dropping Knowledge, DroppingKnowledge.org

Earth First! Journal**,** EarthFirstJournal.org. The *Earth First! Journal* publishes a directory of environmental activist organizations, organizers, and associations.

Eco-Action, Eco-Action.Org; Eco-Action.Net

The Environment Directory, WebDirectory.com

Fairness and Accuracy in Reporting, FAIR.org

Global Action Network, Montreal, Canada; GAN.CA

Good Green Witch, GoodGreenwitch.blogspot.com. Rhonda De Felice is an environmental and sustainable living activist and educator.

The Green Pages, TheGreenPages.CA.
Greenpeace International, Greenpeace.Org/International
Green Volunteers, GreenVolunteers.Org
Philadelphia Independent Media Center, phillyimc.org.
Mindfully, Mindfully.Org
The National Environmental Directory, EnvironmentalDirectory.Net.
Neighborhoods Online, NeighborhoodsOnline.Net
Northwest Earth Institute, 317 SW Alder, Ste. 1050, Portland, OR 97204; NWEI.Org
Old Dog Documentaries, OldDogDocumentaries.Com
Oxygen Collective, POB, 533, Ashland, OR 97520; O2Collective.Org
Pacifica Radio, Pacifica.Org
Portland Independent Media Center, Portland.IndyMedia.Org
Protest.Net, protest.net
Radio 4 All, Radio4All.Org.
Radio-Locator, radio-locator.Com
Resist, Inc., ResistInc.Org
Robin Wood, RobinWood.DE. European environmental concerns.
Rocky Mountain Peace and Justice Center, POB 1156, Boulder, CO 80306; RMPJC.Org
Take Part, TakePart.com
Vermont Law School's Environmental Law Center, POB 96, Chelsea St., South Royalton, VT 05068; VermontLaw.Edu

• Hunger and Homelessness

"Credit crunch? The real crisis is global hunger. And if you care, eat less meat: A food recession is under way. Biofuels are a crime against humanity, but – take it from a flesh eater – flesh eating is worse… While 100m tonnes of food will be diverted this year to feed cars, 760m tonnes will be snatched from the mouths of humans to feed animals – which could cover the global food deficit 14 times. If you care about hunger, eat less meat."

– Journalist George Monbiot, London's *Guardian*, April 15, 2008

"True compassion is more than flinging a coin to a beggar; it comes to see that an edifice which produces beggars needs restructuring."

– Martin Luther King, Jr.

"Even if it's a little thing, do something for those who have need of a man's help, something for which you get no pay but the pivilege of doing it. For, remember, you don't live in a world all your own. Your brothers are here too."

– Albert Schweitzer

"Great indeed is the power acquired through austerity to endure hunger. But greater still is the power of those who relieve the hunger of others."

– Tirukkural 23:225

GRAIN grown for livestock is the primary farm crop on every continent and uses more land, water, and resources to grow than food not grown for farm animals.

Over two thirds of the farmland in Central America is used to grow livestock feed. About two thirds of the grain in Russia is fed to farm animals.

On the land used to produce the beef that would provide the daily food needs of one person, the daily food needs of more than 15 people could be met by growing fruits and vegetables.

> "Industrial agriculture has told the world a big lie, which means the corporations that run it have told the people a big lie, including the governments who have supported them. The lie is that industrial agriculture feeds people. Industrial agriculture feeds profits. People are going hungry. A billion people are hungry today because chemical farming does not let them eat the food they grow; instead they have to pay back the debt."
>
> – Vandana Shiva, author of *Soil Not Oil* and *Earth Democracy*

As the people on the planet are becoming increasingly dependant on corporations to grow their food the food shortage issues are becoming worse; multi-national corporations are genetically engineering seeds that need chemicals made by the same companies; the variety of food plants is being reduced; the soil is being degraded by monocropping and farming chemicals; broad-based food recalls are becoming more common; and family farmers are going out of business as corporate farm companies, genetically engineered seed companies, and corporations and/or governments are controlling food and land prices as well as trade routes.

> "If you can't feed a hundred people, then feed just one."
>
> – Mother Teresa

Grow a food garden. Compost your kitchen scraps. Plant native fruiting trees and bushes, including on wildlands. Nurture wild edibles. Support local organic farmers. Follow a plant-based diet, and eat organically.

> "It's not enough to have lived. We should be determined to live for something. May I suggest that it be creating joy for others, sharing what we have for the betterment of personkind, bringing hope to the lost and love to the lonely."
>
> – Leo Buscaglia

Ample Harvest, AmpleHarvest.org
Food First, FoodFirst.org
Food Forward, FoodForward.org
Food Not Bombs, FoodNotBombs.net
Food Not Lawns, FoodNotLawns.com
The Give Blog, thegiveblog.com. Suja Thomas and Scott Bahr live frugally and give their money to charities.

The Give Project, TheGiveProject.org. Among their projects: giving out fresh organic juices to homeless people on skid row in downtown Los Angeles.
The Hunger Project, THP.org
KitchenGardeners.org
Skip 1, Skip1.org
Urban Organic Gardener, UrbanOrganicGardener.com. Mike Lieberman's blog
Yards to Gardens, y2g.org

• INTENTIONAL COMMUNITIES

COMMUNES and Intentional Communities exist within towns and cities as well as in the countryside. They are quickly becoming popular with those involved in sustainable solutions. It is less expensive and more environmentally friendly for a group of people to live collectively and share facilities than it is for them to live apart and each have their own facilities. This is especially true if they are involved in growing some of their own food, and preparing it together.

Global EcoVillage Network, EcoVillage.org
Intentional Communities Magazine, Communities.ic.org
Lost Valley, LostValley.org
Radical Caring, DSame.com/radicalcaring.html
Raw Communities, RawCommunities.com. A growing list of raw food intentional communities around the world

• TRAVEL

"Thank God men cannot fly, and lay waste the sky as well as the earth."

– Henry David Thoreau

IF you plan on traveling, check the state-by-state and country-by-country listings in this book to see if there are places you can stay. Or the retreat listings. Happycow.net and SoyStache.com also list many places where vegetarians would feel comfortable staying. Check MeetUp.com for events happening in the town of your destination.

The travel industry creates enormous amounts of pollution. From airlines to hotels and from taxis to rental cars, the travel industry is very slowly starting to work on ways to clean up its act.

One way the travel industry pollutes is through its food. Tons of plastics and throwaway eating utensils are used every day by the airline industry. The hotel industry also causes massive amounts of pollution by not using recycled paper tissue, they don't recycle, they use enormous amounts of environmentally unfriendly cleaning materials, use chlorine products in their pools, dispose of hundreds of thousands of mattresses every year, construct and decorate their facilities using environmentally unsafe and nonsustainable materials, and use toxic pesticides, insecticides, weed killer and fertilizers in their landscaping.

If you travel, seek ways to reduce your impact on the planet. If you choose to travel by car remember that sharing car rides is always less polluting than traveling singularly. Check out the Internet rideshare boards that I've listed below.

Adventure Center, Adventure-Center.com
Better World Club, 20 NW 5th Ave., #100, Portland, OR 97210; BetterWorldClub.com.
Eco Club, EcoClub.com
Eco Tourism, EcoTourism.org
Eco Travel, EcoTravel.com
Eco Travel Specialists, EcoTravelSpecialists.com
Gaiam, Gaiam.com
Global Exchange, GlobalExchange.com
Green Earth Travel, VegTravel.com
Green Hotels, GreenHotels.com
Green Seal, GreenSeal.org/FindaProduct/Index.cfm
Happy Cow, happycow.com
Kind Ride Share, KindRideShare.net
Kind Ride Share, KindRideShare.org/kindrideshare
Responsible Travel, ResponsibleTravel.com
SoyStash, soystach.com
Stars Rainbow Ride Board, StarsRainbowRideBoard.org
Vegetarian Resource Group, VRG.org.

• Money and Investing

"I make myself rich by making my wants few."
– Henry David Thoreau

SOME seem to think that if you are rich you must be destroying the planet. But if you participate in socially responsible investing (SRI), you can play a part in making better choices to protect Earth, although it certainly does have its limits.

While there were people always seeking to avoid investing in companies involved in questionable activities, such as the slave trade, SRI became more common in the 1960s when people didn't want to invest in companies that had military contracts, such as Dow Chemical, manufacturer of napalm used in the Vietnam War. In recent decades people have avoided investing in companies associated with South Africa's apartheid government, and also in the seriously corrupt diamond trade, and, because of modern-day slavery in much of the chocolate market. Presently investors are avoiding companies that invest in those that directly or indirectly are associated with slave farms in Africa; in companies that have anything to do with military contracts; in companies involved in genetic engineering of genetically engineered food plants; in companies involved in irradiation of foods; and in companies that have a large influence in factory farming, in major causes of global warming, and in destruction of the environment – such as the petroleum, coal, natural gas, and nuclear power industries. Also, people interested in SRI avoid stocks in tobacco, alcohol, weaponry, and companies that use animals in lab testing.

> "Whether you know it or not, your money is talking. The question is, do you agree with what it is saying? A key factor in Sustainable and Responsible Investing is using the power of our voices to improve the way business is done. Through the shareholder process, your investments can convey your values and concerns to top management, thus changing the way that major corporations impact their employees, our communities and the natural environment. This is known as shareholder activism."
>
> – Gregory Wendt of Green Business Networking, GregWendt.com

Because more and more people are becoming aware of global warming and war issues, there is a whole lot more money going into companies that are involved in less destructive activities. Many of the funds that focus on SRI are producing respectable long-term financial returns (but, lately, the short term investments are less desirable). One reason for this is that companies focusing on socially responsible practices are less likely to get sued, and are more likely to pay and treat their workers in a responsible manner.

> "Try not to become a man of success, but rather try to become a man of value."
>
> – Albert Einstein

If you have money to invest, research the growing number of financial organizations that seek to invest in such things as solar energy (solar electric generating plants, rather than solar panel companies [because solar panels use rare earth minerals, which are obtained by radically ruinous mining operations]), organic farming, nontoxic cosmetics, industrial hemp, and vegan food companies. Look to invest in companies that donate part of their profits to environmental and wildlife protection. Move your money into a "green bank" or credit union focused on environmentally responsible investing.

I encourage people to move their accounts to a credit union, and avoid banks.

One of the most common ways to invest is through a mutual fund. These are funds that invest in a diversified group of companies. Listed below are mutual funds that focus on companies identified as socially responsible. Your initial investment in a mutual fund may be as little as a few hundred dollars, then you agree to put a certain amount of money into the account every month. The mutual fund managers maintain the account by deciding which stocks to invest in, and when to sell them. Investing in a mutual fund instantly diversifies your money and saves on trading commissions paid when you invest in individual stocks. Be sure to investigate if the mutual fund invests in companies that are in tune with your ideas of green.

If you have a 401(k) retirement plan, check to see if they offer socially responsible investing options. If they do not, inquire if they are planning to start providing this option. You might help this happen by providing a list of 401(k) plans that are involved in SRI. (Check the details of your 401(k) plan to see if it is secure from being pilfered by your company or embezzled by company management. Keep an eye on quarterly statements that may detail unexplained dips in balance, changes to investments you did not authorize, and changes in investment managers. The company president may be the sole manager of the account, and able to take "loans" from the account that may never be repaid. The fidelity bond insurance may cover 10 percent or less of the plan's assets. Annual independent audits don't have to be done on 401(k) plans of smaller companies, so problems may take years to be discovered. You may find that other types of savings plans are more secure, and more likely to qualify as SRI.)

Do you have a lot of money? Invest directly in companies that are considered to be environmentally green, and then donate any profits to an organization that works to protect and preserve wild plants, land, water, and animals. Write a will that includes a gift to an environmental charity, such as organizations working to protect the forests of the planet.

Establishing a gift fund or a foundation can turn you into a philanthropist. Gift funds, which are offered through a limited number of mutual fund companies, are less expensive to start and maintain than foundations. Gift funds also have tax and other benefits that foundations do not.

Before you invest in anything, research where your money is going. Avoid investing in companies involved in weaponry, nuclear power; petroleum exploration; tar sands mining; natural gas; genetic engineering of food plants; the irradiation of food; farming chemicals; factory farming; pharmaceutical drugs; the grain industry; chocolate farming that uses slaves; the fur trade; the diamond trade; vivisection; or lumber.

Avoid investing in U.S. government bonds, else you may be helping to fund war, nuclear bombs, and the military/industrial complex. Municipal bonds are likely a much safer investment because they are usually used to fund local citizen projects. But municipal bonds may also fund highways and power plants.

When you purchase stock in a company you are allowed to vote on corporate policy. In this way you can work to make a company more environmentally responsible. It's called "shareholder activism." It has worked in some cases, such as by getting office supply chains to start selling recycled paper.

There are investment funds that work to purchase into companies with histories of bad environmental policy. They do this with the goal of making the companies more environmentally friendly by changing its policies. But some funds don't always engage in this even when they say it is their goal. If you invest in funds that claim they are working to be shareholder activists, make sure the funds stick to their word.

Some of the following may be helpful when seeking to invest your money in socially and environmentally responsible ways. Also, publications such as *Mother Jones*, *Utne*, and *E Magazine* often carry advertisements from investment companies focused on investing in environmentally friendly ways – at least more environmentally friendly than most companies.

Please look into the slow money movement promoted by the Slow Money Alliance. Access: slowmoneyalliance.org.

As You Save, AsYouSow.org. Promotes corporate social responsibility.
Business Ethics Magazine, Business-Ethics.com
Calvert Financial Group, Bethesda, MD; CalvertGroup.com. Mutual funds.
Chittenden Bank, Brattleboro, VT; SociallyResponsible.Chittenden.com
Citizens Funds, Portsmouth, NH; CitizensFunds.com. Mutual funds.
Clean Yield, Greensboro, VT; CleanYield.com. Asset management.
Coalition for Environmentally Responsible Economies, Ceres.org
Domini Social Investments, Providence, RI; Domini.com. Mutual funds.
Dreyfus Corporation, Dreyfus.com. Mutual funds.
Ethical Investing, EthicalInvesting.com
First Affirmative Financial Network, Colorado Springs, CO; FirstAffirmative.com. Asset management.
Green Century Funds, Boston, MA; GreenCentury.com. Mutual funds.
Green MBA, GreenMBA.com
Green Money Journal, Santa Fe, NM; GreenMoneyJournal.com
Interfaith Center on Corporate Responsibility, New York, NY; ICCR.org
Investor Responsibility Research Center, Washington, DC; IRRC.org
KLD Research & Analytics, Inc., Boston, MA; KLD.com. Compiles and maintains profiles on 3,000 U.S. companies. Keeps information on global industry practices. Maintains socially responsible investing indexes.
Latino Community Credit Union, 219 West Main St., POB 25360; Durham, NC 27702; CoOperativaLatina.org
National Green Pages of Co-Op America, 1612 K St., NW, Ste. 600, Washington, DC 20006; CoOpAmerica.org. Contains a financial section for those interested in socially responsible investing.
Natural Investment Services, NaturalInvesting.com
Neuberger Berman Mutual Funds, New York, NY; NB.com
New Alternatives Fund, Melville, NY; NewAlternativesFund.com. Mutual funds.
Parnassus Investments, San Francisco, CA; Parnassus.com. Mutual funds.
Pax World Funds, New York, NY; PaxFunds.com. Mutual funds.
Pension Rights Center, PensionRights.org.

Permaculture Credit Union, 4250 Cerrillos Rd., Santa Fe, NM 87592; PCUOnline.org. Offers savings accounts, various types of loans, and a Visa card.

Portfolio 21, Progressive Investment Management, Portland, OR; Portfolio21.com. Mutual funds.

Principle Profits, Amherst, MA; PrincipleProfits.com. Asset management.

Progressive Asset Management Network, Oakland, CA; ProgressiveAssetManagment.com

Progressive Investor monthly newsletter, SustainableBusiness.com

Real Money bimonthly newsletter on socially responsible investing, Co-Op America; RealMoney.com

Rocky Mountain Humane Investing, GreenInvestment.com. Customized portfolios.

Self-Help Credit Union, Durham, NC; Self-Help.org

ShoreBank Pacific, Ilwaco, WA; Eco-Bank.com

Slow Money Alliance, slowmoneyalliance.org. People contributing to a grassroots, non-profit seed fund supporting small food enterprises and local food systems, building the nurture capital industry, connecting investors to their local economies, and building the nurture capital industry. Started by Woody Tasch to teach people to avoid investing in industrial agriculture.

Sierra Club Mutual Funds, San Francisco, CA; SierraClubFunds.com

Social Investment Forum, Washington, DC; SocialInvest.org. Trade organization for socially responsible investing.

SRI World Group, Brattleboro, VT; SRIWorld.com; and SocialFunds.com

Trillium Asset Management, TrilliumInvest.com

Gregory Wendt, GregWendt.com

Winslow Green Growth Fund, Portland, ME; WinslowGreen.com

• TOXEMIAN

> "And Man created the plastic bag and the tin and aluminum can and the cellophane wrapper and the paper plate, and this was good because Man could then take his automobile and buy all his food in one place and He could save that which was good to eat in the refrigerator and throw away that which had no further use. And soon the earth was covered with plastic bags and aluminum cans and paper plates and disposable bottles and there was nowhere to sit down or walk, and Man shook his head and cried: 'Look at this Godawful mess.'"
>
> – Art Buchwald, 1970

PEOPLE ask me where I got the word "toxemian." It's this simple: I made it up to describe people who are living unsustainable lifestyles, and to label the lifestyles, cultures, and individual practices that are damaging to Earth.

Now I hear that other people are starting to use my word.

> "Will urban sprawl spread so far that most people lose all touch with nature? Will the day come when the only bird a typical American child ever sees is a canary in a pet shop window? When the only wild animal he knows is a rat - glimpsed on a night drive through some city slum? When the only tree he touches is the

cleverly fabricated plastic evergreen that shades his gifts on Christmas morning?

– Frank N. Ikard, North American Wildlife and Natural Resources Conference, Houston, March 1968

"The packaging for a microwavable 'microwave' dinner is programmed for a shelf life of maybe six months, a cook time of two minutes and a landfill dead-time of centuries."

– David Wann, Buzzworm, November 1990

"Oh Beautiful for smoggy skies, insecticided grain,
For strip-mined mountain's majesty above the asphalt plain.
America, America, man sheds his waste on thee,
And hides the pines with billboard signs, from sea to oily sea."

– George Carlin

"Our modern industrial economy takes a mountain covered with trees, lakes, running streams and transforms it into a mountain of junk, garbage, slime pits, and debris."

– Edward Abbey

• Resonation of Instinct

WHEN I was ten, walking alone on my way home from school one early spring day, I stepped on the last bits of ice that were undermined by water running in the street gutter. As I stepped on these little shelves of ice they collapsed into the thin stream of water. Those that wouldn't easily break got stomped on. As they collapsed, they splashed water onto me – which was part of the fun of it.

As I walked along I noticed that the water was turning pink. Looking ahead I saw a thin stream of red that had slowed alongside the street gutter. I wondered why someone had spilled a bunch of red paint. With my eyes I followed the streak of red and saw that it was running in a very thin line down the middle of a driveway of a neighbor's house. Walking up to the driveway, I stopped. My breath left me.

The only time I had seen large animals was at the zoo and on my relatives' dairy farm. But I had never seen a deer up close.

That day I did.

My absent neighbors had returned from a hunting trip. Maybe they were inside taking showers.

I stood alone trying to understand what my eyes were seeing.

Hanging by its hind legs from the backyard tree next to the driveway was a large deer. Its limp body had given up the ghost. Someone had slit through its neck so deeply that its head looked to be hanging from a bit of flesh. Its face on the nearly decapitated head looked to be painted red. Its snout dripped with blood into a puddle on the lawn.

With my eyes, I followed the blood from the puddle, down the driveway, past my feet, and into the street gutter, where it turned the water from the melting ice a bloody pink.

I walked away with a memory I knew I would never forget.

Where I grew up there were wild berry bushes and cherry and other fruit trees. I often saw birds eating the berries and cherries, and they seemed to do so with great pleasure. When you see animals enjoying themselves by doing such things as feasting on wild berries, or playing with their young, you realize that they are beings that feel pleasure, establish relationships, and care for each other. Observing these behaviors displayed in wild animals has helped to make me want to protect them from harm.

Animals are not simple stimulus response mechanisms. It has been proved that the brains of animals release hormones in relation to the thoughts they are displaying; this is similar to how human brains function.

Ethologists are scientists who study animal behavior. Throughout the years those working in this field have conducted numerous studies concluding that animals have memories, show affection, romance their lovers, establish community standards, and role play among themselves; are aware of their behavior as compared to others; experience moods and express emotions of eagerness, jealousy, excitement, compassion, distress, guilt, sadness, depression, and joy; mourn for their dead; have preferences; understand reasoning; are able to remember where they buried things; can experience post-traumatic stress; show favoritism, socialize, teach their young, form intention, practice intimidation tactics, anticipate needs, are cautious, display an understanding of cause and effect, gather observations and make conclusions from them, are able to do simple math; cooperate with the agreements of others; communicate desires; plan strategies, and sometimes hide things from others. They not only form friendships, but their health deteriorates if they do not experience physical and mental stimulation. From ants that cultivate fungus farms, to animals that protect and care for the young of other species, and to dolphin that guard humans from sharks, to New Caledonian crows that fashion hooks to forage for bugs, to bee birds in Africa that know how to lead badgers and humans to beehives, wildlife is made up of active thinkers who display individual personalities and various levels of understanding, and clearly show that they each have a consciousness.

Koko, a gorilla living at the Gorilla Foundation in Northern California, has learned sign language to the point of recognizing over 1,000 signs, as well as thousands of English words.

Animals deserve to live freely on this planet we share. Free from animal farming and free from being experimented on in laboratories. Their habitat needs to be protected, and large parts of it need to be restored so they can survive and prosper.

Witnessing the damage humans have done to wildlife sickens me. Vast areas of Earth and wildlife have been violated by humans in the pursuit of making money, conducting warfare, using tremendous resources on folly, and simply selfishly disrespecting the treasures of Earth and Nature. All throughout the world humans have violated the wild animal kingdom. Within human society many more billions of animals are violated by animal farming, by the exotic animal trade, and in scientific experimentation. All of these activities rob nature, create bad energy, and damage all forms of life on Earth.

> "Suffering is suffering, whether experienced by animals or humans. The physiological process is identical."
> – Professor Mirko Bagaric, Head of Deakin Law School

The way farm animals are treated, the drugs they are given, the unnatural foods they are fed, the toxic chemicals they are treated with, and the conditions they live in make them stressed, depressed, confused, angry, frightened, and diseased. It is no wonder why the rates of degenerative diseases are so high in countries where the most factory farmed meat is consumed. People who are eating meat are eating stress, confinement, depression, frustration, confusion, repression, anger, fright, poisonous farming chemical residues, and disease.

By consuming a vegan diet rich in raw fruits and vegetables while living intentionally, a human can release the energies and illness they have absorbed into their system through their previous consumption of meat, eggs, and dairy products. The longer people consume a diet that is free of meat, eggs, and dairy, the more they will improve not only their own life, but those of the people and animals around them. As their body absorbs a higher quality of nutrients it spins a new fabric of molecules and they resonate with a new level of energy that is attuned to and that will attract vibrant health.

The book, *Old MacDonald's Factory Farm*, by C. David Coats contains a preface about the absurdity of man. It tells of how it is an odd world where humans inflict so much pain on animals; then kill and eat the animals, which makes humans ill, then, in an attempt to "cure" themselves of the diseases formed by eating the animals, they turn to toxic chemical drugs produced by the pharmaceutical industry, which spends hundreds of millions of dollars developing the drugs and testing them on tortured animals in outrageous laboratory experiments. Many of the drugs people take also contain ingredients that are derived from animals killed in slaughterhouses. (See *Naked Empress*, by Hans Ruesch; PETA.Org; and the books *Mad Cowboy* and *No More Bull*, by Howard Lyman, MadCowboy.Com.)

Not only does following a raw vegan diet protect animals from exploitation, it also protects wildlife, wildlands, the oceans, lakes and rivers, and Earth. This is because a raw vegan diet has a much lower impact on Earth than that of the standard American diet (SAD) that consists of meat, dairy, eggs, and highly polluting junk food. It starts with the fact that most food grown on the planet is being fed to farmed animals, and most resources used to grow food, including land, water, and fuel, is used to grow food for farmed – confined – animals being raised to kill. This may come as a surprise to those who thought that there is a food shortage on the planet. As I stated earlier, humans could not possibly consume all of the food that is growing on Earth. There is more than enough food to feed every human on the planet. The largest part of the problem is that most food grown on the planet is used to feed farm animals so that the rich countries can have their meat and dairy products.

> "I can't imagine that if you're putting something in your body that is filled with fear or anxiety, or pain, that that isn't somehow going to be inside of you."
> – Ellen Degeneres

When we refuse to eat animals, dairy products, and eggs, and instead subsist on a plant-based diet rich in raw fruits and vegetables, we are agreeing to live more in tune with Nature. We are not participating in the terrible resource-heavy and pollution-rich animal-killing industries of factory farms and slaughterhouses. We are not part of the tremendously fossil fuel-dependant monocropped GMO grain farming industry using mass quantities of toxic farming chemicals to grow more than 75 percent of its products to feed unnatural diets to billions of incarcerated and drugged animals on meat farms. We are not a part of the fishing industry that kills billions of fish and hundreds of thousands of sea mammals and birds every year. We are not supporting fish farms that are decimating coastal areas, killing wildlife, and using a variety of drugs and toxic chemicals to grow billions of catfish, tilapia, salmon, carp, and other harmless creatures in crammed pens. We are not supporting the rape of the oceans to provide unnaturally high-protein feed for farmed animals that are naturally vegan and that would never eat ocean creatures. We are not part of the egg industry, which kills billions of male chicks soon after birth simply because they can't produce eggs. We are not part of the dairy industry, which kills millions of baby male cows every year so that the mothers' milk can be taken and sold as human food. We are not part of the ranching industry that collectively kills millions of wolves, bears, lions, foxes, groundhogs, raccoons, predator birds, and other wild animals every year. We are not part of an industry that is cutting down the rainforests, sending species into extinction, and ruining the lives of poor people to provide land for cattle-grazing and growing more grain to feed to farmed animals to support the global fast food industry that greatly contributes to human disease. We are not supporting the killing of billions of animals every year. We are cutting down on our use of fossil fuels, water, and land. We are less dependant on corporations and their supermarketing. We are more likely to be of a healthy weight, and to experience fewer of the common chronic and degenerative diseases. When we follow a diet that does not contain anything that was born or hatched, and especially if we grow some of our food and compost our kitchen scraps into soil, we are helping to protect wildlife, wildlands, forests, the oceans, lakes, marshes, streams, and rivers, and Earth.

Nature and animals can teach us things simply by being part of our existence.

> "There are some barbarians who will take this dog, that so greatly excels man in capacity for friendship, who will nail him to a table, and dissect him alive. And what you discover in him are the same organs of sensation you have in yourself."
>
> – Voltaire, *Philosophical Dictionary*

Centuries of writing from all areas of the planet, among the people who didn't know that others existed, and who had no way of communicating with people on other continents, have recorded events where humans have communicated with animals. Native people from various continents even include their communicative thoughts with animals and Nature as part of their spiritual practices. An example is that of the Native Americans who include in their prayers an acknowledgment of a spiritual connection to animals such as deer, bears, wolves, serpents, fish, and birds. Writers of novels and songs often include references of communicating with animals and Nature in their works.

Animals are tuned into an energy that humans ignore, don't seem to consider, think of as impossible, or don't believe they can tune into. Where hope falters, possibilities fail.

Migratory birds often fly away at the same time of year, returning to the same spots year after year. Fish, such as salmon, do the same thing. Whales, sea turtles, and even butterflies do the same. Animals seem to know where they are and where they are going. Dogs and cats removed from their owners often find their owners, even when the owners move to new homes miles away. Farm animals have escaped from their confinement only to be found later at distant farms where their babies had been sold off.

A magnetic field that wraps the earth, the alignment of the stars, the angle of Sun and the moon, the smells of different regions of Earth, polarized ultraviolet light patterns, and other factors may play a part in migration. But there are also factors that guide living things that seem to be tuned into a resonance or energy – an invisible power.

Is this energy field, or a connection to instinct and Nature, something humans are missing out on by eating such unhealthful foods and living in a way that is disconnected from Nature? I believe so.

> "Would Nature have placed our very means of survival – food – in mobile animals, another mammal's skin, and under a hen, or in 260,000 varieties of plants spread over Earth?"
>
> – Rex Bowlby, author of *Plant Roots: 101 reasons why the human diet is rooted exclusively in plants*

• You Are Earth

> "Lack of awareness of the basic unity of organism and environment is a serious and dangerous hallucination."
>
> – Alan Watts

> "The Earth is not dying, it is being killed. And the people who are killing it have names and addresses."
>
> – Utah Phillips

> "Experiencing our own dynamic nature can be the first step towards understanding the dynamic nature of all living systems."
>
> – Adam Wolpert

SOME people look in books as they seek the mysteries and magic things of life. I see the mysteries and magic when I look at the plants, animals, soil, rivers, ocean, and sky. But they are not as they should be.

I see Earth weeping, the wildlife aching, and the people wandering. They are torn from each other by the selfishness that has ravaged the planet. It is a disconnection from nature that has ripped a wound into the spirits of humanity, wildlife, and the living planet. It continues to hemorrhage as commercial society perpetuates a lifestyle dependent on toxic chemicals, cutting down forests, massive mining, burning tremendous amounts of fossil fuels, incarcerating and killing billions of animals, and placing value on collecting money and high-priced belongings.

> "We abuse the land because we regard it as a commodity belonging to us. When we see land as a community to which we belong, we may begin to use it with love and respect."
>
> – Aldo Leopold

In its collective mind, humanity has devalued nature, wildlife, and the sanctity of a planet that breathes and lives and that is being killed by the infestation of greed.

You and everything that you see around you is an expression of energy. The expression has arranged substances into a pattern that makes up the structures of everything.

We are beings made up of magnetically-charged energy fields and we exist on a sphere that also has currents of electricity flowing through it. There are other fields of electricity streaming through the air and in and out of everything surrounding us.

The substances that make up your tissues are recycled from something else. They may have once existed in other people, and in animals, plants, rocks, and soil, and in the air and water you have taken in. Some of the substances inside you existed in dinosaurs, in ancient forests and desert cacti, in wildflowers and fruiting trees, in seaweed and ferns, in eagles and finches, in whales and walruses, in lizards and snakes, and in snails, ladybugs, caterpillars, mosquitoes, and butterflies.

The patterns in which the substances in your body are arranged allow for your body to function as a living being ruled by your spirit. As directed by your spirit you are animated.

Because you continually cast off the outer cells of your skin, grow and lose hair, and are putting forth gasses and waste through your skin, lungs, and eliminative organs while also taking in oxygen, water, and food substances, you are constantly interacting with your environment in a way that makes you part of the environment.

You are a system of substances that are always moving in and out of the different forms of life and in and out of the terrain of the planet. Because there is a continuous flow of substances from outer space falling to the planet, including meteorites and solar electron neutrinos, you are part of the galaxy.

You are sun, stars, planets, soil, rock, mountains, valleys, lakes, rivers, streams, oceans, plants, animals, fungi, bacteria, and air. You are part of the flow of nature and nature is a part of you.

You are the environment. When you are neglecting the environment, you are neglecting yourself. When the environment suffers, you suffer.

Is your consciousness paying attention to the environment and how you impact the environment? If not, it is time to wake up.

Be a part of the solution.

> "There's not a single scientific peer review paper published in the last 25 years that would contradict this scenario: Every living system of Earth is in decline. Every life support system of Earth is

in decline. And these together constitute the biosphere. The biosphere that supports and nurtures all of life. Not just our lives, but perhaps 30 million other species that share this planet with us."

– Ray Anderson

"Man's attitude toward nature is today critically important simply because we now have acquired a fateful power to alter and destroy nature. But man is part of nature, and his war is inevitably a war against himself."

– Rachel Carson

"When we try to pick anything out by itself, we find it hitched to everything else in the universe."

– John Muir

"Some day the earth will weep, she will beg for her life, she will cry with tears of blood. You will make a choice, if you will help her or let her die, and when she dies, you will die too."

– John Hollow Horn, Oglala Lakota, 1932

"Humankind has not woven the web of life. We are but one thread within it. Whatever we do to the web, we do to ourselves. All things are bound together. All things are connected."

– Chief Seattle

THE health of the planet reflects the health of the people living on it. The planet is in its current state of destruction because people have made unwise and unenlightened choices that have resulted in this unfortunate end result. To get a better end result people need to make a better beginning.

Great things have been accomplished in the past. Great things can be accomplished now to turn around the state of the planet.

We are living in a time when we can do tremendous good to improve the condition of wildlife and the environment.

It all starts where you live, by making better choices in your daily life that protect, restore, and nurture nature.

When we realize our kinship with wildlife and our need for a healthful environment we rediscover our connection to and reliance on nature.

Since we are all reliant on the same things, everyone should be involved in protecting what we all need: a healthful environment.

As you work to improve your health, work to improve the health of Earth. On some level, be involved in creating a sanctuary of nature. Welcome the birds, bees, butterflies, beetles, and insects. Protect it as a place for wildlife to play and make their homes.

Find organizations in your community and region that work to protect the environment and the wilds of nature. Select an organization for which you can do volunteer work and/or financially support through any type of donation you can give. Commit to sending a certain amount of money per month to an organization that works to protect nature, even if it is what you consider to be a very small amount.

Through improving your health by following a plant-based, vegetarian diet, you also improve the health of the planet. As each person works to improve their own life to live more in tune with nature, the health of the planet will improve.

The time to do it is now.

Plant trees.

Protect wildlife, wildlands, and the water bodies of Earth, which are all one with us.

Just as a seed never sees the flower, some people who work to restore nature will never see the benefits of their actions. A person who restores land that was once a forest, and plants the trees, may never live to see the trees grow into forests where wildlife lives and raindrops gather into a creek that feeds a river traveling into a distant ocean.

I encourage people to work to protect and restore the natural environment because I recognize our communion with nature, and am aware that nature's health is our health.

While I was growing up I spent a lot of time outside. I liked to sleep beneath the tapestry of stars, which fascinated me. I liked being among the trees, to feel the cool ground beneath my bare feet, to smell the woods after a summer rain, and to swim in rivers and lakes.

I recently found out that the woods where I spent a lot of time while I was growing up had been cut down so that a large parking lot could be put in. The pathways I walked as a child are now paved in concrete. The berry bushes and fruiting trees I ate from have been cut down. There are no longer any birds playing in and picking fruit and berries from the trees and bushes there. There are no bees or butterflies dancing among the wildflowers. And the bunnies, field mice, toads, and snakes have lost their homes. Instead, there is pavement and parked cars.

I think now is more important than ever to realize that we are Earth. As each of our lives depends on Earth, the planet is like the central part of the brain for the human race.

As is with the pineal gland of the brain, the health of the planet collectively can be improved by people eating more healthfully, thinking more positively, and generating positive energy fields throughout the vast landscape of the planet.

> "You must teach your children that the ground beneath their feet is the ashes of your grandfathers. So that they will respect the land, tell your children that the earth is rich with the lives of our kin.

Teach your children what we have taught our children, that the earth is our mother. Whatever befalls the earth befalls the sons of the earth."

– Native American Wisdom

"I tell you truly, you are one with the Earthly Mother; she is in you, and you in her. Of her were you born, in her do you live, and to her shall you return again. It is the blood of our Earthly Mother which falls from the clouds and flows in the rivers; it is the breath of our Earthly Mother which, whispers in the leaves of the forest and blows with a mighty wind from the mountains; sweet and firm is the flesh of our Earthly Mother in the fruits of the trees; strong and unflinching are the bones of our Earthly Mother in the giant rocks and stones which stand as sentinels of the lost times; truly, we are one with our Earthly Mother, and he who clings to the laws of his Mother, to him shall his Mother cling also."

– The Essene Gospel of Peace

Allegheny Defense Project, 311 Pitt St., Pittsburgh, PA 15221; alleghenydefense.org
Amazon Alliance, AmazonAlliance.org
Animal Rights Community, AnimalRightsCommunity.com
Animal Rights International, POB 1292, Middlebury, CT 06762; ARI-Online.org
Animals Australia, AnimalsAustralia.org
Auroville, India; auroville.org
Byron Environment Center, byronenvironmentcentre.asn.au
Cairns and Far North Environment Centre, Australia; cafnec.org.au
California Wilderness Coalition, CalWild.org
Care for the Wild International, CareForTheWild.org
Cascadia Wildlands Project: POB 10455, Eugene, OR 97440; CascWild.org
Circle of Life Foundation, POB 6783, Albany, CA 94706**;** circleoflife.org. Founded by Julia Butterfly Hill, who spent two years living in a redwood tree to save it.
Conservation Council of Western Australia, City West Lotteries House 2 Delhi Street, West Perth, Western Australia, 6005; ConservationWA.asn.au
The Coral Reef Alliance, 351 California St, Ste. 650, San Francisco, CA, 94104, USA; coralreefalliance.org
Earth First!, POB 324, Redway, CA 95560; EarthFirst.org
Earth First! Australia, POB 1270, Albany Western Australia 6330 EarthFirst.org.au
Earth First! Journal, POB 3023, Tucson, AZ 85702-3023; EarthFirstJournal.org
Earth Garden Magazine, POB 2, Trentham, VIC 3458, Australia; earthgarden.com.au. Magazine for sustainable living
Earth Island Institute, 300 Broadway, Ste. 28, San Francisco, CA 94133; EarthIsland.org
Earth Justice, EarthJustice.org
EarthSave, Earthjustice 426 17th St., Oakland, CA 94612; EarthSave.org
Endangered Species Coalition, POB 65195, Washington DC, 20035 USA; givengain.com
End Mountaintop Removal, Appalachian Voices, 191 Howard St, Boone, NC 28607; ILoveMountains.org
Farm Animal Reform Movement, 10101 Ashburton Ln., Bethesda, MD 20817; FarmUSA.org

Farm Sanctuary, Farm Sanctuary National Headquarters, 3100 Aikens Rd. Watkins Glen, NY 14891; P.O. Box 150; FarmSanctuary.org
Food Not Bombs, P.O. Box 424, Arroyo Seco, NM 87514, USA; FoodNotBombs.net
Food Not Lawns, 31139 Lanes Turn Rd., Coburg, OR 97408; FoodNotLawns.com
Friends of Clayoquot Sound, Box 489, 331 Neill St, Tofino BC V0R 2Z0, Canada; FOCS.ca
Green Peace, 702 H Street, NW, Ste. 300, Washington, D.C. 20001, USA; GreenPeace.org/usa
Habitat Works, 3436 Foothill Blvd., Ste.130, La Crescenta, CA 91214; HabitatWork.org
Heal the Bay, 1444 9th St., Santa Monica, CA 90401, USA; HealTheBay.org
In Defense of Animals, 3010 Kerner Blvd., San Rafael, CA 94901, USA; IDAUSA.org
International Rivers Network, 1847 Berkeley Way, Berkeley, CA 94703; InternationalRivers.org
Kahea, The Hawaiian Environmental Alliance, POB 270112, Honolulu, Hawai'i 96827-0112; Kahea.org
Mendocino Environmental Center, POB 299, 106 W. Standley St., Ukiah, CA 95482; MECGrassRoots.org
Natural Resources Defense Council, 40 West 20th St., New York, NY 10011; NRDC.org
Nature in the City, POB 170088, San Francisco CA 94117-0088; NatureInTheCity.org
New England Anti-Vivisection Society, 333 Washington St., Ste. 850, Boston, MA 02108-5100; NEAVS.org
No Veal, POB 15, Watkins Glen, NY 14891; NoVeal.org
The Ocean Project, POB 2506, Providence, RI 02906; TheOceanProject.org
Ohio Valley Environmental Coalition, POB 6753, Huntington, WV 25773-6753; OHVEC.org
Oregon Wild, 5825 North Greeley, Portland, OR 97217-4145; OregonWild.org
The Paw Project, PO Box 445, Santa Monica, CA 90406-0045; PawProject.org
People for Puget Sound, 911 Western Ave., Ste. 580, Seattle, WA 98104; PugetSound.org
Rising Tide Australia, POB 290, Newcastle, 2300; RisingTide.org.au
Rising Tide UK, 62 Fieldgate St., London E1 1ES England; RisingTide.org.uk
Save Bio Gems 40 West 20th St., New York, NY 10011; SaveBioGems.org
Save Happy Valley, POB 9263, Te Aro, Wellington, New Zealand; SaveHappyValley.org.nz
Society for Ecological Restoration International, SER.org
Turtle Survival Alliance, TurtleSurvival.org
United Mountain Defense, UnitedMountainDefense.org
Voice For Animals, VoiceForAnimals.net
Western Mining Action Network, WMAN-Info.org
The Wilderness Society of Australia, Australia; Wilderness.org.au
Wild Lands Project, WildLandsProject.org
Wildlife Watch, WildWatch.org
Woodstock Farm Animal Sanctuary, Woodstock, NY; WoodstockFAS.org
Urban Organic Gardener, UrbanOrganicGardener.com. Mike Lieberman's blog
Yards to Gardens, y2g.org
Zero Waste Alliance, ZeroWaste.org

"The meat industry is one of the most destructive ecological industries on the planet. The raising and slaughtering of pigs, cows, sheep, turkeys and chickens not only utilizes vast areas of land and vast quantities of water, but it is a greater contributor to greenhouse gas emissions than the automobile industry."

– Paul Watson, SeaShepherd.org

"I don't understand why asking people to eat a well-balanced vegetarian diet is considered drastic, while it is medically conservative to cut people open and put them on cholesterol-lowering drugs for the rest of their lives."

– Dr. Dean Ornish

"I became a vegetarian because I was persuaded that Life is as valid for other creatures as it is for humans. I do not need dead animal bodies to keep me alive, strong and healthy. Therefore, I will not kill for food."

– Scott Nearing

"When I was old enough to realize all meat was killed, I saw it as an irrational way of using our power, to take a weaker thing and mutilate it. It was like the way bullies would take control of younger kids in the schoolyard."

– River Phoenix

"As I cannot kill, I cannot authorize others to kill. Do you see? If you are buying from a butcher you are authorizing him to kill – to kill helpless, dumb creatures which neither you nor I could kill ourselves."

– Paul Troubetzkoy

"In all the round world of Utopia there is no meat. There used to be. But now we cannot stand the thought of slaughterhouses. And it is impossible to find anyone who will hew a dead ox or pig. I can still remember as a boy the rejoicing over the closing of the last slaughterhouse."

– Herbert G. Wells, *A Modern Utopia*

Don't eat animals.

Plant food gardens and fruiting tree orchards.

Part 2

• Raw Restaurants, Delis, Markets, Farmers' Markets, Orchards, Chefs, Retreats, Training, Publications, and Web Sites

IF you know of any additions or changes to the following list of restaurants, cafes, delis, and natural foods markets, please send the updated information to: information (at) sunfoodliving.com, or snail mail:

John McCabe
C/O Carmania Books
POB 1272
Santa Monica, CA 90406-1272
Office: Information@SunfoodLiving.com

INCLUSION in this book does not mean the author endorses the products, services, practices, or philosophy of the company, organization, or its founders, owners, or employees.

• U.S. Alabama

Check MeetUp.com for raw food meetups.

The Cardinal Rose Organic Grocery, 9255 Pleasant Grove Rd., Albertville, AL; 256-891-3869; cardinalroseorganicgrocery.com

Dayspring Natural Foods, 223 Opelika Rd., Auburn, AL; 334-821-1965

Earth Fare, 1550 Opelika Rd., Ste. 3; Auburn, AL 36830; earthfare.com. Market.

Earth Fare, 5900 – C University Dr., NW, Huntsville, AL 35906; earthfare.com. Market.

Fairhope Health Foods, 280 Eastern Shore Shopping Ctr., Fairhope, AL; 251-928-0644

Fountain City Health Foods, 111 S. Memorial Dr., Prattville, AL; 334-361-7550

Garden Cove Produce, 628 Meridian St., N., Huntsville, AL; 256-534-COVE; gardencoveproduce.com

Golden Temple Natural Grocery & Café, 1901 11th Ave., S., Birmingham, AL; 205-933-6333

Health Concepts Organic Health Food Store, 1901 Wise Dr., Dotham, AL; 334-673-2444; ShopHealthConcepts.com

Health Wise Foods Market, 5147 Atlanta Hwy., Montgomery, AL 36109; 866-788-9473; HealthWiseFoods.com

Peachtree Natural Food, 1625 E. University Dr., Ste. 116, Auburn, AL; 334-821-7749; peachtreenaturalfoods.com

Raw Life Foods, 1714 W 3rd St., Montgomery, AL 36106

TBO Deli, 5510 Hwy. 280, Birmingham, AL 35242; 205-995-8888. Raw living food lunch specials. Organic juice & smoothies.

Virginia's Health Foods, 3170 Dauphin St., Ste. B, Mobile, AL; 251-479-3952; va-fairhopehealthfoods.com

• U.S. ALASKA

Check MeetUp.com for raw food meetups.

Cactus Flats, 338 Mission Rd., Kodiak, AK; 907-486-4677

Cooper Specialities, POB 4117; Soldotna, AK; 907-265-5686; AlaskaBreadBakers.com. Sells non-GMO seeds, grains, and legumes, and raw honey.

Natural Pantry Health Food Store, 3801 Old Seward Hwy, Anchorage, AK; 907-770-1444; natural-pantry.com

Organic Alaska, 3404 Willow St., Anchorage, AK 99517; 907- 770-2779; OrganicAlaska.com. This is a wholesale price club that orders foods and organic items from the same suppliers to natural foods stores.

Organic Oasis Health Foods, 2610 Spenard Rd., Anchorage, AK; 907-277-7882

Rainbow Foods Market, 224 4th St., Juneau, Alaska 99801; 907-586-6476; Rainbow-Foods.org

Smoky Bay Natural Foods, 248 W. Pioneer Ave., Homer, AK; 907-235-7252

Sunshine Health Foods Store, 410 Trainor Gate Rd., Fairbanks, AK; 907-456-5433

• U.S. ARIZONA

Check MeetUp.com for raw food meetups.

24 Carrots, 61 40 West Chandler Blvd., #2, Chandler, AZ 85226; 24CarrotsJuice.com. Vegan raw.

Amelia's Garden Green Grocer & Café, 305 S. Main St., Snowflake, AZ 85937; 928-536-2046; ameliasgardenhealth.com

Aqua Vita Natural Foods Market, 2801 N. Country Club Rd., Tucson, AZ 85716; aquavitanaturals.com

Bisbee Food Cooperative, 72 Erie St., Bisbee, AZ 85603; 520-432-4011; 520-432-9014

Blue Nile Café, 933 E. University Dr., Ste. 112, Tempe, AZ 85281; 480-337-1113; bluenilecafe.net. Some raw food.

Chakra 4 Herbs & Tea House; 4773 N. 20th St., Phoenix, AZ 85016; 602-283-1210; chakra4herbs.com/aboutus.asp. Vegetarian and vegan. Some raw food options, including salads, nut cheeses, wraps, raw chocolate. Bulk herbs. Oils. Elixirs. Teas.

Chef Sara's Raw Vegan Academe and Café, 6602 E. Cave Creek Rd., Cave Creek, AZ 85331; 480-760-3387. Raw, organic, gluten free cuisine. Chef Sara Siso.

Chocola Tree, Roots, 1595 West Hwy. 89A, Sedona, AZ 86336; 928-282-2997; blisscafe.wordpress.com. Open 7 days. Free wireless.

Chocola Tree, Hillside, 671 Hwy. 179, E-ST1, Sedona, AZ 86336; ChocolaTreeCafe.com. Raw café.

Consipre, 901 N. 5th St., Phoenix, AZ 85004; ConspirePhx.com. All vegan with some raw foods.

Food Conspiracy Co-op, 412 N. 4th Ave., Tucson, AZ 85705; 520-624-4821; FoodConspiracy.org

Healthy Habit Health Foods, 6029 N. 7th St., Phoenix, AZ 85014; 602-252-

6000; healthyhabithealthfoods.com

In The Raw, 143 S. Higley Rd., Gilbert, AZ 85296; RawsomeBar.com.

Loving Hut, 3515-A W. Union Hills Dr., Glendale, AZ 85308; 602-978-0393. Vegan restaurant.

Magpie Natural Foods Co-op & Buying Club, 500 West Gurley St., Prescott, AZ 86301; 520-778-5880

Mount Hope Foods Naturally, 853 S. Main St., Cottonwood, AZ 86326; 928-634-8251; mounthopefoods.com

Natural Life Health Center, 4841 E. Speedway, Tucson, AZ 85712; 520-795-7862; NewLifeHealth.com

New Frontiers Natural Marketplace, 1112 W. Iron Springs Rd., Prescott, AZ 86305; 928-445-7370

New Frontiers Natural Marketplace, 1420 W Highway 89A, Sedona, AZ 86336

North Valley Organics, 17042 N. 38th Ave., Glendale, AZ; 602-751-0553

Pomegranate Café, 4025 E. Chandler Blvd., Ste. 28, Phoenix, AZ. Vegetarian and vegan with some raw.

Pure Joy Living Foods, 320 Smelter Ave., Patagonia AZ 85634; PO BOX 431, Patagonia AZ 85634; purejoyplanet.com. Elaina Love's products, recipes, classes, retreats, workshops and services

Sierra Vista Farmers Market, East Wilcox Dr. & South Carmichael Ave., Sierra Vista, AZ 85635**;** SierraVistaFarmersMarket.com

Sunflower Farmer's Market, 245 E. Bell Rd., Phoenix, AZ 85022; 602-218-4949; sfmarkets.com

Tree of Life Café, 686 Harshaw Rd., POB 778, Patagonia, AZ 85624; 520-394-2589; TreeOfLife.nu; Call for reservations.

Whole Foods Market, 10810 N. Tatum Blvd., Phoenix, AZ 85028; 602-569-7600. Salad bar and some raw deserts.

Vivapura, 320 Smelter Ave., POB 431, Patagonia, AZ 85624-0431; 877-787-6457; Vivapura.net. Not a restaurant. This is a company that produces and distributes raw food products. Chris Whitcoe.

• U.S. ARKANSAS

Check MeetUp.com for raw food meetups.

Ebenezer Hills Healthfood Store, RR2 Box 128, Clarksville, AR 72830-9545; 479-754-3927. Small store with fresh produce and some other raw items.

The Eureka Market, 121 East Van Buren, Ste. B, Eureka Springs, AR; 479-253-8136; eurekamarketfoods.com

Summercorn Foods, 1410 Cato Springs Rd., Fayetteville, AR 72701; 501-521-9338; SummerCorn.com. Natural foods store.

The Olde Towne Store, 113 N. Jefferson Ave., El Dorado, AR; 870-862-1060; theoldetownestore.com

Ozark Natural Foods Co-op, 1554 N. College Ave., Fayetteville, AR 72703; 479-521-7558; OzarkNaturalFoods.com. Natural foods store.

Roger's Natural Health Food Store, 310 N. 13th St., Rogers, AR; 479-637-3316

• U.S. CALIFORNIA

Check MeetUp.com for raw food meetups.

Adama, 428 Chapala St, Santa Barbara, California 93101; adamavegan.com. Vegan. Opened in 2011. In an old house. Fresh juices. Will accommodate gluten-free upon request. Closes breifly in late afternoon.

Alameda Natural Grocery, 1650 Park St., Alameda, CA 94501-7389; 510-865-1500

Alive Veggie, San Francisco, CA 94123; AliveVeggie.com. Catering.

Almond Street Natural Foods, 5267 Almond St., Paradise, CA 95969; 530-877-5164; almondstreet.net. Market.

Aptos Natural Foods, 7506 Soquel Dr., Aptos, CA 95003; 831-685-3334

Arcata Co-op, 811 I St., Arcata, CA 95521-6123; 707-822-5947; northcoastco-op.com

The Art of Food, 1825 Del Paso Blvd., #2, Sacramento, CA 95815; theartoffoodcafe.blogspot.com; thegreenboheme2.blogspot.com. Raw food café. Chef Richard Hemsley.

Au Lac, 16563 Brookhurst St., Fountain Valley, CA 92708 (Orange County); 714-418-0658; AuLac.com. Vegan restaurant with half raw menu. Some consider this to be the best raw restaurant. Chef Ito is a graduate of the Living Light Culinary Institute in Fort Bragg, California.

Au Naturaw, 206 N. Broadway, Ste. A, Santa Ana, CA 92701; AuNatuRaw.com. Raw café. Opened 2012. Marchell Williams, proprietor.

Baagan, 910 Pleasant Grove Blvd., Ste. 160, Roseville, CA 95678; Baagan.com. Vegan cafe. Some raw food on menu, including salads, smoothies, and deserts.

Bautista Organic Date Ranch, POB 726, Mecca, CA 92254-0726; 7HotDates.com; KissMe (at) 7HotDates.com. The Bautista family has a mail-order date company so they can sell the dates they grow directly to the public. In 2004, Enrique Bautista was paralyzed in a car accident while driving home from a farmers' market. Their mail order biz helps them. See the Web site for ordering information. These are good people.

Belicious Green Smoothies, Santa Monica, CA; BeliciousSmoothies.com. Fully-stocked mobile raw vegan smoothie truck with staff available for events and farmers' markets around Los Angeles. Began business January 2011. Laura Rose.

Berkeley Bowl Marketplace, 2020 Oregon St., Berkeley, CA 94703; 510-843-6929; berkeleybowl.com. This is a market with a very large produce section. It has a reputation for being a place with aggressive shoppers who are food intellectuals, and who have been known to get into arguments. Some consider this to be the best produce market in the world.

Berkeley Natural Foods, 1336 Gilman St., Berkeley, CA 94706

Better Life Cuisine, Santa Monica. Café opened in summer 2009, but closed in 2012 and their kitchen continues supplying retail to local natural foods stores. Yanet Gil Martinez.

Better Life Organic Produce, 1400 E. Olympic Blvd., L.A, CA 90021; 213-623-0640. Source to buy cases of organic produce for lower price than markets. Closed Sundays.

Beverly Hills Juice Company, 8382 Beverly Blvd, L.A., CA 90048-2631; 323-655-8300; BeverlyHillsJuice.com. Raw, organic juices. Also sold down the street on Beverly at Erewhon natural foods store.

The Bliss Bar, Santa Monica, CA and Ashland, OR; theblissbar.org; email: activate (at) theblissbar.org. Has a traveling raw food café available for events. Their packaged chocolate and other foods are sold in many natural foods stores.

Bliss Café, 1025 Chorro St., San Luis Obispo, CA 93401; blisscafeslo.com

Bloom Cafe, 5544 West Pico Blvd, Los Angeles, CA 90019; BloomCafe.com; 323-934-6900. Some raw food on vegan menu.

BriarPatch Co-op Market, 290 Sierra College Dr., Grass Valley, CA 95949; briarpatch.coop

Buffalo Whole Foods, 598 Castro St., San Francisco, CA 94114-2512; 415-626-7038. This is a little healthfood store on the corner.

Café Gratitude, CA 94110; 415-824-4652; CafeGratitude.com. Several locations around the San Francisco Bay area, including Berkeley, San Rafael, Oakland, Santa Cruz, and Cupertino. Mostly raw and some cooked vegan food is served at Café Gratitude restaurants. The owners are authors of popular recipe books.

Café Gratitude, 639 N. Larchmont Blvd., Los Angeles, CA; cafegratitude.com. Mostly raw restaurant. This location scheduled to open in March 2011.

Café Gratitude, Rose Ave., Venice CA. Opening 2012.

Café Chakra Living, Ojai, CA; fullchakra.com. Classes and supplies.

Chico Natural Foods, 818 Main St., Chico, CA 95928-5708; 530-891-1421; 530-891-1713; ChicoNatural.net

Community Market, 1899 Mendocino Ave., Santa Rosa, CA 95401-3628; 707-546-1806; SRCommunityMarket.com

Co-Opportunity Natural Foods Market, 1525 Broadway, Santa Monica, CA 90404; 310-451-8902; CoOpportunity.com. All customers welcome, members and non. Great for bulk raw ingredients, including herbs. Also has a made-to-order juice counter at deli. Lots of organic produce. Better prices than any natural foods market in Los Angeles region. Open 7 A.M. to 10 P.M. every day.

Corners of the Mouth Natural Foods, 45015 Ukiah Street. POB 367, Mendocino, CA 95460; 707-937-5345. Small healthfood store in this very small beachside village town. Very helpful staff.

Cornucopia Natural Foods, 26135 Carmel Rancho Blvd., Carmel, CA 93923; 831-625-1415

Cru 1521 Griffith Park Blvd., Los Angeles, CA 90026; 323-667-1551; CruSilverlake.com. Rachel Carr. Across from little park. Farmers' Market held on same street once per week. Mostly raw gourmet full service restaurant in this older part of town. Very much considered to be one of the best raw restaurants. They also have a Good Karma Truck that travels around to various events serving vegan food that is mostly raw. Join them on Facebook.

Date People, POB 808, Niland, CA 92257; DatePeple.net; 760-359-3211. They grow and sell organic dates.

Davis Food Co-op, 620 G Street, Davis, CA 95616; 530-758-2667;

DavisFood.coop.

Rick and Karin Dina, Santa Rosa, CA; RawFoodEducation.com

Earl's Organic Produce, 2101 Jerrold Ave., Ste. 100, San Francisco, CA 94124; earlsorganic.com. Place to purchase cases of organic fruits and veggies. Site contains map of some organic farms in California.

Earthbar, myearthbar.com. Several locations around the L.A. area. Sells some packaged raw foods. Also makes smoothies and juices. Located inside Equinox fitness studio gyms.

Earthbeam Natural Foods Organic Grocery, 1399 Broadway, Burlingame, CA 94010; 650-347-2058; earthbeamfoods.com. Next to Que Se Raw raw café.

Earhtly Juices, 664 El Camino Real, Tustin, CA; EarthlyJuiceCart.com; Raw.

El Cerrito Natural Foods, 10367 San Pablo Ave., El Cerrito, CA 94530; 510-526-1155

Elderberries, 7564 Sunset Blvd., West Hollywood, CA 90046; 323-798-4557. Vegan café with some raw food items.

Elf Café, 2135 W. Sunset Blvd., Echo Park, CA 90026-3124 (Los Angeles); 213-484-6829. Elfcafe.com. Some raw foods. Also, catering. Contact: Astara. ElfCafe (at) gmail.com.

Elliott's Natural Foods, 8063 Greenback Ln., Citrus Heights, CA 95610; 916-726-3033; elliottsnaturalfoods.com

Erewhon Market, 7660-B Beverly Blvd., L.A., CA 90036; 323-937-0777; ErewhonMarket.com. Erewhon has a large raw food section. While some of their products are lower priced, many are priced high, especially higher than the Santa Monica Co-op several miles to the west.

Euphoria Loves Rawvolution (known as ELR), 2301 Main St., Santa Monica, CA 90405; 310-392-9501; EuphoriaLovesRawvolution.com. Matt and Janabai Amsden. Matt is the author of the *RawVolution* recipe book and is a musician. Janabai is a working actress landing roles in Los Angeles theatres. Café often has live music nights. Bohemian feel. WiFi bar with stools and plugs, and also a few outside tables. Juice bar window on the side of the building.

Eureka Co-op, 25 4th St., Eureka, CA 95501-0331; 707-443-6027; northcoastco-op.com/eureka.htm

Eureka Natural Foods, 1450 Broadway St., Eureka, CA 95501; 707-442-6325; 800-603-8364; eurekanaturalfoods.com. Medium-sized natural foods store.

Evolution Fast Food, 2965 5th Ave. (at Quice), San Diego, CA 92103; EvolutionFastFood.com. Vegetairan restaurant with vegan and some raw items on menu. Has a drive-through window. Some of their packaged products are sold at various markets.

The Farmer and The Cook, 339 W. El Roblar, Ojai, CA 93023; 805-640-9608; farmerandcook.com. Farm-based grocery and restaurant with some raw selections.

Fat Uncle Farms, 5924 Daliey St., Goleta, CA 93117; funclefarms.blogspot.com; funclefarms (at) gmail.com. Raw almonds.

Figueroa Produce Market, 6312 North Figueroa St., Los Angeles, CA 90042 (Echo Park); figueroaproduce.com. In addition to produce, they also sell some raw food products, including packaged vegan cheeses and ice cream. However, this isn't a vegetarian store.

Follow Your Heart, 21825 Sherman Way, Canoga Park, CA 91303. Popular, long-time natural foods store juice bar, and a full-service old restaurant inside the store with raw options. Also has sidewalk patio.

The Food Bin, 1130 Mission St., Santa Cruz, CA 95060

Fresh in Topanga, 1704 N. Topanga Cyn. Rd., Topanga, CA 90290. Mostly vegan store and café with juice and smoothies. Also sells produce, a variety of raw honeys and some raw dairy cheese. Will be serving teas and coffees. Outside seating area. Very, very casual. Opened 2012. May be closing on Wednesdays.

Fruit Gallery, 1 Westminster Ave., Venice, CA 90291; 310-452-3034; fruitgallery (at) yahoo.com; Nina Marie Merced; small juice and smoothie bar and market with some fresh and packaged raw and foods

Golden Carrot, 1621 Imola Avenue West, Napa, CA 94559-4795; 707-224-3117

Good Earth Market, 1966 Sir Francis Drake Blvd., Fairfax, CA 94930; goodearthnaturalfoods.net

Good Karma Vegan 37 S. 1st St., San Jose CA 95113; 408-294-2694. Between San Fernando & Santa Clara.

Good Mood Food, Huntington Beach, CA; 714-377-2028; GoodMoodFood.com. Sells some packaged foods in various stores, formerly had a restaurant

Good To Go Restaurant, GoodToGoRestaurants.com. Vegetarian, vegan, and some raw vegan dishes.

Gracias Madre, 2211 Mission St., San Francisco, CA 94110; gracias-madre.com/web. Opened by Terces and Matthew Engelhart of Café Gratitude in 2010. Vegan Mexican food with some raw options.

Grass Roots Natural Foods Store, 2040 Dunlap Dr., South Lake Tahoe, CA 96150-6448; 530-541-7788

The Green Boheme, 1825 Del Paso Blvd, Sacramento, CA 95815; thegreenboheme.com. Raw vegan. Del Paso Heights neighborhood.

Harvest House Natural Foods, 2395 Monument Blvd. M, Concord, CA 94520; 925-676-2458; harvesthouse.com

Health Habit Market, 1906 Vista Del Lago Dr., Valley Springs, CA 95252; health-habit.com.

Henry's Market, 1011 North San Fernando Blvd., Burbank, CA 91504-4329; 818-566-4089

Henry's Market, 21821 Ventura Blvd., Woodland Hills, CA 91364; henrysmarkets.com

Henry's Market, Rancho Temecula Town Ctr., 39606 Winchester Rd., Temecula, CA 92591; 951-694-3680; henrysmarkets.com

Hip, A Vegetarian Joint, 928 E. Ojai Ave., Ojai, CA 93023; hipvegancafe.com.

Isla Vista Food Co-op, 6575 Seville Rd., Isla Vista, Santa Barbara, CA 93117; 805-968-1401; islavistafoodcoop.blogspot.com/; 8am to 11pm everyday. Small, but very well run food co-op in the center of Isla Vista, the area next to UC Santa Barbara. College students galore.

Jimbo's Naturally Organic Food Retailer, 1633 S. Centre City Pkwy., Escondido, CA 92025; 760-489-7755; jimbos.com

Jimbo's Naturally Organic Food Retailer, 10511 4 S Commons Dr., Ste. 155, San Diego, CA 92127; jimbos.com

Jimbos Naturally Organic Food Retailer, 1923 Calle Barcelona, Carlsbad, CA 92009; 760-334-7755; jimbos.com

Jimbo's Naturally Organic Food Retailer, 12853 El Camino Real, San Diego, CA 92130; 858-793-7755; jimbos.com

Judahlicious Cafe, 3906 Judah, San Francisco, CA 94122-1121; 415-66-juice; Judahlicious.com. Mostly raw food in this café next to the Other Avenues natural foods store. Short walk to beach.

Juicy Ladies, 22423 Ventura Blvd., Woodland Hills, CA 91364; juicyladies.com. Organic juices, food and products. Also does events catering.

Juicy Lucy's 703 Columbus Ave., San Francisco, CA 94133-2701; 415-786-1285. Juices.

Matthew Kenney Cuisine, 395 Santa Monica Place Mall, Santa Monica, CA 90401; MatthewKenneyCuisine.com. Restaurant and chef school. Opened fall 2012.

Kind Kreme, 3701 Cahuenga Blvd., Studio City, CA 90068; KindKreme.com. Mollie Angelheart's raw, vegan ice cream parlor. Her parents own the Café Gratitude restaurant chain in San Francisco. This is next to Sunpower Natural Café at 3711 Cahuenga Blvd.

KindKreme, 1700 W. Sunset Blvd., LA, CA 90026; KindKreme.com

KindKreme, 319 S. Arroyo Pkwy., Pasadena, CA 91105; KindKreme.com.

Koral's Tropical Fruit Farm, POB 13, Vista, CA 92085; 760-631-0200. Barry Koral, owner. Barrykoral (at) hotmail.com.

Lassen's Natural Food Store, 4308 California Ave., Bakersfield, CA 93309; 661-324-6990; lassens.com

Lassen's Natural Food Store, 2207 Pickwick Dr., Camarillo, CA 93010; 805-482-3287; lassens.com

Lassen's Natural Food Store, 5154 Hollister Ave., Goleta, CA 93111; 805-683-7696; lassens.com

Lassen's Natural Food Store, 3471 Saviers Rd., Oxnard, CA 93033; 805-486-8266; lassens.com

Lassen's Natural Food Store, 1790 S. Broadway, Santa Maria, CA 93454; 805-925-2432; lassens.com

Lassen's Natural Food Store, 2857 E. Thousand Oaks Blvd, Thousand Oaks, CA 91362; 805-495-2609; lassens.com

Lassen's Natural Food Store, 4071 E. Main St., Ventura, CA 93003; 805-644-6990; lassens.com

L.A. Vegan Crepe, 930 S. Robertson, Beverly Hills, CA 90035. Open late 2012.

Lazy Acres Market, 302 Meigs Rd., Santa Barbara, CA 93109-1984; 805-564-4410; LazyAcres.com. Large, busy natural foods store.

Leaf Organics, 11938 W. Washington Blvd., Los Angeles, CA 90066; LeafOrganics.com. Reopened in June 2010 after a name change from Leaf

Cuisine and change in business plan. Mostly raw with some cooked vegan. Owned by Rod Rotundi. He is also the author of a book on green living and making raw foods. Rod (at) LeafOrganics.com.

Lifefood Organic, 1507 N. Cahuenga Blvd., Hollywood, CA 90028; LifeFoodOrganic.com; AnnieJubb.com. Soups, salads, smoothies. Annie Jubb is an author of a popular raw recipe book. Although most are, some of her foods are not vegan: contain dairy, such as goat milk. Some sprouted hemp seed bread used on sandwhiches, but raw options available.

Living Light Café, 301-B North Main St., Ft. Bragg, CA 95437; 707-964-2420; RawFoodChef.com. This café and the adjoining retail store are part of Cherie Soria's Living Light Culinary Institute, the top school for individuals, chefs, and instructors of raw vegan cuisine. They also offer a nutritional science and nutrition educators program. Holds annual Living Light Chef Showcase: Hot Chefs, Cool Kitchen! An event highlighting some of the best raw food chefs on the planet – streamed live over the internet. Soria is the author of *Raw Food Revolution Diet.* Graduates of her school own or work in raw restaurants and teach classes all over the world. Subscribe to the free eneweslter by accessing the Web site and entering your email address into the subscription box.

The Living Temple, 7310 Center Ave., Huntington Beach, CA 92647; thelivingtemple.com. Store and meeting center selling some raw food products. Various alternative health and conspiracy theory presentations are given here.

Living Tree Community Foods. LivingTreeCommunity.com. This is a raw foods products company that distributes their products to natural foods stores and restaurants, and through the Internet.

Locali Conscious Convenience, 5825 Franklin Ave., L.A., CA 90028 (Hollywood); 323-466-1360; localiyours.com. Sells some raw food products, including vegan cheeses and ice creams.

Jillian Love, JillianLove.com; RawYogaRetreats.com; RawYogaJedi.com. Sanoma, CA.

Brian Lucas, 310-460-9253; ChefBeLive.com; BeLiveLight.com. Known as "Chef BeLive." Considered among the top gourmet raw chefs. Has written an ebook of his recipes. Catering, events, and restaurant consulting.

Lydia's Organics, 31 Bolinas Rd., Fairfax, CA 94930; lydiasorganics.com. A raw food restaurant, catering company, and mobile restaurant. Also sells packaged products at natural foods stores.

Madeleine Bistro, 18621 Ventura Blvd., Tarzana, CA 91356; 818-758-6971; MadeleineBistro.com. Some raw dishes on the menu of this vegan restaurant.

Main Squeeze, 2727 Main St., Santa Monica, CA; SqueezeOnMain.com; 310-399-9914. Fresh juices and smoothies. Opened 2012. John and Guru.

MAKE, Matthew Kenney Cuisine, 395 Santa Monica Place Mall, Santa Monica, CA 90401; MatthewKenneyCuisine.com. Restaurant and chef school. Opened fall 2012.

Mary's Secret Garden, 100 S. Fir St., Ventura, CA 93001; 805-641-FOOD; MarysSecretGarden.com. Vegan restaurant with many raw items on menu.

Check website for potentially newer, larger location. Ventura County. Mary is a real Earth mother who is happy to make the food she serves. Get a hug.

Millenium Restaurant Hotel California, 580 Geary, San Francisco, CA 94102; 415-345-3900; Some raw dishes.

Mooi Food, mooifood.com. Stephen Hauptfuhr. Juice, smoothie, salad, ice cream bar in downtown L.A. to open 2012 at 8th and Main. Formerly had a restaurant in Echo Park, which is now a vegan restaurant called Sage.

Mother's Market, 1890 Newport Blvd., Costa Mesa, CA 92627; 949-631-4141; MothersMarket.com. Mother's Markets are known for being raw friendly.

Mother's Market, 19770 Beach Blvd., Huntington Beach, CA 92648; 714-963-6667; MothersMarket.com

Mother's Market, 2963 Michelson Dr., Irvine, CA 92612; 949-752-6667; MothersMarket.com

Mother's Market, 24165 Paseo De Valencia, Laguna Woods, CA 92653; 949-768-6667; MothersMarket.com

Mountain Song Natural Food Market, 314 N. Mt. Shasta Blvd., Mount Shasta, CA 96067; 530-926-3391; mountainsong.biz

Mike Mullen, raw chef, deserts, event catering. 415-283-7045. OmMikeOm (at) gmail.com

MylkMan.com. A raw vegan almond/coconut mylk delivery service in Los Angles. Jeff Leaf, proprietor.

Natural Grocery Company, 1336 Gilman St., Berkeley, CA 94706; 510-526-2456; NaturalGrocery.com

Natural Grocery Company, 10367 San Pablo Ave, El Cerrito, CA 94530; NaturalGrocery.com

Nature Mart, 2080 Hillhurst Ave., Los Angeles, CA 90027 (Los Feliz); 323-660-0052; naturemart.com. Oldschool natural foods store. Good produce section. Many bulk foods and packaged raw food products, including raw vegan cheeses and ice creams.

Naturewell Market, 3824 West Sunset Blvd., L.A., CA 90026 (Silverlake); 323-638-5894. Some raw food products, including packaged foods and raw vegan ice cream.

Nelson's Living Gourmet, Los Angeles; NelsonsLivingGourmet.com. Makes raw vegan burgers, pizzas, and other products sold at some stores in Los Angeles area. Nelson Tynes Chipman.

Nevermore Farm, nevermorefarm (at) gmail.com. Source for raw almonds.

New Leaf Community Market, 1210 41st Ave., Capitola, CA 95060; 831-479-7987; newleaf.com

Ocean Beach People's Organic Food Co-op, 4765 Voltaire St., San Diego, CA 92107-1733; 619-224-1387; OBPeoplesFood.coop. Large, busy, popular natural foods store.

118 Degrees, 2981 Bristol St., B5, Costa Mesa, CA 92626; Shop118Degrees.com. A full-service raw restaurant that also serves wine.

One Life Natural Foods, 3001 Main St., Santa Monica, CA 90405-5317; 310-392-4501. Organic juice bar inside store, and cold case with packaged raw salads, deserts, kombucha, etc. Two blocks to beach.

Open Source Organics, 7107 Sunset Blvd., LA, CA 90046; OpenSourceOrganics. Grab-n-go café. Juices, smoothies, deserts, simple raw vegan meals. Small patio area.

Optimum Natural Foods, 633 Trancas St., Napa, CA 94558-3084; 707-224-1514

Other Avenues Community Food Store, 3930 Judah St., San Francisco, CA 94122-1121; 415-661-7475; OtherAvenues.org. Very raw friendly natural foods store. Next to Judalicious, a raw and vegan cafe. Short walk to beach.

Patti Jane's Raw Cuisine, Pacific Grove, CA , 93950; pjsrawcuisine.com.

PC Greens, 22601 PCH, Malibu, CA 90265; 310-456-0353. This is a natural foods market that sells some raw food items.

Peace Pies, 4230 Voltaire St., Ocean Beach, CA 92107; peacepies.com. Raw vegan café.

Planet Earth Eco Café, 509 Pier Ave., Hermosa Beach, CA 90254; planetearthecocafe.com

Planet Raw, 6th & Broadway, Santa Monica, CA 90401; PlanetRaw.com. Raw restaurant started by chef and author Jimmy Juliano Brotman.

Premier Organics, 2342 Shattuck Ave., #342, Berkeley, CA 94704; 510-875-2146; premierorganics.org. Produces Artisana nut butters, coconut spreads, and other raw foods.

Que Se Raw Se Raw, 1160 Capuchino Ave, Burlingame, CA 94010; 650-400-8590; QueSeRawSeRaw.com. Raw café. Monday - Friday 10am - 4pm, Saturdays 10am - 2pm, Sundays closed. Alicia Parnell. Next to Earthbeam natural foods store. When the café is closed, the packaged foods can be purchased at Earthbeam.

Questa Food Co-op, 745 Francis St., San Luis Obispo, CA 93401; 805-544-7928

Rainbow Acres Market, 13208 W. Washington Blvd, L.A. (Marina del Rey), CA 90066; 310-306-8330. Large, rambling, busy indie natural foods store. Helpful staff.

Rainbow Bridge Market, 211 E. Matilija St., Ojai, CA 93023; 805-646-4017; RainbowBridgeOjai.com. Natural foods store centrally located in this charming little liberal town in the hills. Small deli café with interior and exterior seating.

Rainbow Grocery Market, 1745 Folsom St., San Francisco, CA 94103-3711; 415-863-0620; RainbowGrocery.coop. Large and busy worker-owned co-op natural foods and general kitchen store with lots of raw bulk items.

Raw Café Muse, UCB Art Museum, 2625 Durant Ave., Berkeley, CA 94720; 510-548-4366. RawCafeMuse.com

Raw Daddy, Corporate office: 33 Baytree Way, San Mateo, CA 94402; 650-280-9412. rawdaddyfoods.com. rawdaddy.blogspot.com. Not a restaurant. Sells raw food with a "fast food concept" at the Sunnyvale Farmers' Market on Saturdays from 9:00am to 1:00pm, and other locations. James Hall.

Raw Done Tastefully, Marina del Rey, CA; RawDoneTastefully.com. Raquel Smith teaches raw food courses.

Raw Energy, 2050 Addison, Berkeley, CA 94704; 510-665-9464. Between Shattuck and Milvia.

Raw Food Central, RawFoodSebastopol.com. Kathryn Ackland. Classes, meetings, events.

RawPeople.com, 6352 Corte Del Abeto, Ste. H, Carlsbad, CA 92011; rawpeople.com. An online raw foods store.

Raw Star Café, 306 Pico Blvd., Santa Monica, CA 90407; Bryan Au, proprietor. RawBryan (at) Hotmail.com.

Real Food Daily, 514 Santa Monica Blvd., Santa Monica, CA 90401; 310-451-7544; realfood.com. Organic heated vegan cuisine with some raw items on menu, including fresh juices. Mostly cooked food with heavy reliance on tofu and seitan.

Real Food Daily, 414 N. La Cienega Blvd., Los Angeles, CA; 310-289-9910; realfood.com. Organic heated vegan cuisine with some raw items on menu, including fresh juices. Mostly cooked food with heavy reliance on tofu and seitan.

Real Raw Live, 5913 W. Franklin, Hollywood, CA 90028 (Hollywood); 866-563-4545; RealRawLive.com. To-go juice bar with some to-go packaged raw foods along with nutritional supplements that aren't so raw. Next to Bourgeois Pig Coffee House.

Rejuice, 3238 Pico Blvd., Santa Monica, CA 90405. Next to Trader Joe's. Juice bar. Owned by actress Elisabeth Rohm.

Sacramento Natural Foods Co-op, 1900 Alhambra Blvd., Sacramento, CA 95816; 916-455-2667

Santa Barbara Certified Farmers' Markets, sbfarmersmarket.org/events.php

Santa Monica Farmers' Market, Arizona at 3rd, Wednesdays. While there are a variety of farmers' markets in Santa Monica, the largest by far is this one on Wednesday mornings that takes up four city blocks. A smaller version takes place at the same location on Saturday morning. On Sunday there is the Main Street Farmers' Market at Ocean Park Blvd., which is festive with live music.

Santa Rosa Community Market, 1899 Mendocino Ave., Santa Rosa, CA 95401-3628; 707-546-1806; srcommunitymarket.com

Seed Restaurant, Santa Rosa, CA; SeedRestaurant.com. Raw vegan restaurant planned.

Shojin, 333 S. Alameda St., St. 310, Los Angeles, CA 90013-1735; 213-617-0305. Organic Japanese vegetarian café with some raw items.

Silverlake Juice Bar, 2813 W. Sunset Blvd., L.A., CA 90026.

Smiling Dog Yoga Vegan Café, 1227 Archer St., San Luis Obispo, CA 93401; 805-546-9100; smilingdogyogaslo.com.

S&S Produce, 1924 Mangrove Ave., Chico, CA 95926-2340; ssproduce.net.

Staff of Life Groceries, 1266 Soquel Ave., Santa Cruz, CA 95062; 831-423-8632; staffoflifemarket.com

Stanford Inn, Raven's Restaurant, Coast Hwy. and Comptche Ukiah Rd., Mondocino, CA 95460; stanfordinn.com. Mostly vegan restaurant with some raw options.

Sun Cafe, 3711 W. Cahuenga Blvd., Studio City, CA 91604; 818-308-7420; suncafe.com. Sells supplies and premade items. Mostly a grab-n-go location. Next to the politically active KPFK 90.7 radio station. Two doors down is Mollie Angelheart's raw, vegan ice cream parlor.

The Sunflower Café, 1435 N McDowell Blvd., Ste. 100, Petaluma, CA 94954; TheSunFlowerCenter.org. Lydia Kindheart. Opened 2012. Lydia is known for her packaged foods, Lydia's Organics.

Sunrise Natural Foods, 2160 Grass Valley Hwy., Auburn, CA 95603; 530-888-8937; sunrisenaturalfoods.net

Sunrise Natural Foods, 1950 Douglas Blvd., Roseville CA, 95661; sunrisenaturalfoods.net

Sunshine Health Foods, 415 Morro Bay Blvd., Morro Bay, CA 93442; 805-772-7873

Thrivin' Edibles, 1600 Dell Ave, Campbell, CA 95008; 408-712-5000; ThrivinEdibles.com. Raw food catering, take-out, and delivery. Patti Searle.

212 Pier Coffee House, 212 Pier, Santa Monica. Coffee house that also has raw chocolate and kombucha and organic teas. Not all vegetarian. Free WiFi. Open 24 hours. Owns Main Squeeze juice bar on Main Street a few blocks away.

Ukiah Natural Foods, 721 South State St., Ukiah, CA 95482-5815; 707-462-4778; UkiahCoop.com

Vardo, 235 Main St., Venice, CA; 310-664-9696. Vegan Mediterranean, some raw on menu. Women like the Latin guy who runs the place, he's a raw dish too.

Vegan Traders, POB 330, Santa Monica, CA 90406; vegantraders.com. A distributor of raw food products to natural foods stores around Southern California. Risa Freeman.

Vegetable Delight Restaurant, Raw Vegan Fusion Bar, 17823 Chatsworth St., Granada Hills, CA 91344; RawSheedsFusionChef.com; VegetableDelight.com. Chef Rawsheed opened this in February 2013.

Veggie Vibes, San Diego; VeggieVibes.net. Gourmet raw vegan and cooked vegan food delivery by Perkunas, who grew up in Peru.

WE Juice for Joy Experience, TheWEConference.com. Kaci Christian, founder, leads quarterly 10-day juice fasting and teleclass with Chef Xian. The WE Conference is a women's empowerment organization base on compassionate principles that promotes health, wellness, compassion, love and peace via plant-based nutrition.

Weyu Le, weyu-le.com. weyule.net. Erica. Makes raw vegan cheeses and ice cream.

The Whole Wheatery Natural Foods Store, 44264 North 10th St. W, Lancaster, CA 93534; 661-945-0773; thewholewheatery.com

Wildberries Marketplace, 747 13th St., Arcata, CA 95521; 707-822-0095; wildberries.com

Jason Wroble, Los Angeles, CA, USA; jasonwrobel.com/jw; 310-383-0445; mintcreativity (at) gmail.com. Event catering.

Vital Heat, 326 Lincoln, Venice, CA 90291; VitalHotSauce.com. Jonathan Snell makes organic raw hot sauce by hand.

Zephyr Vegetarian Café, 340 E. Fourth St., Long Beach, CA 90802; 562-435-7113. Mostly organic, vegetarian restaurant with some raw food items on menu.

• U.S. COLORADO

Check MeetUp.com for raw food meetups.

Amazing Grace Organic Grocery, 213 Lincoln Ave., Breckenridge, CO 80424; 970-453-1445

Boulder Farmers' Market, Boulder, CO. Saturdays 10 am-2pm; Wednesdays 4-8 pm, 13th St. between Arapahoe and Canyon.

Durango Natural Foods, 575 E 8th Ave., Durango, CO 81301; 970-257-8129; DurangoNaturalFoods.com. Market.

First Bite Kitchen, FirstBiteKitchen.com. A helpful Web site. Also offers seminars, classes, dinners. A raw kitchen sharing a space with Dental Health of Boulder. Focus on a pH balanced diet.

Fort Collins Food Co-op, 250 East Mountain Ave., Fort Collins, CO 80524; 970-484-7448; FTCFoodCoop.com

Freshies, 34500 Hwy. 6, Edwards, CO 81632; Freshies.us. Raw food café and delivery.

Hardin's Natural Foods, 31424 Hwy. 92, Hotchkiss, CO 81419; 970-872-3019; hardinsnaturalfoods.com

High Plains Food Co-op, 7900 E Union Ave., Ste 200, Denver, Colorado 80237 80111; highplainsfood.org

Huajatollas Food Co-op, 106 County Road 632, Gardner, CO 81040; 719-746-2314

Leaf, 2010 16th St, Boulder, CO 80302; LeafVegetarianRestaurant.com. Some cooked, some raw vegan and vegetarian. Tom Warnke.

Bridgette Mars, BrigitteMars.com. Chef and author in Boulder, Colorado

Mountain People's Co-op, 30 E. First St., POB 161, Nederland, CO 80466; 303-258-7500

Nature's Oasis Market, 300 S. Camino Del Rio, Durango, CO 81301; 970-247-1988; shopnaturesoasis.com

Pachamama Organic Farm, 10771 N 49th St, Longmont, CO 80503; PachaMamaFarm.com. Freshly-picked produce. Culbertson family

Raw Denver, RawDenver.com; info (at) rawdenver.com. Has information about various Colorado raw foods groups, including Raw Utopia, Boulder Raw, and meetup groups in Boulder, Fort Collins, and Colorado Springs.

Raw Heavens, 1309 E. 3rd Ave., Durango, CO 81301. Food, juice bar, and some packaged foods.

Sammy's Organics, 830 Arcturus Dr., Colorado Springs, CO 80905; 719-471-3348; sammysorganics.com

Tasty Harmony, 130 Mason St., Ft. Collins, CO 80521; 970-689-3234; tastyharmony.com. Jill Steinhauser. Mostly vegan. High percentage of raw foods, including fresh-made nut cheeses, nut milks, deserts, and entrees.

Three Little Figs, Boulder, CO; ThreeLittleFigs.com. Vegan information.

Turtle Lake Refuge, 848 E. 3rd Ave., Durango, CO 81301; 970-247-8395; TurtleLakeRefuge.org. Katrina Blair.

Valley Food Co-op, 3211 Main St., Ste. G, Alamosa, CO 81101; 719-589-5727; ValleyFoodCoop.com

• U.S. CONNECTICUT

Check MeetUp.com for raw food meetups.

Alchemy Juice Bar, 203 New Britain Ave., Hartford, CT 06106; 860-246-5700; AlchemyJuiceBar.com. Imani and John.

Catch A Healthy Habit Café, 39 Unquowa Rd., Fairfield, CT 06824-5015; 203-292-8190; catchahealthyhabit.com; Glen Colello

Chester Sunday Market, 23 Main St, Chester, CT 06412; chestersundaymarket.com. Farmers' market. Summer through autumn.

Citrus Juice Bar Café, 27 Broadway Ave., Mystic, CT 06355; citrus-juice-bar.com.

Garden of Light Natural Foods, 2856 Main St., Glastonbury, CT 06033; 860-657-9131

Garden of Light Natural Foods, 395 W. Main St., Avon, CT 06001; GardenOfLight.net

Garden of Light Natural Foods, 375 Park Ave., East Hartford, CT 06108

Health in a Hurry, 1891 Post Rd., Fairfield, CT 06824; healthinahurry.net. Some raw on menu.

The Stand Juice Company, 31 Wall St., Norwalk, CT 06850; 203-956-5670; raw foods, salads, juices, smoothies; TheStandJuice.com

The Stand Juice Company, 87 Mill Plain Rd., Fairfield, CT 06824; TheStandJuice.com

Willimantic Food Co-op, 91 Valley St., Willimantic, CT 06226; 860-456-3611; WillimanticFood.coop

• U.S. DELAWARE

Check MeetUp.com for raw food meetups.

Good Earth Market & Organic Farm, 31806 Good Earth Ln., Clarksville, DE 19970; GoodEarthMarket.com

Harvest Market Natural Foods, 7417 Lancaster Pike, Hockesisn, DE 19707; HarvestMarketNaturalFoods.com.

Mona's Health Foods, 1802 Marsh Rd., Wilmington, DE 19810

Nature's Way, 74 E Glenwood Ave., Smyrna, DE 19977-1002

Newark Natural Foods Cooperative, 280 E Main St., Ste. 105, Newark, DE 19711; 302-368-5894; NewarkNaturalFoods.coop

Open Cupboard Natural Food, 202 High St., Seaford, DE 19973

Rainbow Earth Foods, 220 Rehoboth Ave., Rehoboth Beach, DE 19971-2134; RaonbowEFoods.com

• U.S. DISTRICT OF COLUMBIA, WASHINGTON

Check MeetUp.com for raw food meetups.

Elizabeth's Gone Raw; Elizabethsgoneraw.com. Raw vegan restaurant. Elizabeth Petty

Everlasting Life Market, 2928 Georgia Ave., NW, Washington, DC 20001; 202-232-1700; EverlastingLife.net. Vegan.

Java Green Organic Eco Café, 1020 19th St., NW, Washington, DC 20036; javagreen.net. More and more raw food items keep appearing on their expanding menu.

The Juice Joint, 1025 Vermont Ave NW, Washington D.C., DC 20005; juicejointcafe.com.

Khepra's Raw Food Juice Bar, 402 H St. NE, Washington, DC 20002; KhepraRawBar.com

Secrets of Nature Restaurant, 3923 S. Capitol St., SW; Washington, DC; 202-562-0041; secretsofnaturehealth.com. Vegan restaurant with both cooked and raw food on menu.

Senbeb Natural Food Co-op, 6224 3rd St NW Map.38e0e06

Washington, DC 20011 5922 Georgia Ave., NW, Washington, DC 20011; 202-723-5566. Specializes in vegan and vegetarian food with a raw food presence, including in their bulk foods, deli, and juice bar.

Wellness Cafe, 325 Pennsylvania Ave. SE, Washington, DC 20003; 202-543-2266; wellnesscafedc.com. Variety of vegan and vegetarian foods, including fresh smoothies.

Yes Organic Market, 1825 Columbia Rd., NW, Adams Morgan, Washington, DC 20009; 202-462-5150; yesorganicmarket.com.

Yes Organic Market, 3809 12th St., NE, Brookland, Washington, DC 20017; 202-546-9850; yesorganicmarket.com.

Yes Organic Market, 658 Pennsylvania Ave., SE, Capital Hill, Washington, DC 20003; 202-546-9850; yesorganicmarket.com.

Yes Organic Market, 3425 Connecticut Ave., NW, Cleveland Park, Washington, DC 20008; 202-363-1559; yesorganicmarket.com.

• U.S. FLORIDA

Check MeetUp.com for raw food meetups.

Ada's Natural Foods Market, 4650 South Cleveland Ave., Ft. Meyers, FL 33907; 239-939-9600; adasnatural.com

Amelia Island Organics, 436 N. Fletcher Ave., Fernandina Beach, FL. 32034; OrganicCoop.com/Amelia. All organic produce buying club. Contact: Trey Abernethy.

Boca Raton Green Market, Royal Palm Place, at South Federal Hwy & South Mizner Blvd., Boca Raton, FL 33432. Weekly farmers' market.

Café 118, 153 East Morse Blvd., Winter Park, FL 32789; 407-389-2233; cafe118.com. Living foods restaurant and juice bar.

Choices Café, 379 SW 15th Rd., Miami, FL 33129; MyChoicesCafe.com. Vegan, raw.

Christopher's Kitchen, 4783 PGA Blvd., Palm Beach Gardens, FL 33418; 561-318-6191; ChristophersKitchenFL.com. Christopher Slawson. Opened 2011.

Coconut Grove Farmers Market, 3300 Grand Ave, Miami, FL 33133; GlaserOrganicFarms.com/market.html. Presented by Glaser Organic Farms.

Darbster Vegetarian Restaurant, 8020 South Dixie Hwy., West Palm Beach, FL 33405; Darbster.com. Lake Worth raw food MeetUp group meets here.

Deer Run Bed & Breakfast, 1997 Long Beach Rd., Big Pine Key, FL 33043; deerrunfloridabb.com. A vegan bed & breakfast hotel.

Dining In The Raw, 800 Olivia St., Key West, FL 33040. 305-295-2600. Vegetarian, vegan and raw dishes. Rita Romano, author of *Dining in the Raw.*

Essentials For Life Market, 2106 Flora Ave., Ft. Myers, FL 33907; 239-939-2529; MyEssentialsForLife.com.

Ethos Vegan Kitchen, 1235 N. Orange Ave., Ste. 101; Orlando, FL 32804; ethosvegankitchen.com. Vegan, cooked and raw.

Ever'man Natural Foods Market, 315 W. Garden St., Pensacola, FL 32502; 850-438-0402; Everman.org.

Food and Thought, 2132 Tamiami Trail North, Naples, FL; FoodAndThought.com. Organic produce. They own a farm where they grow some of what they sell. It isn't a vegetarian store. But, in addition to fresh, organic produce, they have some packaged raw food and some raw food options in their deli.

Food Without Fire, Miami Beach, FL; 305-674-9960; Email: sunshine_ph (at) hotmail.com.

The Garden, Shoppes of Lake Village, Hwy. 441, Leesburg, Florida; 352-314-0909. Inside My Father's Garden natural foods store.

Glaser Organic Farms, 19100 SE 137th Ave., Miami, FL 33177; 305-238-7747; GlaserOrganicFarms.com. They also offer food preparation classes, and they have a weekly raw street market, Green Market, on Saturday.

Grass Root Organic Catering, POB 853, Tampa, FL; TheGrassRootLife.com. Spencer and Sabrina.

Green Wave Café, 5221 West Broward Blvd., Plantation, FL 33317; GreenWaveCafe.org. Lisa Valle is a graduate of Cherie Soria's Living Light Culinary Institute in Fort Bragg, California.

Happy Healthy Human, 1869 South Patrick Drive, Indian Harbour Beach, FL 32937; happyhealthyhuman.com. HappyHealthyHuman (at) gmail.com. Raw café. Organic produce. Owner: Jason Santini.

Help Yourself Foods, 829 Fleming St., Key West, FL 33040

Hippocrates Institute, 1443 Palmdale Court., W. Palm Beach, FL 33411; 561-471-8876; HippocratesInst.com. This is a health retreat center rooted in the teachings of the late Dr. Ann Wigmore.

Jessica's Organic Farm, 4180 47th, Sarasota, FL 34235; jessicasorganicfarm.com

Juice Therapy Café, 8220 Griffin Rd., Davie, FL 33328. Opened 2011.

Kissimmee Organic Co-op, 4830 Lake Cecile Dr., Kissimmee, FL 34746; 407-870-9839. Market.

Le Bistro De Vie, 353 Plaza Dr #2, Eustis, FL, 32726. Opened 2010.

La Vie En Raw Café, 3808 SW 8th St., Coral Gables, FL 33134; 305-444-3826; lavieenrawcafe.com; info (at) lavieenrawcafe.com. Opened in 2010. Also offers chef training. Sabina Torrieri.

Leafy Greens Café, 1431 Central Ave., St. Petersburg, FL 33705; 727-289-7087; LeafyGreensCafe.com; Denise (at) LeafyGreensCafe.com.

Lifefood Gourmet, 1248 SW 22nd St., Miami, FL 33145; 305-856-6767, Lifefoodgourmet.com. All raw. John Schott, proprietor.

Little River Co-op, 3218 Palmetto Rd., Wimauma, FL 33598; 702-995-1092; Market.

Live Food Experience, LiveFoodExperience.com. Raw food chefiing and training by Adam Graham.

Mayat's Healthy & Easy Recipes, Miami, FL 33168; mayatshealthyrecipes.com. Yoga, raw food, and positive lifestyle coaching.

Natural Food Co-op, 14750 M.L.K. Blvd., Dover, FL 33527; 813-659-0349. Market.

Nature's Acre, naturesacre.com. This isn't a restaurant. But a small farm planted with a wide variety of fruiting trees, tropical and subtropical edible plants, and some vegetables. They hold potlucks and full moon gatherings.

Nuage Café, 5903 W. Hillsboro Blvd., Parkland, FL 33067; nuagecafe.org. Organic, raw. Theirry Brouwers, owner.

Organica Food Co-op, 470 2nd St. N, Ste. C, Safety Harbor, FL 34695; 727-804-7229

The Organic Jungle Restaurant, 2500 N Highway A1A, Indialantic, FL 32903; JungleOrganic.com; 321-773-5503. Organic food in organic market. Dinner, lunch, and Sunday brunch.

The Present Moment Cafe, 224 W. King St., St. Augustine, FL 32084-4144; 904-827-4499; ThePresentMomentCafe.com. Yvette and Nathan Schindler

Raw Food Underground, Lake Worth, FL; RawFoodUnderground.com

Rawkstar Café, 32522 U.S. Hwy. 19 N, Palm Harbor, FL 34683; RawkStarCafe.com. Adam and Karen.

Rawsome Eats, Boynton Beach, FL; RawsomeEats.com.

Robert Is Here Fruit Stand, 19200 SW 344th St, Homestead, FL 33034; RobertIsHere.com. Robert started his stand when he was a child. Now he owns a farm. Good place to get fruit.

Shakti Life Kitchen, POB 331874, Atlantic Beach, FL 32233; shaktilifekitchen.com. Valerie.

Souther's Natural Food Co-op, 14750 Martin Luther King Jr. Blvd., Dover, FL; 813-659-0349

Sublime Restaurant, 1431 N. Fed. Hwy., Ft. Lauderdale, FL 33304; 954-539-9000; SublimeVeg.com. Some raw.

The Sugar Apple, 917 Simonton St., Key West, FL 33040; sugarapplekeywest.com. Natural foods store with a vegan café.

Sunseed Food Co-op, Inc., 6615 N. Atlantic Ave., Cape Canaveral, FL 32920; 321-784-0930; SunseedFoodCoop.com. Market.

Thrive, 1239 Alton Rd., Miami Beach, FL, 33139; ThriveVegan.com. A mostly raw café.

Vida de Café, 120 8 Ave., St. Pete Beach, FL 33706; vidadecafe.com. Vegan and raw cuisine.

Vitality Bistro, 301 N. Baker St., #106, Mount Dora, FL 32757Mr. Dora, FL; VitalityBistro.com. Closed Sunday and Monday. Opened in 2012. Tenanda Madhi, owner.

Zenergy Truck, ZenergyTruck.com. A mobile raw vegan restaurant.

• U.S. GEORGIA

Check MeetUp.com for raw food meetups.

Arden's Garden, 985 Monroe Dr. NE, Atlanta, GA 30308; ardensgarden.com. Juice and smoothies.

Arden's Garden, L5P, 1117 Euclid Ave., Atlanta, GA 30307; ardensgarden.com. Juice and smoothies.

Arden's Garden, buckhead, 3757 Roswell Rd. (near Johnny's Hideaway), Atlanta, GA 30342; ardensgarden.com. Juice and smoothies.

Arden's Garden, East Point, 3113 Main St, Atlanta, GA 30344; ardensgarden.com. Juice and smoothies.

Arden's Garden, Kirkwood, 2005 Hosea Williams Blvd., Atlanta, GA 30317; ardensgarden.com. Juice and smoothies.

Brighter Day Natural Foods, 1102 Bull St., Savannah, GA 31401; 912-236-4703; brighterdayfoods.com

Chef T, Atlanta, GA; superiorlifestyle.org. Chef T makes vegan and raw food. He caters, does private chefing, and provides total food services.

Daily Groceries Food Co-op, 523 Prince Ave., Athens, GA 30601; 706-548-1732.

Earth Fare, 1689 S. Lumpkin St., Athens, GA 30606; earthfare.com. Market.

Earth Fare, 368 Fury's Ferry Rd., Ste. 3, Martinez, GA 30907; earthfare.com. Market.

Garden of Eat'n Natural Foods Market, 140 S.W. Broad St., Jesup, GA 31545; 912-588-9696

Higher Ground Market, 2555 J Warren Road, Cornelia, GA 30531; 706-776-3488.

Island Natural Market, 204 Retreat Village, Saint Simons Island, GA 31522; 912-634-0394

Licious Dishes; e-liciousdishes.com. Raw food company.

Life Grocery Natural Food Co-op & Café, 1435 Roswell Rd., Marietta, GA 30062; 770-977-9583. LifeGrocery.com.

Living Food Delights, 465 Blvd SE, Ste. 201A, Atlanta, GA 30312; 404-635-1133

Loving It Live, 2796 E. Point St., E. Point, GA 30344; 404-765-9220; LovingItLive.com

Natural Marketplace, 69 North Main St., Jasper, GA 30143; naturalmarketplace.net

Nuts and Berries, 4274 Peachtree Rd., NE, Brookhaven, GA 30319; nutsnberries.com. Market. Small café with salads and vegan food.

Rainbow Grocery, 2118 N. Decatur Rd., Atlant, CA 30033; RainbowGrocery.com. Oldest organic market in Atlanta. Café with smome vegan and veggie food.

Return to Eden, 2335 Cheshire Bridge Rd., Atlanta, GA 30324; return2eden.com. Market. Some packaged and some fridge case raw foods.

R. Thomas Deluxe Grill, 1812 Peachtree St., NW, Atlanta, GA 30309; rthomasdeluxegrill.net. This place isn't vegan or vegetarian, but they have some vegan and vegetarian food, and, oddly enough, some raw food on the menu. They also have smoothies and juices.

Sevananda Food Co-op, 467 Moreland Ave. NE, Atlanta, GA 30307; 404-681-2831; Sevananda.coop.

Tassilis Raw Reality, 1059 R.D. Abernathy Blvd., Atlanta, GA 30310; tassilisrawreality.com

• U.S. Hawaii

Check MeetUp.com for raw food meetups.

Alive & Well Market 340 Hana Hwy., Kahului, Maui, HI 96732; 808-877-4950

Banyan Tree Santuary, 73-4464 Kohanaiki Rd., Kaulua Kona, Big Island, HI 96740; banyantreesanctuary.com. Healing sanctuary run by raw vegans. 3.3 acres, 200 fruit trees, organic carden, yoga, medication, workshops, massage. Contact: Raybo: iamrg51 (at) gmail.com

Blossoming Lotus Restaurant, 4504 Kukui St., Kaapa, Kauai, HI 96746; 808-822-7678; BlossomingLotus.com

Down to Earth, 525 South King Street, Honolulu, Hawaii 96826, Oahu; 808-947-7678; downtoearth.org

Down to Earth, 98 - 129 Kaonohi Street, Aiea, Hawaii 96701, Oahu; 808-488-1375; downtoearth.org

Down to Earth, 01 Hamakua Drive, Kailua, Hawaii 96734, Oahu; 808-262-3838; downtoearth.org

Down to Earth, 305 Dairy Rd, Kahului, Hawaii 96732, Maui; 808-877-2661; downtoearth.org

Down to Earth, 1169 Makawao Avenue, Makawao, Hawaii 96768, Maui; 808-572-1488; downtoearth.org

Greens & Vines Raw Vegan Restaurant, 909 Kapiolani Blvd., #8, Honolulu, HI 96814; e-licousdishes.com

Hawaiian Moons Natural Foods, 2411 S. Kihei Rd., Kihei, Maui, Hawaii; 808-875-4356; hawaiianmoons.com

Roger Haeske, RogerHaeske.com; LightningSpeedFit.com; PushUpBlaster.com

Kalani Oceanside Retreat, RR2 Box 4500, Pahoa, Big Island, HI 96778; kalani.com. South of the town of Pahoa, on the coast. This is not a restaurant, but is an intentional community that accepts paying guests that can stay in cabins with either shared or private rooms, or camp on the big lawn in a tent. It is very casual, like summer camp for adults. Several yoga rooms on different parts of the large property. Sunday dance church with DJs. Large pool that is clothing op after dinner. Sauna. Massage rooms staffed by MTs. Their community café is buffet with shared tables on large porch, often has raw items on the menu. Many yoga retreats are held here. Before your stay, notify them that you are a raw vegan, and they will be sure to accommodate your dietary choices.

Hoku Whole Foods, 951 Kipuni Way, Kapaa, HI; 808-821-1500; hokuwholefoods.com

Kokua Market Natural Foods Co-op, 2643 S. King St., Honolulu, HI 96826; 808-941-1922; kokua.coop.

Island Naturals Market & Deli, 303 Makaala St., Hilo, Hawaii 96720 (Big Island); 808-935-5533; islandnaturals.com.

Joy's Place 1993 South Kihei Rd., Kihei, Maui, HI 96753-7834; 808-879-9258

Mana Foods Market, 49 Baldwin Ave., Paia, Maui, HI 96779; 808-579-8078; ManaFoodsMaui.com. Raw items in deli.

Mandala Garden 29 Baldwin, Paia, Maui, HI 96779; 808-579-9500

Renee Loux Morgan, EuphoricOrganics.com. Chef, author, and TV personality who lives in Maui, Hawaii.

Papaya's Natural Foods, 4-831 Kuhio Highway Kapa'a, HI 96746 Kauai; 808-823-0190; papayasnaturalfoods.com

Papaya's Natural Foods, 5-5161 Kuhio Highway, POB 219, Hanalei, Kauai, HI 96714 (north shore location); 808-826-0089**;** papayasnaturalfoods.com. Store and café.

Pahoa Natural Foods Market, Kuna St., Big Island, HI 96778; 808-965-8322

• U.S. IDAHO

Check MeetUp.com for raw food meetups.

Boise Consumer Co-op, 888 W. Fort St., Boise, ID 83702; 208-472-4500; BoiseCoop.com. Market.

Capital City Public Market, N 8th St, Boise, ID 83702; CapitalCity{ublicMarket.com. Farmers' market. Seasonal.

Glow Live Food Café, 380 Washington Ave., #105, Ketchum ID 83340; 208-725-0314; opening summer 2008

Mercia's Natural Foods Market, 1511 Fillmore St. N., Twin Falls, ID; 208-734-0665; merciasnaturalfoods.com**.**

Moscow Food Co-op, 121 E. 5th St, Moscow, ID 83843; 208-882-8537; MoscowFood.coop. Market.

Mountain Nutrition Market, 6769 South Main, Bonners Ferry, ID; 208-267-3748

Nature's Nook Health Food Store, 160 E. Valley River Dr., Rexburg, ID; 208-356-5284

Pilgrim's Market Natural Foods Store, 1316 N. 4th St., Coeur d'Alene, ID 83814; 208-676-9730; pilgrimsmarket.com

Wealth of Health Natural Food Store, 1725 W. Broadway, Idaho Falls, ID 83401; 208-542-0015; wealthofhealthnutrition.com

• U.S. ILLINOIS

Check MeetUp.com for raw food meetups.

Borrowed Earth Café, 970 Warren Ave., Downers Grove, IL 60515; 630-795-1729; borrowedearthcafe.com; Raw and mostly organic. 30 minutes west of Chicago.

Chicago Diner 3411 N. Halsted, Chicago, IL 60657; 773-935-6696; VeggieDiner.Com. Vegan diner with some raw options.

Chowpatti, 1035 S, Arlington Heights Rd., Arlington Heights, IL 60005; Chowpatti.com. International vegetarian cuisine restaurant with raw options.

Common Ground Food Co-op, 1 Lincoln Sq. Village, Urbana, IL 61801; 217-352-2214; CommonGround.coop. Market.

Cornucopia Natural Foods, 89 S Seminary St., Galesburg, IL 61401; 309-342-3111

Duck Soup Co-op, 129 E. Hillcrest Dr., DeKalb, IL 60115; 815-756-7044; DuckSoupCoop.com.

Earth's Healing Café, 1942 West Montrose Ave, Chicago, IL 60613; EarthsHealingCafe.com. Organic raw vegan. Gluten- and wheat-free.

Fruitful Yield, 214 N. York Blvd., Elmhurst IL. Market.

Fruitful Yield, 130 West Golf Rd., Schaumburg, IL. Market.

Golden Pacific, 5252 N. Broadway, Chicago, IL; sells young coconut and some frozen exotic fruit

Go Raw Chicago, GoRawHaveFun.com. Site for raw food information in Chicago. Lenette Nakauchi.

Great Taste Café, 355 East Grand Avenue, Chicago IL 60611; gfreev.com. Organic, with some raw items on menu.

The Green Grocer, 1402 W. Grand, Chicago, IL 60622; 312-624-9508; GreenGrocerChicago.com

Green Spirit Living, Chicago, IL. Linda Szarkowsky is a graduate of Living Light Culinary Institute and teaches classes in raw food cuisine. Linda (at) GreenSpiritLiving.com.

In the Raw, 483 Central Ave., Highland Park, IL 60035; 847-432-9999; InTheRawHP.com. Co-ownders Matthew Kenny and Beth Taussig. Open 2012.

Karen's Fresh Corner, 1901 N. Halsted Ave., Chicago, IL 60614; 312-255-1590; KarynRaw.com

Neighborhood Co-op Grocery, 1815 W. Main St., Carbondale, IL 62901; 618-529-3533; Neighborhood.coop.

New Leaf Natural Grocer, 1261 W. Loyola Ave., Chicago, IL 60626; 773-743-0400; NewLeafNatural.net. Natural foods store with raw food products.

South Suburban Food Co-op, 21750 Main St., Matteson, IL 60433; 708-747-2256; SouthSuburbanFoodCoop.com

Straddle Creek Food Co-op, 112 Market St., West, Mt. Carroll, IL 61053; 815-244-2667

True Nature Health Foods, 6034 N. Broadway St., Chicago, IL 60660; 773-465-6400; TrueNatureFoods.com.

• U.S. INDIANA

Check MeetUp.com for raw food meetups.

Autumn Whispers Health Foods Store, 18 N. Indiana St., Mooresville, IN; 317-831-7817; autumn-whispers.com

Back to Basics Organic Market & Café, 1307 S. Heaton (Hwy. 35), Knox, IN; 574-772-2345; backtobasicsorganics.com

Bloomingfoods Market & Deli 3220 E. 3rd St., Bloomington, IN 47401; 812-336-5400; BloomingFoods.coop

Centre-In Food Co-op, 314 S. Main St., Goshen, IN 46526; 219-534-2355

Clear Creek Food Co-op, 701 West National Rd., Earlham, Richmond, IN 47374; 765-983-1547; ClearCreekCoop.org

Creekside Outpost Organic Café and Natural Foods Store, 614 Hausfeldt Ln., New Albany, IN 47150-2223; 812-948-9118; creeksideoutpost.com

Down to Earth Market, 14678 State Rd. 23, #A, Granger, IN; 574-271-1497

Georgetown Market, 4375 Georgetown Rd., Indianapolis, IN; 317-293-9525; georgetownmarket.com

Lost River Market & Deli, 26 Library St., Paoli, IN 47454; 812-723-3735; LostRiverCoop.com

Maple City Market, 314 S. Main St., Goshen, IN.

Paradise Organics Natural Food and Lifestyle Store, 2700 SR 261, Newburgh, IN 47630-8634; 812-842-0820; paradiseorganics.net

Plainfield Cooperative Buying Club, 8364 E. County Rd., 801 S., Plainfield, IN 46168; 317-834-1141

Rainbow Blossom Market, New Albany Market, 3003 Charlestown Crossing Way, New Albany, IN 47150; RainbowBlossom.com

Raw, Chicago French Market, 131 North Clinton St., Chicago, IL 60661; frenchmarketchicago.com. Carole Jones and Polly Gaza. Monday through Saturday. Indoor booth market.

River City Food Co-op, 116 Washington, Evansville, IN 47713; 812-423-1183; RiverCityFoodCoop.org

Three Rivers Food Co-op's Natural Grocery, 1612 Sherman St., Fort Wayne, IN 46808; 260-424-8812; 3RiversFood.coop

Yah's, 2347 E 75th St, Chicago, IL 60649; yahscuisine.com. Vegan, raw and cooked. Juices. Smoothies.

• U.S. Iowa

Check MeetUp.com for raw food meetups.

Everybody's Whole Foods, 501 N. 2nd St., Fairfield, IA; 641-472-5199; everybodyswholefoods.com

Fresh Café & Market, 1721 25th Street, #110, Des Moines, IA 50266; FreshCafeMarket.com. Smoothies, juice bar, food.

John's Natural Foods, 326 5th St., Ames, IA; 515-233-1280; johnsnaturalfoods.com

Mustard Seed Community Farm, 366 W Ave., Ames, IA 50014; mustardsedfarm.org. A CSA farm.

New Pioneer Co-op, 498 1st Ave., Coralville, IA 52241; 319-358-5513; NewPi.com.

New Pioneer Co-op, 22 South Van Buren St., Iowa City, IA 52240; 319-338-9441; NewPi.com.

Oneota Community Food Co-op, 415 West Water St., Decorah, IA 52101; 563-382-4666; oneotacoop.com

Wheatsfield Cooperative Grocery, 413 Douglas Ave., Ames, IA 50010; 515-232-4094; Wheatsfield.coop

• U.S. Kansas

Check MeetUp.com for raw food meetups.

Café Gratitude, 333 Soutwest Blvd., Kansas City, MO 64108; gratitudekc.com. The first Café Gratitude to open outside of California.

Community Mercantile, 901 Iowa St., Lawrence, KS 66044; 785-843-8544; TheMerc.coop. communitymercantile.com.

Prairieland Market, 138 S. 4th, Salinas, KS 67401; 785-827-5877

The Raw Body Twins, Susan and Stacey, POB 26311, Shawnee Mission, KS 66225-6311; TheRawBodyTwins.com. Raw food coaches and motivational life advisers.

Topeka Natural Food Coop, 503 SW Washburn Ave., Topeka, KS 66606; 785-235-2309; GeoCities.com/TopekaFoodCoop

• U.S. Kentucky

Check MeetUp.com for raw food meetups.

Amazing Grace Whole Foods and Nutrition Center, 1133 Bardstown Rd., Louisville, KY; 502-485-1122; amazinggracewholefoods.com

Bardstown Road Farmers' Market, 1722 Bardstown Rd, Louisville, KY 40205; bardstownroadfarmersmarket.com

Good Foods Market & Café, 455-D Southland Dr., Lexington, KY 40503; 859-278-1813; GoodFoods.coop

Green Apple Foods Store, 150 Raliegh Dr., Elizabethtown, KY; 270-982-7753

Heath Health Foods, 2006 Lone Oak Rd., Paducah, KY; 270-534-4977; heathhealthfoods.com

Healthy Alternative Natural, 7508 Mall Rd., Florence, KY 41042; 859-282-5888

Jing Masters, 3738 Lexington Rd., Louisville, KY 40207; jingmasters.com. Superfood elixir bar. Inside Rainbow Blossom.

Lexington Farmer's Market (Southland), 318 Southland Dr, Lexington, KY 40503; lexingtonfarmersmarket.com.

LifeBar, 3738 Lexington Rd., Louisville, KY 40207; LIfeBarLouisville.com

Otherworld Food Co-op, Inc., 1865 Celina Rd., Burkesville, KY 42717; 270-433-7400

Rainbow Blossom Market, St. Matthews Market, 3738 Lexington Rd., Louisville, KY 40207; 502-896-0189; RainbowBlossom.com

Rainbow Blossom Market, Middletown Market, 12401 Shelbyville Rd., Louisville, KY 40243; 502-244-2022; RainbowBlossom.com

Rainbow Blossom Market, Springhurst Market, 3608 Springhurst Blvd., Louisville, KY 40241; 502-339-5090; RainbowBlossom.com

• U.S. Louisiana

Check MeetUp.com for raw food meetups.

Charlestown Farmers' Market, 1001 Ryan St., Lake Charles, LA 70601

Columbia Street Natural Food Store, 415 N. Columbia St., Covington, Louisiana; 985-893-0355

Horn of Plenty Natural Food Store, 623 East Ascension St., Gonzales, Louisiana; 225-644-6080; hornofplenty.org

Oil Center Health Foods, 326 Travis St., Lafayette, Louisiana; 337-269-0144

Organically Yours Health and Natural Foods Store, 2901 Kaliste Saloom Rd., Lafayette, Louisiana; 337-989-1500

Out of Eden Health Market, 7007 Hwy. 182 E, Morgan City, Louisiana; 985-380-3155

Pure Foods & Health Natural Food Store, 138 W. Prien Lake Rd., Lake Charles, Louisiana; 337-905-7873; purefoodsandhealth.com

Sunshine Garden Health Food Store, 124 N. Jefferson Ave., Covington, Louisiana; 985-893-1463

Sunshine Health Foods Store, 3011 Airline Dr., Ste. E, Bossier City, Louisiana; 318-746-9788; sunshinehf.com

Sunshine Health Foods, 5751 Youree Dr., Shreveport, Louisiana; 318-219-4080; sunshinehf.com

Surrey's Café & Juice Bar, 1418 Magazine St., New Orleans LA 70130; SurreysCafeAndJuiceBar.com. Juices, wheatgrass.

Vegetarian Shop Health Food Store, 4201 W. Esplanade Ave., Metairie, Louisiana; 504-454-2306

• U.S. Maine

Check MeetUp.com for raw food meetups.

Aimee's Livin' Magic store, 254 Cider Hill Rd., York, ME 03909; 207-409-0899; AimeesLivinMagic.com

Belfast Co-op, 123 High St., Belfast, ME 04915; 207-338-2532; Belfast.coop

Blue Hill Co-op Community Market, 4 Ellsworth Rd., POB 1133, Blue Hill, ME 04614; 207-374-2165; BlueHill.coop

Fare Share Market, 443 Main St., Norway, ME 04268; 207-743-9044; FareShareCoop.org

Fresh off the Farm, 495 Commercial St., Rockport, ME 04856; 207-236-3260

Good Tern Natural Foods Co-op, 750 S. Main St., Rockland, ME 04841; 207-594-8822

Hampden Natural Foods, 108 Main Rd. South, Hampden, ME 0444; 207-862-2500; hampdennaturalfoods.com

The Juice Cellar, 9 beaver St., Ste. D, Belfast, ME 04915; TheJuiceCellar.com. Raw smoothies and juice bar, raw snacks, plus coffee and tea.

Maine Seaweed Co., POB 57, Steuben, ME 04680; 207-546-2875; alcasoft.com/seaweed. Source for raw seaweeds.

Morning Dew Natural Foods Grocery, 19 Sandy Creek Rd., Bridgton, ME 04009; 207-647-4003; morningdewnatural.com

One Earth Natural Food Store, 191 Emery Mills Rd., Shapleigh, ME 04076; 207-636-2500

Red Hill Natural Foods, 29 Hartford St., Rumford, ME 04276; 207-369-9141

Rising Tide Co-op, 15 Coastal Marketplace Dr., Damariscotta, ME 04543; 207-563-5556; RisingTide.coop

Royal River Natural Foods, 443 US Rte. 1, Freeport, ME 04032; 207-865-0046; rrnf.com

Uncle Dean's Good Grocery, 80 Grove St., Waterville, ME 04901; 207-873-6231; uncledeans.com

• U.S. Maryland

Check MeetUp.com for raw food meetups.

Bethesda Co-op, 6500 Seven Locks Rd., Cabin John, MD 20818; 301-320-2531

Cheverly Community Market, Cheverly Community Center, 6401 Forest Rd, Cheverly, MD 20785; CheverlyCommunityMarket.com. Farmers' market.

Common Market Co-op, 5728 Buckeystown Pike Unit 1-B, Frederick, MD 21704; 301-663-3416; CommonMarket.coop

David's Natural Market & Cafe, 5430 Lynx Ln., Columbia, MD 21044; 410-730-2304; davidsnaturalmarket.com

David's Natural Market & Cafe, 1523 – E Rock Spring Rd., Forest Hill, MD 21050; davidsnaturalmarket.com

David's Natural Market & Cafe, 871 Annapolis Rd., Gambrills, MD 21054; davidsnaturalmarket.com

Everlasting Life Healthfood Store; 9185 Central Ave., Capitol Heights, MD 20743-3845; 301-324-6900. Also has vegan and raw on café menu.

Glut Food Co-op, 4005 34th St., Mt. Rainier, MD 20712; 301-779-1978; Glut.org

Great Sage Restaurant, 5809 Clarksville Square Dr., Clarksville, MD 21029; 443-535-9400. Great-Sage.com. Organic vegetarian, with some raw items on menu.

Greenbelt Consumer Cooperative, 121 Centerway, Greenbelt, MD 20770; 301-474-0522

Liquid Earth Café, 1626 Aliceanna St., Baltimore, MD 21231; 410-276-6606; LiquidEarth.com. Vegetarian café, organic juices

Maryland Food Co-op, B-0203 Stamp Student Union University, College Park, MD 20742; 301-314-8089. Membership buyers club.

My Organic Market (MOMs), 6824 Race Track Rd., Bowie, MD 20715; myorganicmarket.com

My Organic Market (MOMs), 5273 Buckeystown Pike, Frederick, MD 21703; myorganicmarket.com

My Organic Market (MOMs), 7351 Assateague Dr., 190, Jessup, MD 20794; myorganicmarket.com

My Organic Market (MOMs), 11711 Parklawn Dr., Ste. B, Rockville, MD 20852; 301-816-4944; myorganicmarket.com

My Organic Market (MOMs), 9827 Rhode Island Ave., College Park, MD 20740; myorganicmarket.com

Natural Zing, 1851 Florence, Mt. Airy, MD; 301-703-4116; MAIL: Natural Zing, POB 749, Mount Airy, MD 21771; naturalzing.com. Lots of raw food items. Also have raw potlucks.

Ocean City Organics Inc., 11944 Ocean Gateway, Ocean City, MD 21842-9506; 410-213-9818. Food and green household items.

OK Natural Foods, 11 W. Preston St., Baltimore, MD 21201-5716; 410-837-3911

Purée Juice Bar, 4903 Elm St., Bethesda, MD 20804; PureeJuiceBar.com/hello.html. Organic juices and some raw foods.

Roots Market, 5805 Clarksville Sq. Dr., Clarksville, MD 21029; 443-535-9321; rootsmkt.com

Silver Spring Food Co-op, 8309 Grubb Rd., Silver Spring, MD 20910; 240-247-2667; silverspring.coop

Takoma Park Food Co-op, 201 Ethan Allen Ave., Takoma Park, MD 20912; 301-891-2667; TPSS.coop

Vegetable Garden, 11618 Rockville Pike, Rockville, MD 20852-2703; 301-468-9301; TheVegetableGarden.com. Vegan with some raw.

The Village Co-op, 2429 Saint Paul St., Baltimore, MD 21218; Baltimorevillage.org.

The Yabba Pot, 2433 St. Paul St., Baltimore, MD 21218-5125; 410-662-8638; TheYabbaPotCafe.com. Some raw menu items.

Zia's Café/Juice Bar/Catering, 13 Allegheny Ave., Towson, MD 21204; ziascafe.com; info (at) ziascafe.com. Daniela Troia, owner. Luke, manager. Smoothie, juice bar, café that also does catering and wholesale vegan and raw menu items. Their raw deserts and entrees are available at local natural foods stores. This is NOT an all vegan or an all vegetarian, or an all raw restaurant. Some meat served.

• U.S. MASSACHUSETTS

Check MeetUp.com for raw food meetups.

Chianti's Restaurant, 286D Cabot St., Beverly, MA 01915; 978-921-2233. Italian restaurant that serves raw food meals when customers call ahead first. Proprietor Richard Marino, is into raw food, and hosts raw dinners.

All the Best Natural Foods Store, 1 Pleasant St., Cohasset, MA 02025; 781-383-3005

Artichoke Food Co-op, 800 Main St., Worcester, MA 01610; 508-752-3533; ArtichokeCoop.org

Berkshire Co-op Market, 42 Bridge St., Great Barrington, MA 01230; 413-528-9697; BerkShireCoop.org

Common Sense Wholesome Food Market, 53 Main St., Plymouth, MA 02360; 508-732-0427; commonsensemarket.com

Cornucopia Foods Market, 150 Main St., #8, Northampton, MA 01060; 413-586-3800; CornucopiaFoods.net

Green Fields Market, 144 Main St., Greenfield, MA 01301; 413-773-9567; GreenFieldsMarket.coop.

The Greenhouse Natural Foods Market, 558 Summer St., Barre, MA; 978-355-3481

Green Street Natural Food, 164 Green St., Melrose, MA; 781-662-7741; greenstreetnaturalfood.com

Harvest Co-op Markets, 581 Massachusetts Ave., Cambridge, MA 02139; 617-661-1580; Harvest.coop

Harvest Co-op Markets, 57 South St., Jamaica Plain, MA 02130; 617-524-1667; Harvest.coop

Karma, 48 Main St, Northampton, MA 01060; bekarma.com. Vegetarian and vegan, cooked and raw available. Juices and elixirs. Also has massage studio.

Leverett Village Co-op, 180 Rattlesnake Gutter Rd., Leverett, MA 01054; 413-367-9794

The Living Earth Store & Café, 232-234 Chandler St., Worcester, MA 01609-2980; 508-753-1896; lefoods.com

Naked Earth A Whole Foods Market, 2655 Main St., Foster Sq., Brewster, MA; 508-896-5071; nakedearthmarket.com

Organic Garden Café, 294 Cabot St., Beverly, MA 01915; 978-922-0004;

Organic Rainbow, 267 Rantoul St., Beverly, MA 01915; 978-927-4600; theorganicrainbow.com

Other Side Cafe, 407 Newbury St., Boston, MA 02115-1801; 617-536-8437. Some raw items on menu.

Prana Café, 292 Centre St., Newton, MA 02458; 617-527-7726; thepranacafe.com. Down the street from Prana Power Yoga. Taylore and Phillipe.

Rawbert's Organic Café, 294 Cabot St., Beverly, MA. 978-922-0004; OrganicGardenCafe.com

Revitalive Health and Wellness, 128 High St., Newburyport, MA 01950; 978-462-1488. Quick-serve raw food cafe.

River Valley Market, POB 1245, Northampton, MA 01061; 802-722-4212; RiverValleyMarket.coop

Roots Natural Foods, 100 Crawfort St., Unit 7, Leominster, MA; 978-534-7668; rootsnaturalfoods.com

Roslindale Farmers Market, Boston, MA 02131; roslindale.net.

Second Nature, 15 Greenhalge St., Worcester, MA 01604; livesecondnature.com. Educational seminars, consultations, raw foods, and more. Kimberli A. Almonla. LiveSecondNature (at) Gmail.com.

Tropical Foods Supermarket, 2102 Washington St., Boston, MA 02119; TropicalFoods.net. Specialty store selling unusual foods from around the world.

Wild Oats Cooperative, 248 Main St., Route 2, Colonial Shopping, Williamstown, MA 01267; 413-458-8060

• U.S. MICHIGAN

Check MeetUp.com for raw food meetups.

Arbor Farms Market, 2103 W. Stadium, Ann Arbor, MI; 734-996-8111; arborfarms.com

Brighton Food Cooperative, 2715 West Coon Lake Rd., Howell, MI 48843; 517-546-4190

The Bulk Food Barn Buying Club, 3306 Flushing Rd., Flint, MI 48504; 810-720-9161

Cacao Tree Café, 204 W 4th St, Royal Oak, MI 48067; CacaoTreeCafe.com. Raw vegan menu. Gluten-free. Juices, smoothies, wheat grass, deserts. Also, soups and salads.

Cass Corridor Food Co-op, 456 Charlotte St., Detroit, MI 48201; 313-831-7452

Choice Foods Co-op, Royal Oak, MI 48073

Dibbleville Food Cooperative, Fenton, MI 48430

East Lansing Food Co-op, 4960 Northwind, East Lansing, MI 48823; 517-337-1266; ELFCo.coop

Flint Farmers' Market, 420 E Boulevard Dr, Flint, MI 48503; flintfarmersmarket.com

Green Tree Grocery Natural Foods Co-op, 214 N. Franklin, Mount Pleasant, MI 48858; 989-772-3221

Grain Train Natural Food Market, 220 E. Mitchell St., Petoskey, MI 49770; 231-347-2381; GrainTrain.coop

Hartland's Nutrition Connection Cooperative, 1898 Korte St., POB 530, Hartland, MI 48353; 810-632-7952

Hillsdale Family Food Co-op, 31 N. Broad, Hillsdale, MI 49242; 517-439-

1397

Inn Season Café, 500 East Fourth St., Royal Oak, MI 48067; 248-547-7965; theinnseasoncafe.com. Vegetarian/vegan with some raw options.

Ionia Natural Food Co-op, Healthy Basics 2, 576 State St., Ionia, MI 58846

Keweenaw Food Co-op, 1035 Ethel Ave., Hancock, MI 49930; 906-482-2030; Keweenaw.coop

Living Zen Organics, Detroit Zen Center, 11464 Mitchell St., Hamtramck, MI 48212; detroitzencenter.org/livingzen.htm. Info (at) detroitzencenter.org. Providing raw food Friday and Saturady. They also sell their raw products at Detroit Eastern Farmers' Market,, Ann Arbor Farmers' Market, Natural Food Patch in Ferndale, Goodwells in Detroit, and Harvest Health in Grand Rapids.

Marquette Food Co-op, 109 West Baraga Ave., Marquette, MI 49855; 906-225-0671; MarquetteFood.coop

New Territory Market Cooperative, 132 Water St., Benton Harbor, MI 49022; 616-926-9391

Northwind Natural Foods Co-op, 116 S. Suffolk St., Ironwood, MI 49938; 906-932-3547

Oryana Food Cooperative, 260 E. 10th St., Traverse City, MI 49684; 231-947-0191; Oryana.coop

People's Food Co-op & Café Verde, 214-216 N. 4th Ave., Ann Arbor, MI 48104; 734-994-9174; PeoplesFood.coop

People's Food Co-op of Kalamazoo, 436 Burdick St. S., Kalamazoo, MI 49007; 616-342-5686; PeoplesFoodCo-op.org

Rainbow Health Foods, 66783 Gratiot Ave., Richmond, MI 48062; 810-727-5475

The Raw Café, 4160 Woodward Ave. Detroit MI 48201; TheRawCafe.om. Corner of Willis Street.

Red Pepper Deli, 116 W. Main St., Northville, MI 48167; 248-773-7671; myspace.com/redpepperdeli. RedPepperDeli (at) Yahoo.com. Full menu organic raw food. Carolyn Simon

Royal Oak Farmers Market, 316 E 11 Mile Rd, Royal Oak, MI 48067; ci.royal-oak.mi.us/portal/community-links/farmers-market. Open all year.

Try It Raw Café, 213 East Maple Rd., Birmingham, MI 48009. Limited seating, mostly take-out concept.

Woodland Food Co-op, 116 N. Main St., Woodland, MI 48897; 616-367-4188

Ypsilanti Food Co-op and River Street Bakery, 312 N. River St., Ypsilanti, MI 48198; 734-483-1520

Zerbo's Health Foods Market, 34164 Plymouth Rd., Livonia, MI; 734-427-3144; zerbos.com

• U.S. Minnesota

Check MeetUp.com for raw food meetups.

Bluff Country Co-op, 121 W 2nd St., Winona, MN 55987; 507- 452-1815; Bluff.coop

Cook County Whole Foods Co-op, Box 813 / 20 E. 1st St., Grand Marais, MN 55604; 218-387-2503; Boreal.org/~foodcoop

Countryside Co-op, POB 262 Hwy. 371 South, Hackensack, MN 56452; 218-675-6865

Crow Wing Food Co-op, 823 Washington St., Brainerd, MN 56401; 218-828-4600; CrowWingFoodCo-op.com

Earth Foods TV, Minnesota, USA; EarthFoods.TV. Ryan. Source for scientifically / evidence-backed nutrition information on fruits, vegetables, sprouts, superfoods, sea vegetables, herbs, seeds, and the like. Sharing juicing recipes, smoothie recipes, testimonials, and videos. Also, EarthFoods on FaceBook.

Eastside Food Co-op, 2551 Central Ave., Minneapolis, MN 55418; 612-788-0950; EastSideFood.coop

Ecopolitan Restaurant, 2409 Lyndale Ave. S., Minneapolis, MN 55405; 612-874-7336; Ecopolitan.com. Raw vegan restaurant.

Everybody's Healthfood Market, 11 1st Street N., Long Prairie, MN 56347; 320-732-3900

Finland Cooperative, Box E, Main St., Finland, MN 55603; 218-353-7389

Good Earth Food Co-op, 2010 8th Street N Centenial Plaza, St. Cloud, MN 56303; 612-253-9290

Granary Food Co-op, 47 NW 2nd St., Ortonville, MN 56278; 320-839-6204

Harmony Food Co-op, 117 3rd St. NW, Bemidji, MN 56601; 218-751-2009; HarmonyCoop.com

Hampden Park Food Co-op, 928 Raymond Ave., St. Paul, MN 55114; 651-646-6686

Harvest Food Co-op, 137 East Front St., Owatonna, MN 55060; 507-451-0340

Just Food Co-op, 612 First Street West, Northfield, MN 55057; 507-650-0106; JustFood.coop

Kandi Cupboard, 412 Litchfield Ave. SW, Willmar, MN 56201; 320-235-9477

Lakewinds Natural Foods, 1917 2nd Ave. S., Anoka, MN 55303; 763-427-4340; LakeWinds.coop

Lakewinds Natural Foods, 435 Pond Promenade, Chanhassen, MN 55317; 952-697-3366; LakeWinds.coop

Lakewinds Natural Foods, 17523 Minnetonka Blvd., Minnetonka, MN 55345; 952-473-0292; LakeWinds.coop

Linden Hills Food Co-op, 2813 W 43rd St., Minneapolis, MN 55410; 612-922-1159; Lindenhills.coo

Mill City Farmers Market, Chicago Ave., Minneapolis, MN 55401; MillCityFarmersMarket.org.

Mille Lacs Area Food Co-op, Main Street, Isle, MN 56342; 320-676-3813

Mississippi Market Natural Foods Co-op, 1810 Randolph Ave., St. Paul, MN 55105; 651-690-0507; MSMarket.coop

Mississippi Market Food Co-op, 622 Selby Ave., St. Paul. MN 55104; 651-310-9499; MSMarket.coop

Moms Food Co-op, 1709 Hwy. 95 E, Cambridge, MN 55008; 763-689-4640

Natural Foods Co-op, 230 N. Sibley Ave., Litchfield, MN 55355; 320-693-7539

Natural Harvest Whole Food Co-op, 505 3rd Street N, Virginia, MN 55792;

218-741-4663; naturalharvest.virginiamn.com

North County Cooperative Grocery, 1929 S 5th, Minneapolis, MN 55454; 612-338-3110; NorthCountryCoop.com

Northwoods Whole Foods Co-op, 125 N. Central Ave., Ely, MN 55731; 218-365-4039

Oak Center General Store Food Co-op, Rt. 1 Box 52BB, Hwy. 63, Lake City, MN 55041; 507-753-2080

Plum Creek Food Co-op, 910 4th Ave., Windom MN 56101; 507-831-1882

Pomme De Terre Food Co-op, 613 Atlantic Ave., Morris, MN 56267; 320-589-4332; PDTFoods.org

Susan Powers, POB 184, Crystal Bay, MN 55323; RawMazing.com. Recipes and blog.

Pure Market Express, 500 N Chestnut St, Chaska, MN 55318**;** PureMarketExpress.com. Gluten-free, dairy-free, sugar-free, vegan, breakfast, lunch, dinner, desert.

Rainbow Food Co-op, 103 South Main St., Blue Earth, MN 56013; 507-526-3603

Raw Food Right Now, POB 22426, Eagan, MN 55122-0426, USA; rawfoodrightnow.com. This is a blog about raw food that is put together by Heidi and Justin Ohlander.

River Market Community Co-op, 221 N. Main St., Stillwater, MN 55082; 651-439-0366; RiverMarket.coop

Rochester Good Food Co-op, 1001 6th St., NW, Rochester, MN 55901; 507-289-9061; RochesterGoodFood.com

Spiral Food Co-op, 307 E 2nd St., Hastings, MN 55033; 651-437-2667

Seward Co-op Grocery & Deli, 2111 East Franklin Ave., Minneapolis, MN 55404; 612-338-2465; Seward.coop

St. Peter Food Co-op & Deli, 119 W. Broadway, St. Peter, MN 56082; 507-934-4880; StPeterFood.coop

Tao Natural Foods & Café, 2200 Hennepin Ave, Minneapolis, MN 55405**;** TaoNaturalFoods.com. Natural foods market, café, and juice bar.

Valley Natural Foods Co-op, 13750 County Road 11, Burnsville, MN 55337; 952-891-1212; ValleyNaturalFoods.com

Wedge Community Co-op, 2105 Lyndale Ave. S., Minneapolis, MN 55405; 612-871-3993; Wedge.coop

Western Prairie Food Co-op, 674 6th St., Dawson, MN 56232

Whole Foods Co-op, 610 E 4th St., Duluth, MN 55805; 218-728-0884; WholeFoods.coop

Wintergreen Food Coop, 1414 West Main St., Albert Lea, MN 56007; 507-373-0386

• U.S. MISSISSIPPI

Check MeetUp.com for raw food meetups.

Hitching Lot Farmers Market, N 2nd Ave & N 2nd St, Columbus, MS 39701. Seasonal since 1976.

Rainbow Whole Foods Co-op Grocery, Deli and Café, 2807 Old Canton Rd., Jackson, Mississippi 39216; 601-366-1602; RainbowCoop.org

Renaissance Natural Foods Store, 104 W. Railroad St., Long Beach, Mississippi; 228-865-9911

Whole Health Connection Natural Foods Store, 221 Williams Ave., Picayune, Mississippi 39466; 601-749-9831; wholehealthconnection.com

• U.S. MISSOURI

Check MeetUp.com for raw food meetups.

Asian Farmers' Market, 81st & Olive, University City, MO. For coconuts.

Bad Seed Farmers' Market, 1909 McGee St, Kansas City, MO 64108; badseedfarm.com. Seasonal farmers' market.

Biver Farms, Brett Palmier, organic farmer and Community Supported Agriculture: OrganicSales1 (at) earthlink.net

Clayton Farmers Market, North Central & Maryland Ave., Clayton, MO; Saturday mornings

Eden Alley Vegetarian Café, 707 W 47th St, Kansas City, MO 64112; edenalley.com. Vegetarian and vegan and raw menu.

Feral Foods, FeralFoods.org. Site for raw foodists in Missouri.

FuD, 813 W 17th St, Kansas City, MO 64108; eatfud.com. Vegan and organic. Opened April, 2010.

Mamma Jeans Market, 1110 E. Republic Rd., Springfield, MO 65807

Mamma Jeans Market, 1727 S. Campbell Ave., Springfield, MO 65807

Natural Way Market 8110 Big Bend Blvd., Webster Groves, MO 63139; 314-961-3541; TheNatWay.com

Natural Way Market 12345 Olive Blvd., Creve Coeur, MO 63141; 314-878-3001; TheNatWay.com

Natural Way Market 468 Old Smizer Mill Rd., Fenton, MO 63026; 636-343-4343; TheNatWay.com

Raw Food Basics, RawFoodBasics.com. Email: rawfoodbasics (at) yahoo.com. Terry Stiers, chef

Sappington Farmers' Market 8400 Watson Rd., St. Louis, MO 63119; SappingtonFarmersMkt.com

Soulard Farmers Market 730 Carrol St., St. Louis, MO 63104; 314-622-4180

VegaDeli, 177 Hilltown Village Ctr., Chesterfield, MO 63017; 307 & 309 Belt Ave., St. Louis, MO 63112; VegaDeli.com. Vegan deli with raw choices on menu. Kosher. Gluten free.

VegaDeli, 307 Belt Ave, St. Louis, MO 63112; vegadeli.com. Vegan and half raw. Kosher. Gluten free.

• U.S. MONTANA

Check MeetUp.com for raw food meetups.

Billy's Organic Food and Lifestyle Health Food, 818 South First, Hamilton, MT; 406-375-9909

Bitterroot Grocery Emporium, 200 Main St., Hamilton, MT; 406-363-2366; bitterrootgroceryemporium.com/store

Bonanza Health Foods Store, 923 Grand Ave., Billings, MT; 406-252-4923

Bozeman Community Food Co-op, 908 W Main St., Bozeman, MT 59715; 406-587-4039; Bozo.coop

Dancing Rainbow Natural Grocer, 9 S. Montana St., Butte, MT; 406-723-

8811

Food Works Natural Market, 412 East Park St., Livingston, MT; 406-222-8223

Good Earth Market, 3115 10th Avenue N, Billings, MT 59101; 406-259-2622

Good Food Store, 920 Kensington, Missoula, MT 59802; 406-728-5823

Good Food Store, 1600 S. 3rd St. West, Missoula, MT; 406-541-3663; goodfoodstore.com

Heart Rock Market Organic and Natural Foods, 321 W. Park Ave., Anaconda, MT; 406-563-5077

Mary's Health Foods, 2564 King Ave., W., Ste. J, Billings, MT; 406-651-0557; maryshealthfood.com

Montana Harvest Natural Foods Health Food Store, 31 S. Willson Ave., Bozeman, MT; 406-585-3777; montanaharvest.net

Mountain Valley Foods, 25 Commons Way, Kalispell, MT; 406-756-1422. Has organic juice bar.

Naturally Good Things Health Food Store, 313 California Ave., Libby, MT; 406-293-6771

Rainbow's End Natural Foods, 910 N. 1st St., Hamilton, MT; 406-363-1626

2 J's Produce, 105 Smelter Ave., NE, Great Falls, MT; 406-761-0134. Large bulk section. Organics and vegetarian food.

Withey's Health Foods, 1231 South Main, Kalispell, MT; 406-755-5260

• U.S. NEBRASKA

Check MeetUp.com for raw food meetups.

Affiliated Food Co-op, Inc., 13th St. & Omaha Ave., Norfolk, NB 68701; 402-371-0555

Chadron Natural Food Co-op, 218 Chadron Ave., Chadron, NB 69337

Happy Heart Specialty Foods, 301 S. Jeffers, North Platte, NB; 308-532-1505

Harvest Health Market and Daily Grind Coffee Shop, 419 N. Main St., Fremont, NB; 402-721-7031

Jane's Health Food, 6103 Maple St., Omaha, NB; 402-558-8911

Open Harvest Natural Foods Co-op, 1618 South St., Lincoln, NB 68502; 402-475-9069; OpenHarvest.com

Winnetoon Mall Co-op, 312 W. Main St., Winnetoon, NB 68789; 402-847-3368

• U.S. NEVADA

Check MeetUp.com for raw food meetups.

Atomic #7, 605 Mall Ring Cir, Henderson, NV 89014; atomicnumber7.com. Alternative ice cream parlor. Vegan options and raw made-to-order.

City of Las Vegas Farmers Market at Bruce Trent Park, 1600 N Rampart Blvd, Las Vegas, NV 89128; lasvegasfarmersmarket.com

Go Raw Café, 2910 Lake East Dr., Las Vegas, NV 89117; 707-254-5382; GoRawCafe.com

Go Raw Café, 2381 E. Windmill Way, Las Vegas, NV 89123; GoRawCafe.com

Great Basin Community Food Co-op, 271 Wonder St., Reno, NV; 775-324-6133; GreatBasinFood.coop

NatuRaw, POB 870, 257 S Moapa Blvd., Overton, NV 89040; NatuRaw.com. Raw products company

Pure Health Foods Store, 7575 W. Washington, #129, Las Vegas, NV 89128; 702-366-9297; purehealthfoodslv.com. Closed Sundays.

Radical Roots Cuisine, 1085 S. Virginia St., Reno, NV 89502; RadicalRootsCuisine.com. Has a Facebook page.

Rainbows End Health Foods, 1100 E. Sahara Ave., Las Vegas, NV 89104; 702-737-1338; rainbowsendlasvegas.com. Healthfood store with specialty raw foods, bulk foods, deli.

U B Raw Inc., 380 Bannock St., Mesquite, NV 89027; 702-346-5029; UBRaw.com; Email: info (at) UBRaw.com. Not a restaurant. Ronnie and Minh provide raw food training.

Vod Deli, 350 W Liberty St, Reno, NV 89501; 775-323-3000. Vegan organic deli

• U.S. NEW HAMPSHIRE

Check MeetUp.com for raw food meetups.

A-Market Natural Foods, 125 Loring St., Manchester NH 03103

Country Life Vegetarian Restaurant, 15 Roxbury St., Keene, NH 03431; 603-357-3975; some raw

Concord Cooperative Market, 24 South Main St., Concord, NH 03301; 603-225-6840; ConcordFoodCoop.coop

Co-Food Stores, coopfoodstore.coop/locations

Hanover Co-op Food Store, 45 South Park St., POB 633, Hanover, NH 03755; 603-643-2667; CoopFoodStore.com

Hanover Co-op: Lebanon, PO Box 633, Hanover, NH 03755; CoopFoodStore.com

Susty's Café, 159 First NH Turnpike, Rte. 4; Northwood NH 03621; 603-942-8425; SustysNorthwood.com. Vegan with some raw options, call first.

• U.S. NEW JERSEY

Check MeetUp.com for raw food meetups.

East Coast Vegan, EastCoastVegan.com

Veg New Jersey, VegNJ.com

Dean's Natural Food Market, 1119 State Rte. 35 N, Ocean, NJ 07712; 732-517-1515; deansnaturalfoodmarket.com

Dean's Natural Food Market, 490 Broad St., Shrewsbury, NJ 07702; DeansNaturalFoodMarket.com.

Energy Bar 307C Orange Rd., Montclair, NJ 07042; 973-746-7003; KHeperFoods.com. Raw food service company. Catering, food classes, packaged foods, demos services, private chefing.

George Street Co-op, 89 Morris St., New Brunswick, NJ 08901; 732-247-8280; GeorgeStreetCoop.com

Good Karma Café, 17 E Front St, Red Bank, NJ 07701**;** goodkarmacafenj.com**.** Raw and cooked vegan food, juices, smoothies, deserts.

Green Acres Health Foods, 1297 Centennial Ave., Piscataway, NJ; 732-562-9088; greenacreshealthfood.com

Healthfair, 625 Branch Ave., Little Silver, NJ 07739; healthfairvitamins.com. Produce and juice bar. Some prepared raw foods.

Healthworks Market, 786 Haddon Ave., Ste. A, Collingswood, NJ 08108-3739

In Good Taste Market, 1301 N Delsea Dr., Vineland, NJ 08360; 609-794-4856.

Kaya's Kitchen, 1000 Main St, Belmar, NJ 07719; kayaskitchenbelmar.com. Organic vegetarian with juice bar. Cooked with raw vegan options. Bohemian vibe. Some live music.

Nature's Corner Natural Market, 2407 Rte 71, Spring Lake Heights, NJ 07762; NaturesCornerNaturalMarket.com.

Organica Natural Foods, 246 Livingston St., Northvale, NJ; 201-767-8182; organicanaturalfoods.com

Purple Dragon Co-op Membership Buying Club, 289 Washington St., Glen Ridge, NJ; 973-429-0391; purpledragon.com

The Rainbow Garden Natural Café, 10 Bridge St., Ste. 6, Frenchtown, NJ; 908-996-2537. Organic vegan café. Lunch. Dinner. Smoothies. Deserts. Take-out.

Karen Ranzi, Ramsey, New Jersey; SuperHealthyChildren.com. Karen coordinates the New Jersey Raw Food Support Network. Karen (at) superhealthychildren.com

RawFullyTempting.com. Hillborough, NJ. "Online café."

Subia's Organic Market, 506 Jersey Ave, Jersey City, NJ 07302; 201-432-7639. Organic vegetarian and raw food, juice bar.

Sussex County Food Co-op, 30 Moran St., Newton, NJ 07860; 973-579-1882; SussexCountyFoods.org

• U.S. NEW MEXICO

Check MeetUp.com for raw food meetups.

Albuquerque Downtown Growers Market, Central Ave SW & 8th St SW, Albuquerque, NM 87102; ABQGrowersMkts.org. Farmers' market.

Body of Santa Fe, 333 Cordova Rd., Santa Fe, NM 87505; 505-986-0362. BodyOfSantaFe.com. Café. Some raw dishes.

Cid's Health Food Market, 623 Paseo Del Pueblo Norte, Taos, NM 87571; 505-758-1148; cidsfoodmarket.com

Down To Earth Nutrition Center Natural Foods Store, 102 N. Missouri Ave., Roswell, NM 88203; 505-623-4883; dtehealth.com

La Montanita Food Co-op: Central, 3500 Central SE Nob Hill Shopping Ctr., Albuquerque, NM 87106; 505-265-4631; LaMontanita.coop

La Montanita Food Co-op: Gallup, 105 E. Coal Ave., Gallup, NM 87301; 505-863-5383; LaMontanita.coop

La Montanita Food Co-op: Santa Fe, 913 West Alameda, Santa Fe, NM 87501; 505-984-2853; LaMontanita.coop

La Montanita Food Co-op: Valley, 2400 Rio Grande Blvd. NW, Albuquerque, NM 87104; 505-242-8800; LaMontanita.coop

Mountain View Market, 1300 El Paseo Road South, Suite M, Las Cruces, NM 88001; 505-523-0436; mountainviewmarket.com.

Raw Soul, Santa Fe, NM. RawSoul.com. Lillian Butler and Eddie Robinson. Formerly owned a restaurant in New York City.

Raw To Go, 105-B Quesnel St., Taos, NM 87571. Behind Rellenos Café. Taamer Fasheh.

Raw Vegan for Life, 2023 Calle Perdiz, Santa Fe, NM 87505; SantaFeLivingFoods.com

Santa Fe Farmers' Market, 1607 Paseo De Peralta, Santa Fe, NM. Saturday 8 am-12 noon.

Semilla Natural Foods, 510 University Ave., Las Vegas, NM 87701-4349; 505-425-8139

Silver City Food Co-op, 520 N Bullard St., Silver City, NM 88061; 505-388-2343; SilverCityFoodCoop.com

Toucan Market, 1701 #1 E. University, Pan Am Plaza, Las Cruces, NM 88001; 505-521-3003; toucanmarket.com

Vegan Santa Fe, 323 Mckenzie St., Santa Fe NM 87501; VeganSantaFe.com. Raw vegan. Also does cakes, pies, and deserts. Ships throughout 48 U.S.. Mariela (at) vegansantafe.com.

• U.S. NEW YORK

Check MeetUp.com for raw food meetups.

Abundance Cooperative Market, 62 Marshall St., Rochester, NY 14607; 585-454-2667; Abundance.coop

Angelica Kitchen, 300 E. 12th St., New York, NY 10003; 212-228-2909; AngelicaKitchen.com. Some raw dishes on menu.

Blossom Restaurant, 187 Ninth Ave. New York, NY 10011; 212-627-1144; blossomnyc.com. Organic vegan, with some raw items on menu. Between 21 St. and 22nd St..

Bob's Natural Foods, 104 W. Park Ave., Long Beach, NY 11561; 516-889-8955; BobsNaturalFoods.com

Boni-Bel Organic Farm Store, 301 Doansburg Rd., Brewster, NY 10509; 845-279-1090

Bonobo's Restaurant, 18 E. 23rd St., New York, NY 10010; 212-505-1200; BonobosRestaurant.com

Bonobo's Annex, 156 West 20th Street, NY, NY 10011-3603; BonbobosRestaurant.com

Café Blossom, 466 Columbus, New York, NY 10024-7407; 212-875-2600; blossomnyc.com. Also has Blossom Restaurant at 187 Ninth Ave., and Cafe Blossom East at 1522 1st Ave. Vegan cafe, not all raw.

Café Blossom East, 1522 1st Ave., New York, NY; 212-988-2221; blossomnyc.com. Also has Blossom Restaurant at 187 Ninth Ave., and Café Blossom at 466 Columbus. Vegan cafe, not all raw.

Cambridge Food Co-op, 1 West Main St., Cambridge, NY 12816; 518-677-5731; cambridgefoodcooop.com

Candle Café, 1307 Third Avenue at 75th St., New York, NY 10021; 212-472-0970; candlecafe.com. Some raw food.

Caravan of Dreams, 405 E. 6th St., New York, NY 10009; 212-254-1613; CaravanOfDreams.net. Vegan. "Extensive raw food options."

Commodities East, 165 1st Ave., New York, NY 10003; 212-260-2600. Natural foods market with produce section.

Community Co-op, 589 E. Albany St., Little Falls, NY 13365-1526; 315-823-0686

Counter Restaurant, 105 1st Ave., New York, NY 10003; 212-982-5870; CounterNYC.com. Vegetarian bistro, wine bar. Grows herbs and vegetables on rooftop garden.

Crown Heights neighborhood, Brooklyn, NY. West Indian stores selling tropical fruits. Especially in summer. Also holds an annual West Indian-American parade or carnival that attracts more than a million people.

Earth Matters, 177 Ludlow St., New York, NY 10002; 212-475-4180; earthmatters.com. Organic market and restaurant between Houston and Stanton. Not vegan. But some vegan and raw options.

Eat Raw, Brooklyn; 866-432-8729; eatraw.com. Online raw food and lifestyle information.

Esperance Co-op, Box 204 Rd. #1, Pattersonville, NY 12066; 518-864-5506

Essex Street Market, 120 Essex St., NY, NY; essexstreetmarket.com. Lower Eastside on Essex between Delancey and Rivington. Large indoor market with multi-ethnic foods in many booths. Some sell exotic fruits. Not all booths are vegan or vegetarian. Monday through Saturday. Closed Sunday.

Euphoria Loves Rawvulution (ELR) Café, 504 East 12th St., NY NY 10009. Opened summer 2011. Also has location in Santa Monica, California.

Exitic Superfoods, exoticsuperfoods.com

5C Café, 68 Ave. C, New York, NY 10009; 212-477-5993; 5culturalcenter.org. At 5th Street. Cultural center and café. Vegetarian food, with some raw.

Flatbush Food Cooperative, 1318 Cortelyou Rd., Brooklyn, NY 11226-5604; 718-284-9717; FlatbushFoodCoop.com

Fine & Raw Chocolate, (mailing address: 151 Kent Ave., Ste. 108, Brooklyn, NY 11211); fineandraw.com. Daniel. Sells chocolate at various markets.

4th Street Food Co-op, 58 East 4th St., New York, NY 10003-8914; 212-674-3623; 4thstreetfoodcoop.org. Membership market.

Gingersnaps Organic, 130 East 7th St., New York, NY 10009; GingerSnapsOrganic.com. Vegan.

Go Natural Health Food Store, 4503 Queens Blvd., Sunnyside, NY 11104

Good Cheap Food, 53 Main St., Delhi, NY 13753; 607-746-6562

Green Market, cenyc.org/greenmarket. This organization runs 46 different farmers' markets in and around New York City. Their website has a downloadable map of all of the farmers' markets, includes a list of dates and hours of operation. Some don't run during the winter months, others are year-round/indoors. "Promotes regional agriculture and ensures a continuing supply of fresh, local produce. Supports farmers and preserves farmland for the future by providing regional small family farmers with opportunities to sell their fruits, vegetables and other farm products."

Green Star Cooperative Market, 701 West Buffalo St., Ithaca, NY 14850; 607-273-9392; greenstar.coop

Greenstar Oasis Market, 215 N Cayuga St., Ithica, NY 14850

Healthfully Organic Food Market, 98 E. 4th St., New York, NY 10003; 212-343-1152; healthfully.com. Between 1st & 2nd Ave. Organic market with lots of raw, organic foods. Also has juice and smoothie bar.

High Falls Food Coop, 1398 State Rd. 213, High Falls, NY 12440; 845-687-7262; highfallsfoodcoop.com

High Vibe, 138 E. 3rd., New York NY 10009; 212-777-6645; HighVibe.com. Raw food supplies.

Honest Weight Food Coop, 484 Central Ave., Albany, NY 12206; 518-482-2667; HonestWeight.coop

Hong Kong Supermarket, 82-02 45th Ave., Queens, New York, 11373. Elmhurst neighborhood at 82nd Street. Fresh fruits and vegetables, including tropical fruit and coconuts. Not a vegetarian place. But many consider this an excellent source for produce. They have other locations in New York.

Hungry Hollow Co-op, 841 Chestnut Ridge Rd., Chestnut Ridge, NY 10977; 845-356-3319; hungryhollow.org.

Jandis Market, 3000 Long Beach Rd., Oceanside, NY 11572; 516-536-5535; Jandis.com. All-vegetarian, compassionate, eco-friendly grocery store, with live food take out.

JivamukTea Café, 841 Broadway, New York, NY 10003 (just below Union Square); 212-353-0214; jivamuktiyoga.com. Yoga studio with a raw food café and other amazing products.

Juice Press, 70 East 1 St., New York, NY 10003. Variety of raw food creations.

Juicy Naam, 27 Race Lane, East Hampton, NY 11937; TheJuicyNaam.us. Juices and food. Giuliana Torre.

Karma Road, 11 Main St, New Paltz, NY 12561; 845-255-1099; KarmaRoad.net. Jenn and Seth.

Lexington Co-operative Market, 807 Elmwood Ave., Buffalo, NY 14222; 716-884-8828; Lexington.coop

Life Thyme Market, 410 6th Ave., New York, NY 10011; 212-420-9099; LifeThymeMarket.com. Raw Food dishes at the deli counter

Liquiteria 170 Second Ave., New York, NY10003; 212-358-0300. Juices and smoothies.

Live Island Café, 201 C East Main St., Huntington, NY 11743; LiveIslandCafe.com. Okima studied at Brenda Kobb's Living Foods Institute in Atlanta.

Live Live, 261 10th St., New York, NY 10009; live-live.com. Food, books, classes, skin care, appliances, live snacks, supplements, raw resources.

Lori's Natural Deli, 900 Jefferson Rd., Rochester, NY 14623; LorisNatural.com.

Lotus Hotel and Live Food Yoga, POB 40, Ithaca, NY 14851; CaspersFarm.com. Opening 2012. Michael Casper.

Manna Foods Natural Foods Store, 171 Mamaroneck Ave., White Plains, NY 10601; 914-946-2233; mannafoodsonline.com

North Country Co-op, 25 Bridge St., Plattsburg, NY 12901; 518-561-5904

One Lucky Duck Pure Juice & Takeaway 125 1/2 E. 17th St., New York, NY 10003-3402; 212-477-7151; oneluckyduck.com

Organic Avenue Boutique, 116 Suffolk St., New York, NY 10002; organicavenue.com

Organic Avenue Boutique, 43 8th Ave, New York, NY 10014; OrganicAvenue.com

Organic Avenue Boutique, 28 Jobs Lane, Southampton, NY 11968; organicavenue.com

Organic Forever, 2053 East Ave., New York, NY 10026; 212-666-3012; OrganicForever.com

Organic Soul Café 6th St. Ctr., 638 E. 6th St., New York, NY 10009; 212-677-1863; Some raw food.

Park Slope Food Co-op, 782 Union St., Brooklyn, NY 11215; 718-622-0560; FoodCoop.com. Location of the monthly Brooklyn Raw food Potluck.

Peacefood Café, 460 Amsterdam Ave., New York, NY 10024; peacefoodcafe.com. Some raw food, some cooked food, and juice bar. Free WiFi. Between 82 and 83, Upper West Side.

Jill Pettijohn, 156 Atlantic Ave, Brooklyn, NY 11201; jillpettijohn.com. Chef and raw cleanse coach.

Potsdam Consumer Co-op, 24 Elm St., Potsdam, NY 13676; 315-265-4630; PotsdamCoop.com

Pure Food and Wine, 54 Irving Pl., New York, NY 10003; 212-477-1010; PureFoodAndWine.com

Queens, NY. Has a neighborhood with Indian stores selling tropical fruits and dates. R train to Roosevelt Ave. and 74th.

Queens Health Emporium, 15901 Horace Harding Expressway. Fresh Meadows, NY 11365; queenshealthemporium.com. Natural foods store.

Quintessence 263 E. 10th St. New York, NY 10009; 646-654-1823; raw-q.com. Raw restaurant.

Raw Food Health Retreat, Moon River, (mailing address: Catherine Rubin, POB 428, Nyack, NY 10960); rawfoodhealthretreat.com

The Raw Spa, 475 Kent Ave., Ste. 801, Brooklyn, NY 11211; 917-664-2952

Raw Star Café, 687 Washington Ave., Brooklyn, NY 11238

Rockaway Raw Café, Blue Firmament Holistic Center. 202 Merrick Rd, Rockville Centre, NY, 11570.

Rockin Raw, rockinraw.com.

Sacred Chow, 227 Sullivan St., New York, NY 10012; 212-337-0863; SacredChow.com. Vegan, not all raw. Kosher.

Sun In Bloom Café, 460 Bergen St., Brooklyn, NY 11217; suninbloom.com. Park Slope neighborhood. Gluten-free, vegan, raw.

Suny Binghamton Co-op, Student Union Suny Binghamton, Binghamton, NY 13905; 607-777-4258

Syracuse Real Food Co-op, 618 Kensington Rd., Syracuse, NY 13210; 315-472-1385; SyracuseRealFood.coop

Teany, 90 Rivington St., New York, NY 10002; 212-475-9190; teany.com. Nice atmosphere and offers 98 varieties of loose leaf tea.

Turquoise Barn, 8052 Country Hwy. 18, Bloomville, NY 13739; 607-538-1235; turquoisebarn.com. Vegetarian, vegan, raw food bed & breakfast on an organic farm, hostel, camping, classes/workshops/apprenticeships, retreats, art gallery & events. All food served is organic, from their gardens, or local when possible. Hiking, biking, swimming, skiing all nearby. Located 3 hours from NYC. Check site for information about events. Area is popular with athelete bikers. Next to the Catskills Scenic Trail. Access: catskillscenictrail.com. Michelle Premura and Michael Milton are proprietors.

Twin Pines Food Co-op - Thrift Shop- Kayak Club, 382 Main St., Port Washington, NY 11050; 516-883-9777

Urban Rustic Market, 236 N. 12th St., Brooklyn, NY 11211; urbanrustic.com. Some freshly made juices and smoothies. This small market specializes in local foods and has a produce section. Not all vegan or vegetarian products.

The V-Spot, 156 Fifth Ave., Brooklyn, NY 11217; 718-622-2275; TheVSpotCafe.com. Vegan with some raw options.

Westerly Natural Market, 913 8th Ave., New York, NY 10019; 212-586-5262; WesterlyNaturalMarket.com. Organic market with lots of raw, organic foods—both packaged and prepared

Yoga In The Raw, Ashtanga Yoga, 71 Main St., New Paltz, NY 12561; yogaintheraw.com. Michael Stein and Angela Starks. Yoga studio, raw food classes and green living seminars.

Yoga Prana Power, 862 Broadway, 2nd Flr., New York, NY 10003 (just above Union Square); 212-460-9642; pranapoweryoga.com. Yoga studio with raw food. Taylor and Phillipe.

• U.S. North Carolina

Check MeetUp.com for raw food meetups, including the Asheville Raw Food MeetUp.

Absolute Organics, LLC, 204 N McDowell St., Charlotte, NC 28204; TheAbsoluteOrganics.com. Organic produce home delivery service. Delivers either weekly or bi-weekly.

Berrybrook Farm Natural Foods Store, 1257 East Blvd., Charlotte, NC; 704-334-6528; berrybrookfarm.com/home.htm. Variety of foods, including fresh smoothies and juices.

Black Mountain Natural Foods, 108 Black Mountain Ave., Black Mountain, NC; 828-669-9813; blackmountainnaturalfoods.com

Butternut Squash, University Square, 133 E W. Franklin St., Chapel Hill, NC 27516. butternetsquashrestaurant.com. Vegetarian, vegan, and raw food are on their menu. Opened in 2009.

Café Harmony, 5645 Creedmoor Rd., Raleigh, NC 27612; 919-510-6910; CafeHarmony.net; Sarah Bogle: CafeHarmony (at) att.net. Organic restaurant with some raw items, snacks, and deserts. Has juice, smoothie, and wheatgrass bar. Two doors down from Harmony Farms market.

Center City Green Market, 101 S Tryon St, Charlotte, NC 28202; CentercityGreenMarket.com. Seasonal farmers' market.

Charlotte Tailgate Market, CharlotteTailGateMarket.com. Local food farmers' market.

Chatam Marketplace, 480 Hillsboro St., Ste.320; Pittsboro, NC 27312; 919-542-2643; ChathamMarketplace.coop

Deep Roots Market, 3728 Spring Garden St., Greensboro, NC 27407; 336-

292-9216; DeepRootsMarket.com

Durham Co-op Grocery, 1101 W Chapel Hill St., Durham, NC 27701; 919-490-0929; DurhamFoodcoop.org

Earth Fare, 66 Westgate Parkway, Asheville, NC 28806; earthfare.com. Market.

Earth Fare, 1856 Hendersonville Rd., Asheville, NC 28803; earthfare.com. Market.

Earth Fare, 178 W. King St., Boone, NC 28607; earthfare.com. Market.

Earth Fare, 12235 N. Community House Rd., Charlotte, NC 28277; earthfare.com. Market.

Earth Fare, 721 Governor Morrison St., Ste. 110; Charlotte, NC 28211; earthfare.com. Market.

Earth Fare, 2965 Battleground Ave., Greensboro, NC 27408; earthfare.com. Market.

Earth Fare, 10341 Moncreiffe Rd., Raleigh, NC 27617; earthfare.com. Market.

French Broad Food Co-op, 90 Biltmore Ave., Asheville, NC 28801; 828-255-7650; frenchbroadfood.coop.

Full Lotus Juice Bar & Café, 716 Ninth St., Durham, NC 27705; fullLotusJuiceBarAndCafe.com

Greenlife Grocery, 70 Merrimon Ave., Asheville, NC 28801-2323; greenlifegrocery.com. Some packaged and fresh raw foods, including in the deli. Also, raw ice cream and pies.

Green Light Café, Ashville, NC; GreenLightCafe.com. Vegan and vegetarian food. Café opened in 2010. Started as a catering company and mobil restaurant.

Harmony Farms, 5653 Creedmoor Rd., Raleigh, NC 27615; Harmony-Farms.net. Organic produce for over 30 years. Nancy and Steve Long, owners. Two doors down from Café Harmony.

Haywood Road Market, 771 Haywood Rd., Asheville, NC 28806; 828-225-4445; HaywoodRoadMarket.org

Healthy Home Market, 5410 East Independence Blvd, Charlotte, NC 28212; HEMarket.com.

Healthy Home Market, 261 Griffith St., Davidson, NC 28036; HEMarket.com.

Healthy Home Market, 2707 South Blvd., Charlotte, NC 28209; HEMarket.com. Has a raw food section.

Healthy Home Market, 16 2nd St. NW, Hickory, NC 28602; HEMarket.com.

Hendersonville Community Co-op, 715 Old Spartanburg Hwy., Hendersonville, NC 28792; 828-693-0505; Hendersonville.coop

Lenore's Natural Cuisine, 164 Ox Creek Rd., Weaverville, NC 28787; lenoresnatural.com. Lenore Baum teaches raw organic vegan classes near Asheville.

Laughing Seed Café, 40 Wall Street, Asheville, NC 28801; 828-252-3445; LaughingSeed.com. Veggie place with some raw options + wine.

Luna's Living Kitchen, 2102 South Blvd., Charlotte, NC 28203; LunasLivingKitchen.com. Raw food restaurant. Juliana Luna is manager/owner. Randy, Andy, Koichi.

North Carolina Raw, ncraw.com

Over The Moon Raw Foods, Charlotte, NC; OverTheMoonRawFoods.com. Raw food catering. Brenda Lee Gambill.

Raw Life Coaching, rawlivecoaching.com

Southwest Asheville Farmers' Market, 718 Haywood Rd., Asheville, NC

Tidal Creek Cooperative Food Market, 5329 Oleander Dr., Ste. 100, Wilmington, NC 28403; 910-799-2667; TidalCreek.coop

Triangle Raw Foods, Durham, NC; trianglerawfoods.com. Raw vegan cuisine truck.

Vegan Girl blog, vegangirl.com

Weaver Street Market, 101 E Weaver St., Carrboro, NC 27510; 919-929-0010

The Xammin' Unbakery, Asheville, NC; FoolInDaRain (at) gmail.com; 828-273-6160. Xam Devesh, owner. Beegan (with vegan option) organic catering business. Handcrafted delights, specializing in deserts. See Xam Devesh on Facebook.com, or xammin.blogspot.com.

• U.S. North Dakota

Check MeetUp.com for raw food meetups.

Amazing Grains Natural Food Market, 214 De Mers, Grand Forks, ND 58201; 701-775-4542

• U.S. Ohio

Check MeetUp.com for raw food meetups.

American Harvest Health Foods, 13387 Smith Rd., Cleveland, OH 44130; 440-888-7727

Bexley Natural Food Co-op, 508 North Cassady Ave., Columbus, OH 43209; bexleynaturalmarket.org; 614-252-3951

Café Sprouts, 55 E. College St., Ste. 1, Oberlin, OH 44074; CafeSprouts.com. Kristen.

Cincinnati Natural Foods, 6911 Miami Ave., Madeira, OH 45243; 513-271-7777.

Cincinnati Natural Foods, 9268 Colerain, Cincinnati, OH 45239; 513-385-7000; cincinnatinaturalfoods.com

Cleveland Food Co-op, 11702 Euclid Ave., Cleveland, OH 44106; 216-791-3890

Clifton Natural Foods, 169 W. McMillan St., Clifton, OH 45219-1316; 513-961-6111

Clintonville Community Market, 200 Crestview Rd., Columbus, OH 43202; 614-261-3663; CommunityMarket.org

Clintonville Farmers' Market, West Dunedin Rd., Columbus, OH 43214; clintonvillefarmersmarket.org. Seasonal farmers' market.

Cooperative Market, 1835 W. Market St., Akron, OH 44313; 330-869-2590.

Coop On Coventry, 1807 Coventry Rd., Cleveland Heights, OH 44118; 216-321-9292

Dharma Deli, 600 E. 2nd St., Dayton, OH 45402; dharmadeli.webs.com. Inside National City 2nd St., Market. Lori Anne "Persephone" Agricola and George Eninger. Some raw items on menu.

Good Food Co-op, Harkness Basement, 113 W. College St., Oberlin OH 44074. On Oberlin campus.

Good N Raw, 11860 Clifton Blvd., Lakewood, OH 44107; 216-521-2225; goodnraw.com. Nicole Tuzzio.

Health Foods Unlimited, 2205 Miamisburg-Centerville Rd., Centerville, OH 45459; 937-433-5100; healthfoodsunlimited.com.

Jungle Jim's, 5440 Dixie Hwy., Fairfield, OH 45104-4108; junglejims.com. Source for tropical fruits, dates, etc.

Jungle Jim's, 4450 Eastgate South Dr., Cincinnati, OH 45245; junglejims.com

Kent Natural Foods Co-op, 151 E Main St., Kent, OH 44240; 330-673-2878; KentNaturalFoods.org

Local Roots, 140 S. Walnut, St., Wooster, OH 44691 (mailing address: POB 1349, Wooster, OH 44691); localrootswooster.com. Natural market.

Loving Café, 6227 Montgomery Rd, Cincinnati, OH 45213; thelovingcafe.com. Vegetarian.

Ms. Julie's Kitchen, 1809 S. Main St., Akron, OH 44301

Mustard Seed Market and Café, Montrose, W. Market Plz, 3885 W. Market St., Akron, OH 44333; 330-666-SEED (7333); MustardSeedMarket.com

Mustard Seed Market and Café, Uptown Solon Shopping Ctr, 6025 Kruse Dr., Solon, OH 44139; 440-519-FOOD (3663); Café: 440-519-3600; MustardSeedMarket.com

Nature's Bin Market, 18120 Sloane Ave. Lakewood, OH 44107; 216-521-4600; Cornucopia-Inc.org

Nature's Goodness, 702 Eleanora Dr., Cuyahoga Falls, OH 44223; 330-922-4567

New Earth Natural Foods, 1605 State Rd., Cuyahoga Falls, OH 44223; newearthnaturals.com; 330-929-2415.

Organic Energy Restaurant and Power Juice Café, 28500 Mills Rd., Suite J, Solon, OH 44139; 440-349-1500; organicenergycafe.com

Phoenix Earth Food Co-op, 1447 W Sylvania Ave., Toledo, OH 43612; 419-476-3211

Rainbow Health Foods, 508 Main St., Hamilton, OH 45013; 513-896-4508

Raisin Rack Natural Foods, 2545 Schrock Rd., Westerville, OH 44709; 614-882-5886; raisinrack.com

Squeaker's Vegetarian Cafe & Health Food Store, 175 N. Main St., Bowling Green, OH 43402; 419-354-7000

Squeaker's Vegetarian Cafe & Health Food Store, 601 N. Main St., Findlay, OH 45840; 419-424-3990.

Susan's Natural World, 8315 Beechmont Ave., Cincinnati, OH, 45255; SusansNaturalWorld.com

Shawna Stursa, Columbus, OH; rawshawna.info. A living foods educator.

Sunflower Natural Foods, 2591 N. High St., Columbus, OH 43202-2555; 614-263-2488.

Weber's Health Foods, 18400 Euclid Ave., Cleveland, OH 44112

Wooster Food Co-op, 138 E. Liberty St., Wooster, OH 44691; 330-264-9797; 330-264-9797; woosternaturalfoods.blogspot.com

Zagara's, 1940 Lee Rd., Cleveland Heights, OH 44118; Zagarasmarketplace.com. Grocery store known for their produce department featuring locally-grown produce.

• U.S. OKLAHOMA

Check MeetUp.com for raw food meetups.

Big Al's Healthy Foods, 3303 E 15th St, Tulsa, OK 74112. Deli offers vegan, vegetarian, and/or all raw.

Family Health Food Store, 1020 W. Main, Durant, OK 74701; 580-924-3214

The Health Food Center, 7301 S. Penn, #D, Oklahoma City, OK 73159; 405-681-6060; thehealthfoodcenter.net

In the Raw Norman, 575 University Blvd., Norman, OK 73069; InTheRawSushi.com. Vegetarian, vegan.

Native Roots Market, 132 West Main St., Norman, OK 73069; 405-310-6300; nativerootsmarket.com

The Oasis Health Food Store, 111 N. Muskogee Ave., Tahlequah, OK 74464; 918-456-1414

Pure Cafe, Tulsa, OK 74135; 918-619-6650; purerawcafe.com. Opened in 2009. Ships raw meals nationwide. Chef Cynthia Beavers. Has an enewsletter. Email is: rawfoodchef (at) yahoo.com.

Raw Intentions, 848 S. Aspen Ave., Broken Arrow, OK 74012. RawIntentions.com. Raw café. Opened 2012. Denise Madeja, proprietor.

Tulsa's Cherry Street Farmers Market, Tulsa, OK 74103; cherrystreetfarmersmarket.com. Seasonal

Veggies Health Advantage Store and Restaurant, 1202 Brookview Dr., Ardmore, OK 73401; 580-226-2424

• U.S. OREGON

Check MeetUp.com for raw food meetups.

Also check: NWVeg.org/Restaurants

Alberta Cooperative Grocery, 1500 NE Alberta St., Portland, OR 97211; 503-287-4333

Ashland Food Co-op, 237 N. 1st St., Ashland, OR 97520; 541-482-2237; AshlandFood.coop

Astoria Cooperative, 1355 Exchange St., Ste. 1, Astoria, OR 97103; 503-325-0027; AstoriaCoop.org

Blossoming Lotus Restaurant, 1713 NE 15th, Portland, OR 97212; 503-228-0048; blpdx.com. Some raw dishes and deserts on menu.

Brooking Natural Food Co-op, 630 Fleet St., POB 8051, Brookings, OR 97415; 541-469-9551

Capella Market, 2489 Williamette, Eugene, OR 97405; 541-345-1014; CapellaMarket.com

Coos Head Food Store, 1960 Sherman (Hwy101), North Bend, OR 97459; 541-756-7264

Cornucopia Natural Foods, 111 NW 6th St., Redmond, OR 97756-9573; 541-548-5911

Dawn Patrol, 108 Hwy 35, Hood River, OR 97031. dawnpatrol97031.blogspot.com

Devore's Good Food Store, 1124 NW Newport Ave., Bend, OR 97701; 541-389-6588

The Feel Good World, Bikram Yoga, John's Landing, 5816 SW Hood Ave., Portland, OR 97239; TheFeelGoodWorld.com; 503-452-1132. Pre-packaged and fresh foods in lobby. Live food kitchen and juice bar and catering kitchen for Cell Rejuvenation Center.

First Alternative Coop, 1007 SE 3rd St., Corvallis, OR 97333; 541-753-3115; FirstAlt.coop

First Alternative Natural Foods Co-op, 2855 NW Grant Ave., Corvallis, OR 97330; 541-452-3115; FirstAlt.coop

Food Fight! Grocery, 1217 SE Stark St., Portland, OR 97214; 503-233-3910, FoodFightGrocery.Com

Food Front Coop, 2375 NW Thurman St., Portland, OR 97209; 503- 222-5658; FoodFront.coop. Keeps increasing their raw food presence.

Food Front Coop SW, 6344 SW Capital Hwy., Portland, OR 97239; foodfront.coop.

Friendly Street Market, 2757 Friendly St., Eugene, OR 97405; 541-683-2079

Good Life Café and Juice Bar, 208 NW 6th St., Old Town Marketplace, Grants Pass, OR 97526. Vegan and vegetarian. Sierra Warrn, owner/operator.

Greater Baker Food Co-op, 2816 10th St., Baker City, OR 97814; 541-523-6281

Growers Market, 454 Williamette, Eugene, OR 97401; 541- 687-1145

Health Food Mart, 259 E. Barnett Rd., Ste. D, Medford, OR 97501

Healthy Living Foods Lending Library and Potlucks Monthly, Jill Divine, Eugene, OR; jdevine (at) yahoo.com

It's Alive!, itsalivefood.com. Raw crackers, pates, and sauerkraut sold in stores.

Kiva Natural Food Store, 125 W 11th Ave., Eugene, OR 97401-3009; 541-342-8666; kivagrocery.com

LifeSource Natural Foods, 2649 Commercial St. SE, Salem, OR 97302; lifesourcenaturalfoods.com.

Livin' Spoonfull, gluten-free-crackers.com/index.html. Makers of gluten-free sprouted seed crackers.

The Market of Choice, 1475 Siskiyou Blvd., Ashland, OR 97520; 541-488-2773; marketofchoice.com. Markets with increasing percentage of organic produce and raw food.

The Market of Choice, 1060 Green Acres Rd., Eugene, OR 97401; 541-344-1901; marketofchoice.com

The Market of Choice, 5639 Hood St., West Linn, OR 97068; 503-594-2901; marketofchoice.com

The Market of Choice, 67 West 29th Ave., Eugene, OR 97405; 541-338-8455; marketofchoice.com

The Market of Choice, 2580 Willakenzie, Eugene, OR 97401; 541-345-3349; marketofchoice.com

The Market of Choice, 1960 Franklin Blvd., Eugene, OR 97403; 541-687-1188; marketofchoice.com

The Market of Choice, 8502 SW Tenwilliger Blvd, Portland, OR 97219; 503-892-7331; marketofchoice.com

Mirador Community Store, 2106 SE Division St., Portland, OR 97202;

miradorcommunitystore.com. Community kitchen with juicing, sprouting, and dehydrating supplies, and books.

Mother's Natural Grocery, 975 2nd St. SE, Bandon, OR 97411; 541-347-4086

Mustard Seed Farms, c/o David & Nancy Brown, 7300 McKay Rd, St. Paul, OR 97137; mustardseedorganic.com. A CSA farm. Good source for organic veggies.

Nature's General Store, 1950 Northeast 3rd St., Bend, OR 97701; 541-382-6732

New Frontier Market, 1101 W. 8th Ave., Eugene, OR 97402; 541-345-7401

New Life Nutrition, 240 2nd SW, Albany, OR 97321; 541-926-1982

New Odyssey Juice Bar, 1044 Willamette St., Eugine, OR 97401; NewOdyssey.us.

New Seasons Market, 3495 SW Cedar Hills Blvd., Beaverton, OR 97005; newseasonsmarket.com.

New Seasons Market, 7300 SW Beaverton-Hillsdale Hwy., Portland, OR 97225; 503-292-6838; newseasonsmarket.com. Prides itself on selling a large variety of locally produced foods and products. Check the Web site for other locations, all in Oregon.

New Seasons Market, 15861 SE Happy Valley Town Ctr. Dr., Happy Valley, OR; newseasonsmarket.com

New Seasons Market Sellwood, 1214 SE Tacoma, Portland, OR; newseasonsmarket.com.

New Seasons Arbor Lodge, 6400 N. Interstate, Portland, OR; newseasonsmarket.com.

New Seasons Mtn. Park, 3 Monroe Parkway, Lake Oswego, OR; newseasonsmarket.com.

New Seasons Market Orenco, 1453 NE 61st St., Hillsboro, OR; newseasonsmarket.com.

New Seasons 7 Corners, 1954 SE Division St., Portland, OR; newseasonsmarket.com

New Seasons Market Concordia, 5320 NE 33rd Ave., Portland, OR; newseassonsmarket.com.

Northwest Veg; NWVeg.org. Vegetarian information, events, resources in the Pacific Northwest.

Oceana Natural Foods Co-op, 159 SE 2nd St., Newport, OR 97365; 541-265-8285; OceanaFoods.org

Oregon Natural Market, 373 SW 1st St., Ontario, OR 97914; 541-889-8714; oregonnaturalmarket.com

Oregon Raw Resources, oregonrawresource.org. Brion Oliver and Kyler Grandkoski's list of Oregon raw resources.

Papa G's, 2314 SE Division St., Portland, OR 97202; 503-235-0244; papagees.com. Organic vegan deli with lots of locally-grown food, and increasing amount of raw, deli style. Organic salad bar.

People's Food Co-op, 3029 SE 21st St., Portland, OR 97202; 503-674-2642; 503--232-9051; Peoples.coop. Juice bar, fresh produce, supplies.

Prasad, Portland, OR; 503-224-3993; prasadcuisine.squarespace.com. Vegetarian. Has some raw food items. Former location of Blossoming Lotus.

Promise Natural Foods, 503 South Main St., Canyonville, OR 97417; 541-839-4167

Proper Eats Market & Café, 8638 N. Lombard Ave., Portland, OR 97203; propereats.org. Vegetarian, vegan, and raw.

Raw and Living Spirit Retreat, Portland, OR; RawAndLivingSpirit.org

Raw Diet Health Revolution Newsletter, therawdiet.com. Mike Snyder's newsletter.

Raw Diet Health Store, Portland, OR; store.therawdiet.com/index.html. Mike Snyder.

Raw Family, POB 172, Ashland, OR 97520; RawFamily.com. This is the wonderful Boutenko family. They are authors of several popular books about raw food, including *Green for Life* and *The Raw Smoothie Revolution* by Victoria Boutenko, and the recipe book *Fresh* by brother and sister Sergei and Valya Boutenko. They also wrote *Raw Family Signature Recipes.* The family has traveled around the world to teach people about raw foods, and often conducts seminars and raw food prep classes. Sergei also has a company that takes people on wild food foraging hikes and adventures, check out HarmonyHikes.com.

Raw Matrix, rawmatrix.net. Makers of organic, raw salads, desserts. Sold at Alberta Co-Op Grocery, People's Food Co-op, and Food Front Co-op. Also, foods to-go or delivery.

Raw Princess Studio, 1511 SW Market Street, Portland, OR 97201; rawprincess.org. Cindy Cummins. Makes and sells raw food items. Conducts juicing gatherings. Has a MeetUp group. Site has blog with recipes.

Raw Vortex, rawvortex.squarespace.com. Is a Website of inspiration and recipes from Kara Maia Spencer of Oregon.

Red Barn Natural Grocery, 357 Van Buren St., Eugene, OR 97402; 541-342-7503; RedBarnNaturalGrocery.com

Sarah's Raw Vegan Cafe, 519 NW Colorado Ave., Bend, OR 97701. Sarah Bornstein, proprietor. Opened 2012. Has Facebook page.

Seaside Health Foods, 144 N. Roosevelt Dr., Seaside, OR 97138; 503-738-3088

Sundance Natural Foods, 748 E. 24th Ave., Eugene, OR 97405-2936; 541-343-9142; SundanceNaturalFoods.com

Toby's Family Foods, 1160 Shelley St., Springfield, OR 97477

Trillium Natural Foods, 1026 South Jetty, Lincoln City, OR 97367-2642; 541-994-5665

• U.S. Pennsylvania

Check MeetUp.com for raw food meetups.

Veg PA, VegPA.net

All the Way Live, 6108 Germantown Ave., Philadelphia, PA 19144; alllivefood.com; 215-821-RAW8 (7298). Empress Nyeisha.

Appalachian Whole Foods Market, 100 W. High St., Carlisle, PA 17013; appalachianwholefoods.com; 717-241-6982

Arnold's Way, 319 W. Main St., Store #4, Rear, Lansdale, PA 19446; 215-361-0116; ArnoldsWay.com

Earthlight Natural Foods, 933 C Ann St., Stroudsburg, PA 18360; 570-424-6760; earthlightnaturalfoods.com

East End Food Co-op, 7516 Mead St., Pittsburgh, PA 15208; 412-242-3598; EastEndFood.coop

The Enchanted Kitchen, 127 S. Pough St., State College, PA 16801; TheEnchantedKitchen.net; april (at) theenchantedkitchen.net. Inside the Lotux Center Yoga.

Everything Natural Under the Sun, 3415 Pleasant Valley Blvd., Altoona, PA 16602; 814-943-6330; livingnaturallyonline.com

Genesee Natural Foods, 5405 Locust Lane, Harrisburg, PA 17109; 717-545-3712

Govinda's Gourmet Vegetarian, 1408 South St., Philadelphia, PA 19146. Some raw food available.

Jar Bar, 113 S. 12th St., Philadelphia, PA 19107; JarBarPhilly.com. Smoothies, juice bar, vegetarian/vegan restaurant.

Kimberton Whole Foods at Mill Town Market, 150 East Pennsylvania Ave., Downingtown, PA 19335; 610-873-8225; kimbertonwholefoods.com. Organic and biodynamically farmed produce.

Kimberton Whole Foods, 2140 Kimberton Rd., Kimberton, PA 19460; kimbertonwholefoods.com.

Kimberton Whole Foods, 239 Durham Rd., Ottsville, PA 18942; kimbertonwholefoods.com.

Kimberton Whole Foods, 1139 Ben Franklin Hwy. East, Douglassville, PA 19518; kimbertonwholefoods.com.

Loving Life Cafe, 717-476-Love; LovingLifeCafe.com. Jody Allen.

Love Street Living Foods, 91 Westwood St., Ste. 1, Pittsburgh, PA 15211, USA; 412-381-1867; LoveStreetLivingFoods.com. Sells raw food supplies.

Mariposa Co-op, 4726 Baltimore Ave., Philadelphia, PA 19143; 215-729-2121

Martindale's Natural Market, 1172 Baltimore Pike, Olde Sprout Shopping Village, Springfield, PA 19064; 610-543-6811; martindalesnutrition.com

Nature's Pantry, 2331 Commercial Blvd., State College, PA 16801; 814-861-5200; naturespantrypa.com

Oasis Living Cuisine, Great Valley Shop. Ctr., 81 Lancaster Ave., Malvern, PA 19355; 610-647-9797; OasisLivingCuisine.com

Raw Can Roll Café, 39 Old Swede Rd., Douglassville, PA 19512; RawCanRollCafe.com. Sheryll Chavarria and Deb Marbaker.

Raw Lifeline, Huntington Valley, PA; 215-947-1510; RawLifeLine.com. Chef Joel Odhner's raw food services and teaching company.

Swarthmore Co-op, 401 Dartmouth Ave., Swarthmore, PA 19081; 610-543-9805; Swarthmore.coop

Weavers Way Cooperative Association, 559 Carpenter Ln., Philadelphia, PA 19119; 215-843-2350; WeaversWay.Coop

Whole Foods Co-op, 1341W. 26th & Brown Ave., Erie, PA 16508; 814-456-0282; WholefoodsCoop.org

• U.S. RHODE ISLAND

Check MeetUp.com for raw food meetups.

Alternative Food Co-op, 357 Main St., Wakefield, RI 02880; 401-789-2240; 401-789-1717; AlternativeFoodcoop.com

Bliss Natural Grocer, 311 Broadway, Newport, RI; 401-608-2322; blissnaturalgrocer.com

Eastside Marketplace, 165 Pitman St., Providence, RI; 401-831-7771; eastsidemarket.com

Food for Thought Natural Foods Store, 140 Point Judith Rd., #32, Narragansett, RI; 401-789-2445

Foodworks, 9 Cedar Swamp Rd., Smithfield, RI; 401-232-2410

Garden Grill, 727 East Ave., Pawtucket, RI 02860 401-726-2826; gardengrillecafe.com

Harvest Natural Foods, 181 Bellevue Ave., Newport, RI; 401-846-8137

• U.S. SOUTH CAROLINA

Check MeetUp.com for raw food meetups.

Earth Fare, 74 Folly Rd. Blvd., Charleston, SC; 843-769-4800; earthfare.com. Market.

Earth Fare, 3312-B Devine St., Columbia, SC 29205; earthfare.com. Market.

Earth Fare, 3620 Pelham St., Greenville, SC 29615; earthfare.com. Market.

Earth Fare, 725 Cherry Rd., Rock Hill, SC 29732; earthfare.com. Market.

14 Carrot Whole Foods Store, 5300 Sunset Blvd., Lexington, SC 29072; 803-359-2920; 14carrot.net

Garner's Natural Market & Café, 60 E Antrim Dr., Greenville, SC 29607; 864-242-4856

Good Life Café, 3681-D Leaphart Rd., West Columbia, SC 29169; GoodLifeCafe.net. Chef Sharon Wright.

Lifeit Café, Greenville, SC 29601; lifeitcafe.com. Vegan cuisine. Supplies and classes by Latrice Folkes.

The Sprout Café, 627 Johnnie Dodds Blvd., Mount Pleasant, SC 29464; 843-849-8554. TheHealthySprout.com. Vegetarian café with some raw items. Mickey and Caroline Brennan.

The Sprout, 627 Johnnie Dodds Blvd., Mount Pleasant, SC 29465; thesproutsc.typepad.com; TheHealthySprout.com

It's Only Natural, 95 Factory Creek Court, See Island Parkway, Beaufort, SC; 843-986-9595; itsonlynaturalsc.com

Upstate Food Co-op, 404 John Holiday Rd., Six Mile, SC 29682; 864-868-3105; upstatefoodcoop.com/

• U.S. SOUTH DAKOTA

Check MeetUp.com for raw food meetups.

Breadroot Natural Foods Co-op, 130 Main St., Rapid City, SD; 605-348-3331; breadroot.com

Carolina First Saturday Market, Greenville, SC 29602; SaturdayMarketLve.com. Seasonal farmers' market.

The Co-op Natural Foods, 2504 S. Duluth Ave., Sioux Falls, SD 57105; 605-339-9506; CoopNaturalFoods.com

Earth Goods Natural Foods, 738 Jennings Ave., Hot Springs, SD; 605-745-7715; earthgoodsnaturalfoods.com

Good Earth Natural Foods, 638 Main St., Spearfish, SD; 605-642-7639

LE Juice, Savannah Hwy. & Daniel St, Charleston, SC 29407; 843-766-8800. Restaurant, juice bar. Kosher and vegan.

Main Street Market Natural Foods Store, 512 Main St., Rapid City, SD; 605-341-9099; themainstreetmarket.com

Natural Abundance Food Co-op, 125 S Main St., Aberdeen, SD 57401; 605-229-4947

The Organic Salad Basket Market, 633 Main St., Hill City, SD; 605-391-2052

The Sprout. Mt Pleasant, SC 29464; thehealthysprout.com. Restaurant.

• U.S. TENNESSEE

Check MeetUp.com for raw food meetups.

Abundant Living Natural Food Store, 855 Keith St. NW, Cleveland, TN; 423-614-7885; abundantlivingorganic.com

Earth Fair, 1814 Gunbarrel Rd., Ste. 100, Chattanooga, TN 37421; earthfare.com. Market.

Earth Fair, 1735 W. State-of-Franklin Rd., Johnson City, TN 37604; earthfare.com. Market.

Earth Fair, 140 N. Forest Park Blvd., Knoxville, TN 37919; earthfare.com. Market.

Earth Fair, 10903 Parkside Dr., Knoxville, TN 37934; earthfare.com; 865-777-3837. Market.

Fresh Life Natural Food Coop, 9101 Glouster Ln., Chattanooga, TN 37416; 423-344-9244

Greenlife Grocery (Two North Shore), 301 Manufacture's Rd., Ste. 105, Chattanooga, TN 37405; 423-702-3700

Harding Health Foods, 4649 Nolensville Pike, Nashville, TN; 615-834-3770

The Health Barn, 3116 East Oakland Ave., Johnson City, TN; 423-283-4719

Heavens to Betsy, 174 Woodmont Ave., Nashville, TN 37205; NashvilleRawFoods.com. Vegan raw and alternative store.

Midtown Food Coop, 2158 Central Ave., Memphis, TN 38104; 901-276-2250

Morningside Buying Club, 215 Morningside Lane, Liberty, TN; 615-563-2353; morningsidefarm.com

Naturally Good Food Market, 4242 Port Royal Rd., Spring Hill, TN; 931-486-3192; naturallygoodfood.com

Nutrition World Natural Food Store, 6201 Lee Hwy., Chattanooga, TN; 423-892-4085; nutritionw.com

Oldfort Co-op, Cleveland, TN; 423-338-4151

Three Rivers Market, 937 North Broadway, Knoxville, TN 37917; 865-525-2069; ThreeRiversMarket.coop

The Turnip Truck Market, 970 Woodland St., Nashville, TN; 615-650-3600; theturniptruck.com

Whole Foods Market, 5022 Poplar Ave., Memphis, TN; 901-685-2293.

• U.S. TEXAS

Check MeetUp.com for raw food meetups.

Alternative Food Co-op, 2611 Boston Ave., Lubbock, TX; 806-747-8740

Barefoot Market, 2187 W. South Loop, Stephenville, TX 76401. Fully stocked health food store and raw food bar. Behind HEB grocery. Opened October 2011.

Beets Café, 1611 W 5th St., Suite 165, Austin, TX 78703; 512-477-2338; beetscafe.com. Chef Sylvia Heisey is a graduate of the Living Light Culinary Institute in Fort Bragg, California.

Best of the Blessed Healthy Food Co-op, 2900 Mistywood Ln, Denton, TX 76209; 940-380-0787

Bliss Raw Café and Elixir Bar, 6005 Berkshire Ln., Dallas, TX 75225; blissrawcafe.com.

Brazos Natural Foods, 4303 S. Texas Ave., Bryan, TX; 979-846-4459; brazosnaturalfoods.com

Casa De Luz Center for Integral Studies, 1701 Toomey Rd., Austin, TX 78704; casadeluz.org. Some raw food served in a buffet style. Macrobiotic place. They have an on-site food garden, and offer classes and seminars. They also have a food store.

Central City Co-op, 2115 Taft, Houston, TX 77006; 713-524-9408; CentralCityCo-op.org

Cornucopia Natural Foods, 1104 – J Thorpe Ln., San Marcos, TX 78666-7126; 800-353-5044. Cornucopianaturalfoods.com

Cupboard Natural Foods & Café, 200 W. Congress St., Denton, TX; 940-387-5386; cupboardnaturalfoods.com

Daily Juice Cafe, 4500 Duval St., Austin, TX 78751; 512-380-9046; DailyJuice.org. Monday through Friday.

Erma's Nutrition Center, 18045 Upper Bay Rd., Nassau Bay, TX; 281-333-4746; ermasnutritioncenter.com

EZRawFood101.com, Austin, TX; Chef Alicia Ojeda

Green Market Natural Foods, 1909 Texoma Pkwy, Sherman, TX 75090; greenmarketnaturalfoods.com

Pat Greer's Kitchen, 412 W Clay St., Houston, TX 77019; 713-807-0101; patgreersrawvegankitchen.com. Raw vegan.

Hail Merry, Dallas, TX; hailmerry.com. Makers of raw granolas distributed nationally (some products contain maple syrup). Angela Lima: ALima (at) hailmerry.com.

Health Food House Market, 4206 N. Ben Jordan, Victoria, TX; 361-573-4711

Healthy Approach Market, 5100 State Hwy. 121, Colleyville, TX; 817-399-9100; healthyapproachmarket.com

Keller Texas Produce Co-op, 1401 Briar Meadow Dr., Keller, TX 76248; 817-284-2433

Lamar Street Green Cafe at Whole Foods 525 N Lamar Blvd, Austin, TX 78703. Deli fridge, sit-down bar and made-to-order menu with some raw items.

Morning Glory Natural Foods, 124 S. First St., Lufkin, TX; 936-637-7481; morninggloryhealth.com

Chef Alicia Ojeda, Austin, TX; EZRawFood101.com

Oxygen Life Spa, The Rudra Ctr., 609 N. Locust St., Denton, TX 76201; OxygenLifeSpa.com

Pearl Farmers' Market, San Antonio, TX 78215; pearlfarmersmarket.com. Pearl Parkway near the Stable lawn

Rawfully Organic Co-op, 11402 Chaucers Oaks Ct., Houston, TX 77082; rawfullyorganic.com. A buyers' co-op of organic fruits and vegetables. Started by Kristina Carillo-Bucaram, KristinaBucaram.com; Kristina (at) RawFullyOrganic.com; FullyRaw.com.

Roy's Natural Market, 6025 Royal Lane, #130, Dallas, TX 75230; 214-987-0213; roysnaturalmarket.com

Sunfire Health Foods, 4915 MLK Jr. Blvd., Houston, TX 77021; 713-643-2884; SunfiredHealthFoods.com

Well Body Natural Foods, 3651 34th St., Lubbock, TX; 806-793-1015; wellbodynaturals.com

Wheatsville Food Co-op, 3101 Guadalupe, Austin, TX 78705; 512-478-2667; Wheatsville.com. Lots of raw food.

Whole Foods Market, 525 N. Lamar, Austin, TX 78703. Store features a raw café bar. This is their headquarters. I don't usually list Whole Foods market in this book, but I take this exception. Whole Foods prices are so high they may as well call themselves Whole Greed. I think it is better to shop at farmers markets and at natural food co-ops, rather than purchase items at a store that is owned by stock investors who could care less about organic foods.

• U.S. UTAH

Check MeetUp.com for raw food meetups.

Ginger's Garden Café, 188 S. Main St., Springville, UT 84663; 801-489-4500; gingersgardencafe.com; some raw food, juices, supplies, books. Bobbie is manager. Connected to Dr. Christopher's Herb Shop.

Good Earth Natural Foods, 500 S. State St., Orem, UT; 801-765-1616; goodearthnaturalfoods.com

Harmons Market, 1189 East 700 South, St. George, UT; 435-628-0411; harmonsgrocery.com

Liberty Heights, 1300 South 1100 East, Salt Lake City, UT; 801-58-FRESH; libertyheightsfresh.com

Moab Community Food Co-op, 111 N 100 West, Moab, UT 84532; 801-259-5712

Moonflower Market, 39 E 100 N, Moab, UT; 435-259-5712

Omar's Rawtopia, 2148 Highland Dr., Salt Lake City, UT 84106; omarsrawtopia.com. Owner, Omar Abou-Ismail.

Sage's Cafe, 473 E. 300 S., SLC, UT 84102; 801-322-3790; SagesCafe.com. Organic vegetarian.

• U.S. VERMONT

Check MeetUp.com for raw food meetups.

Adamant Co-op, 1313 Haggett Rd., Adamant, VT 05648; 802-223-5760;

adamantcoop.org. Small store with local organics when available and that also has pre-order club and special orders.

Brattleboro Food Co-op, 2 Main St., Brookside Plaza, Brattleboro, VT 05301; 802-257-0236; BrattleboroFoodCoop.com

Buffalo Mountain Food Co-op, 14 North Main St., Hardwick, VT 05843; 802-472-6020

City Market - Onion River Co-op, 82 S. Winooski Ave. Ste. 2, Burlington, VT 05401; 802-863-3659; CityMarket.coop

Co-Food Stores, coopfoodstore.coop/locations

Hunger Mountain Co-op, 623 Stone Cutters Wy., Montpelier, VT 05602; 802-223-8000; HungerMountain.com

Middlebury Natural Foods Co-op & Café, 9 Washington St., Middlebury, VT 05753; 802-388-7276

Nutshell Co-op, Box 175, Rte. 100, Wardsboro, VT 05355; 802-896-6032

Putney Food Co-op, 8 Carol Brown Way, Putney, VT 05346; 802-387-5866; PutneyCoop.com

Rail City Market Co-op, 8 S Main St., St. Albans, VT 05478; 802-524-3769

Roo's Natural Foods Market, 2 Lower Main St., E (Rte. 15), Johnson, VT 05656; 802-635-1788. Small, but has organic produce.

Rutland Area Food Co-op, 77 Wales St., Rutland, VT 05701; 802-773-0737

Springfield Food Co-op, 335 River St., Springfield, VT 05156; 802-885-3363

St. J. Food Co-op, 490 Portland St., St. Johnsbury, VT 05819; 802-748-9498; StJFoodCoop.com

Upper Valley Food Co-op, 193 N Main St., White River Junction, VT 05001; 802-295-5804

Vermont Fiddle Heads, 18 Worcester Village Rd. (Rt. 12), Worcester, VT 05682; 802-223-2111; vt-fiddle.com. Raw food café, potlucks, workshops. Accepts orders for bulk raw food items. Packaged raw foods. Source for hemp tea and sprouting bags. Eight miles north of Montpelier, 20 minutes from Stowe.

• U.S. VIRGINIA

Check MeetUp.com for raw food meetups.

Cranberry's Grocery & Eatery, 7 South New St., Staunton, VA; gocranberrys.com

Crozet Natural Foods, POB 634, Crozet, VA 22932

Eats Natural Foods Co-op, 1200 N. Main St., Blacksburg, VA 24060; EatsNaturalFoods.com

Ellwood Thompson's Natural Market, 4 N. Thompson St., Richmond, VA; ellwoodthompsons.com

Fare Share Cooperative, 2132 W. Main St., Richmond, VA 23220

Harvest Market, 7610 Heths Salient St., Ste. 112, Spotsylvania, VA 22553; HrvstMrkt.com; TamisDavid (at) HrvstMrkt.com.

Healthway Natural Foods, 1610 Belle View Blvd., Alexandria, VA; healthwaynaturalfoods.com

Healthy Foods Co-op, 110 W Washington St., Lexington, VA 24450; HealthyFoodsMarket.com

Heritage Health Food Store & Juice Bar, 314 Laskin Rd., Virginia Beach, VA; caycecures.com

Lizz Creative Juices, 915 Lafayette Blvd., Fredericksburg, VA 22401; DeepRootedNutrition.com. Inside the Gallery at 915. Juices, smoothies, elixirs, and some raw snacks. Vegan, gluten free. Elizabeth Howard. DeepRootedNutrition (at) yahoo.com. Opened in 2012. Facebook page is Liz Creative Juices.

My Organic Market (MOMs), 3831 Mt. Vernon Ave., Alexandrea, VA 22305; 703-535-5980; myorganicmarket.com

The Natural Market, 5 Diagonal St., Warrenton, VA 20186

Natural Mercantile Market (MOMs), 341 East Colonial Hwy., Hamilton, VA; 540-338-7080; naturalmercantile.com

Organic Food Depot, 2007 N. Amistead Ave., Hampton, VA; 757-826-6404; organicfooddepot.com

Quenna's Raw And Vegan, 9619 Granby St, Norfolk, VA 23503; 757-714-2396. Raw food and juices.

Rebecca's Natural Food Market, 1141 Emmet St., Charlottesville, VA; 434-977-1965; rebeccasnaturalfood.com

Roanoke Natural Foods Co-op, 1319 Grandin Road SW, Roanoke, VA 24015; 540-343-5652; RoanokeNaturalFoods.coop

Sue's Super Nutrition Market, 3060 S. Main St., Harrisburg, VA; 540-432-9855

Valley Market, POB 23, Staunton, VA 24402-0023; ValleyMarket.org

The White Pig Bed & Breakfast, 5120 Irish Rd., Schuyler, VA 22969; thewhitepig.com. A vegan bed & breakfast that is also an animal sanctuary.

• U.S. WASHINGTON

Check MeetUp.com for raw food meetups.

AmeRAWcan Bistro, 745 St Helens Ave., Tacoma WA 98402; AmeRawCanBistro.com. Darrin and Tina London. While some of their menu is raw and organic, this is not a vegan or vegetarian restaurant. Some of their menu includes cooked meat.

Bear Foods Market, 125 East Woodin Ave, Chelan, WA 98816

Bellingham Co-op, 1220 N. Forest St., Bellingham, WA 98225; CommunityFood.coop.

Blossom Local Natural Grocer, 135 B Lopez Rd., POB 838, Lopez Island, WA 98261

Café Flora, 2901 E. Madison St., Seattle, WA 98112; 206-325-9100; cafeflora.com; Some raw items on menu.

Chaco Canyon Cafe, 4757 12th Ave. NE, Seattle, WA 98105; 206-522-6966; ChacoCanyonCafe.com. Raw restaurant.

Chaco Canyon Café, 3770 SW Alaska St., Seattle, WA 98126; ChacoCanyonCafe.com. Raw restaurant.

CoCoa Banana, 118 Cherry Street, Seattle, WA 98104. cocoabanana.com. Smoothies, juices, salad bar. Monday-Friday 9-4.

Community Food Co-op, 1220 North Forest St., Bellingham, WA 98225; 360-734-8158; CommunityFood.Coop

Cordata Co-op, 315 Westerly Rd., Bellingham, WA 98226

Ferry Food Co-op, 34 N Clark Ave., Republic, WA 99166; 509-775-3754

The Food Co-op, 414 Kearney St., Port Townsend, WA 98368; 360-385-2883; FoodCoop.coop

Good Earth Natural Foods, 500 S. State, Orem, WA 84058

Green Line Organic Health, 12653 NE 85th St., Kirkland, WA 98033

Bruce Horowitz, TheSunKitchen.com. Raw chef classes and catering. LongevityChef.com. RawPermaculture.com.

House of the Sun Raw Bar; 1313 156th St., NE, Ste. 125, Bellevue, WA 98007; houseofthesunrawfood.com. Wholesale kitchen with a take-out window. Products available at various markets. Adam Lewis.

Huckleberry's Fresh Market, 926 S. Monroe St., Spokane, WA 99204; 509-624-1349; huckleberrysnaturalmarket.com

Island Health Foods, 11354 Kallgren Rd. NE, Bainbridge Isle, WA 98110; islandhealthfoods.com

Living Green Natural Food and Apothecary, 630-A Second St., Langley, WA 98260; 360-221-8242; some raw

Lorien Herbs & Natural Foods, 1102 S. Perry St., Spokane, WA 99201

Madison Market/Central Co-op, 1600 E Madison, Seattle, WA 98122; 206-329-1545; MadisonMarket.com

Manna Mills Natural Market, 21705 66th Ave., NE, Wountlake Terrace, WA 98043; MannaNaturalMarket.com

Mill Creek Natural Foods, 4315 Main St., Union Gap, WA 98903; 509-452-5386; millcreekfoods.com

Mother Nature's Natural Foods, 516 1st Ave. N, Seattle WA 98109-4522

Mt Sunflower Natural Market, 358 N. Main St., Colville, WA 99114

Nature's Market, 26011 104th Ave. SE, Kent WA 98030

Northwest Veg; NWVeg.org. Vegetarian information, events, resources in the Pacific Northwest. NWVeg.org/restaurants

Okanogan River Co-op, 21 W 4th Street, POB 591, Tonasket, WA 98855; 509-486-4188

Olympia Food Co-op – East, 3111 Pacific Ave. SE, Olympia, WA 98501; 360-956-3870

Olympia Food Co-op - West, 921 N Rogers, Olympia, WA 98502; 360-754-7666

Omega Nutrition, 6515 Aldrich Rd., Bellingham, WA 98226

Puget Consumers' Co-op – Fremont, 600 N 34th St., Seattle, WA 98103; 206-632-6811; PCCNaturalMarkets.com

Puget Consumers' Co-op – Greenlake, 7504 Aurora Ave. N, Seattle, WA 98103; 206-525-3586; PCCNaturalMarkets.com

Puget Consumers' Co-op, 1810 12th Ave NW, Issaquah, WA 98027; 425-369-1222; PCCNaturalMarkets.com

Puget Consumers' Co-op, 10718 NE 68th St., Kirkland, WA 98033; 425-828-4622; PCCNaturalMarkets.com

Puget Consumers' Co-op, 11435 Avondale Road NE, Redmond, WA 98052; 425-285-1400; PCCNaturalMarkets.com

Puget Consumers' Co-op - View Ridge, 6514 40th St., NE, Seattle, WA

98115; 206-526-7661; PCCNaturalMarkets.com

Puget Consumers' Co-op - Seward Park, 5041 Wilson Ave. S, Seattle, WA 98118; 206-723-2720; PCCNaturalmarkets.com

Puget Consumers' Co-op - West Seattle, 2749 California Ave., SW, Seattle, WA 98116; 206-937-8481; PCCNaturalMarkets.com

Raw Institute of Permaculture Education, RawPermaculture.org.

Raw Vegan Source, Redmond, WA; rawvegansource.com. Raw store, supplies, recipes, and permaculture. By Tom Armstrong and Susan Park.

Sidecar for Pigs Peace Store, 5270 B University Way NE (at 55th), Seattle WA 98105; 206-523-9060; sidecarforpigspeace.com. Store that sells everything vegan, a lot of cooked stuff, but more and more raw food.

Skagit Valley Food Co-op, 202 S. First St., Mount Vernon, WA 98273; 360-336-9777; SkagitFoodCoop.com

Sno-Isle Natural Foods Co-op, 2804 Grand Ave., Everett, WA 98201; 425-259-3798; SnoIsleFoods.coop

Sunny Farms, 261461 Hwy. 101 W, Sequim, WA 98382

Terra Organica, 929 N. State St., Bellingham, WA 98225

Thrive, 1026 NE 65th St., Seattle, WA 98115; 206-334-7111; generationthrive.com. Raw, organic restaurant and supply store. Monika Kinsman. Monika (at) generationthrive.com.

Vegetarians of Washington, VegOfWA.org

Vibrant Health Foods, 1314 Yakima Valley Hwy., Sunnyside, WA 98944

Wenatchee Natural Foods, 222 N Wenatchee, WA 98801; 509-665-9999; wenatcheenaturalfoods.com

Willow's Naturally, 169 Winslow Wy. East, Bainbridge Island, WA 98110

• U.S. WEST VIRGINIA

Check MeetUp.com for raw food meetups.

Good Energy Foods, 214 3rd St., Elkins, WV 26241; 304-636-5169; goodenergyfoods.com

Mountain People's Market, 1400 University Ave., Morgantown, WV 26505; 304-291-6131; mountaincoop.com

Natural Roads Food Co-op, 20 Fairfax Dr., Wheeling, WV 26003; 304-242-8873

• U.S. WISCONSIN

Check MeetUp.com for raw food meetups.

Basic Cooperative, 1221 Woodman Rd., Janesville, WI 53545; 608-754-3925

Café Manna, 3815 N Brookfield Rd, Brookfield, WI 53045; CafeManna.com. Vegetarian and vegan. Cooked and raw. Juices.

Cafe Tarragon, 2352 S Kinnickinnic Ave, Milwaukee, WI 53207; futuregreen.net. Organic vegetariand and vegan raw food. Gluten-free. Inside Future Green Store.

Chequamegon Food Co-op, 215 Chapple Ave., Ashland, WI 54806; 715-682-8251

The Getaway Car Juice Bar & Gallery, 7821 Hwy 42, Egg Harbor, WI 54209. 920-868-3300

Iron River Grocery Co-op, 307 North Main St., Iron River, WI 54847; 715-

372-4264

Island City Food Co-op, 1490 Second Ave., POB 857, Cumberland, WI 54829; 715-822-8233

Kickapoo Exchange Food Co-op, Box 276, 209 Main St., Gays Mills, WI 54631; 608-735-4544

Loving Hut, 165 University Ave, Palo Alto, CA 94301; lovinghut.us/paloalto. Organic vegan.

Main Street Market Whole Foods Co-op, 1 South Main St., Rice Lake, WI 54868; 715-234-7045

Mega Pik N Save, 1201 S Hastings Way, Eau Claire, WI 54701; 715-836-8700; megafoods.com

Menomonie Market Food Co-op, 521 2nd Street East, Menomonie, WI 54751; 715-235-6533; menomoniemarket.org

Natural Alternatives Food Co-op, 241 Main St., POB 377, Luck, WI 54837; 715-472-8084

Nature's Bakery Co-op, 1019 Williams St., Madison, WI 53703; 608-257-3649; naturesbakery.coop

Nature's Pantry Food Co-op, 258 South Knowles St., New Richmond, WI 54017; 715-246-6105

Neighborhood Natural Foods Coop, 320 Main St., POB 35, Iron River, WI 54847; 715-372-4022; basicshealth.com

Outpost Natural Foods Co-op, 100 E Capital Dr., Milwaukee, WI 53212; 414-961-2597; outpostnaturalfoods.coop

Outpost Natural Foods Co-op: Wauwatosa, 7000 W. State St., Wauwatosa, WI 53213; 414-778-2012; outpostnaturalfoods.coop

People's Food Co-op, 315 S 5th Ave., La Crosse, WI 54601; 608-784-5798; pfc.coop

Pine River Food Co-op, 134 W Court St., Richland Center, WI 53581; 608-647-7299

Raw Deal, 544 Broadway S., Menomoni, WI 54751; 715-231-3255; therawdeal.weebly.com. Deli with some raw items.

Riverwest Co-op Grocery & Café, 733 N. Clark St., Milwaukee, WI 53212; 414-264-7933; riverwestcoop.org

Stevens Point Area Food Co-op, 633 Second St., Stevens Point, WI 54481; 715-341-1555

Trillium Natural Foods Community Co-op, 517 Springdale St., Mount Horeb, WI 53572; 608-437-5288

Viola Food Co-op, 110 Commercial St., POB 243, Viola, WI 54664; 608-627-1476

Viroqua Food Cooperative, 609 N. Main St., Viroqua, WI 54665; 608-637-7511; viroquafood.coop

Vita Rawstaurant, 131 N Broadway, Green Bay, WI 54303; 920-884-8482. Raw food. Family-owned.

Whole Earth Grocery, 126 S. Main St., River Falls, WI 54022; 715-425-7971

Willy Street Co-op, 1221 Williamson St., Madison, WI 53703; 608-251-6776; willystreet.coop

Yahara River Grocery Cooperative, 229 East Main St., Stoughton, WI 53589;

608-877-0947; yaharagrocery.coop

• U.S. Wyoming

Check MeetUp.com for raw food meetups.

Alpenglow Natural Foods, 109 E. 2nd St., Casper, WY; 307-234-4196; alpenglownaturalfoods.com

Big Hollow Food Co-op, 119 S. 1st St., Laramie, WY; 307-745-3586; bighollowfc.com

Crazy Lady Farm and Greenhouse, 229 first West/POB 74, Fairview, WY 83119; 307-887-6302. Delivering organic produce baskets to your door, tours of our farm and you-pick. In scenic Star Valley, Wyoming. Charly McOmber, RainbowCottage (at) live.com.

Good Health Emporium, 753 E. Brundage Lane #C, Sheridan, WY; 307-674-5715

Hole in the Wall Health Foods, 152 N. Kimball St., Casper, WY; 307-473-2992

Jackson Whole Grocer, 974 West Broadway, Jackson, WY; 307-733-0450; JacksonWholeGrocer.com**.** Co-op market in downtown.

Pinedale Farmer's Market, North Tyler Ave, Pinedale, WY 82941**;** PineDaleFarmersMarket.org.

Sweet Grass Food Co-op, 169 Esterbrook Rd., Douglas, WY 82633; 307-358-0582

• U.S. Puerto Rico

Check MeetUp.com for raw food meetups.

Natural High Cafe, Freshmart Aguadilla, Plaza Victoria, Route #2, Km. 129.5, Rincon PR 00677; 787-823-1772; NaturalHighCafe.com

• African Continent

Check MeetUp.com for raw food meetups.

Bolo Bolo, 42 Palmer Rd. Muizenberg, Western Cape, South Africa; BoloBolo.co.za. Vegan café and book store. Some raw items on menu.

Eat Your Garden, South Africa; eatyourgarden.co.za. These people will plant an organic garden for you.

Food and Trees for Africa, trees.co.za. Excellent group involved in planting trees and promoting food gardening and permaculture.

Legassi Gardens, Addis Ave., Pokuase Junction, Greater Accra, Ghana, Africa. legassigardens.com. LegassiGardens (at) hotmail.com. Managed vegetarian apartments with vegetarian café.

Living Food for Africa, LivingFoodForAfrica.com. Angie Curtis put this wonderful site together (info (at) livingfoodforafrica.com). Lots of links to various helpful sites, including information on organic food stores, gardening, and more.

MyAfya. myafya.com/therapies/rawfood

Raw Magic Online, RawMagickOnline.com. A blog from Craig de Gouveia of Cape Town.

Soaring Free Superfoods, POB 88, Simonstown 7995, South Africa; superfoods.co.za. Peter and Beryn Daniel. (Peter (at) superfoods.co.za). Raw food chefs who give courses and sell products. Formerly lived in UK.

Space of Love, SpaceOfLove.co.za. Ashleigh Gordon: ashleighgordon (at) googlemail.com. Ian Light: wildvision (at) gmail.com. In 2010, they began holding these Space of Love Gatherings, which are conscious co-created weekends of song, dance, inspiration, sharing, healing, fun and connection. "Talks and workshops offered by us, for us include permaculture, yoga, raw food, storytelling, vision circles, and earth celebrations."

South African Vegan Society, vegansociety.co.za

Tatamoo Raw Vegan Cheese, 3 Regent Square, Woodstock, 7925 Cape Town, South Africa; tatamoo.co.za. Henni van der Westhuizen

Urban Sprout, urbansprout.co.za. This is an interesting site that includes lots of goings on in Africa to help heal the planet. Site includes a green directory.

• AUSTRALIA

Check MeetUp.com for raw food meetups.

About Life Natural Market, 605 Darling St., Rozelle, NSW, 2039, Australia; aboutlife.com.au.

About Life Natural Market, 31-37 Oxford St., Bondi Junction, NSW 2022, Australia; aboutlife.com.au.

Abundant Garden, 191 Petsch Creek Rd., Tallebudgera Valley, QLD 4228, Australia; 1 300 762 292; Info (at) abundantgarden.com.au. Peter and Heather

Academy of Natural Living, Clohey River Health Farm, POB 901, Cairns, QLD 4870, Australia; 07-4093-7989; international +61 7 4051 0177; iig.com.au/anl. John Fielder conducts fasts. When seeking care from any health practitioner, it is wise to check on their background and history, and to ask questions regarding any suggested treatment with the goal of finding what is best for you.

Acres Australia, POB 1822, Noosaville, BC, QLD 4566, Australia; acresaustralia.com.au. National newspaper for sustainable agriculture.

Alchemia Liquid Nutrition AKA **Alive and Wild**, Shop 2, 130 Jonson Street, Byron Bay, NSW 2481, Australia; alchemialiquidnutrition.com; aliveandwild.com.au; 0412 400 085. Vicki Veranese. Info (at) aliveandwild.com. Café. Opened 2010.

Alfalfa House Organic Co-op, 113 Enmore Rd., Enmore, Sydney, NSW 2042; Australia; 029-519-3374; alfalfahouse.org

Alive Organics, Shop 7, 507-515 Walter Rd. East, Morley, WA 6062, Australia; (08) 9377-3880; 08-9371-9908; AliveOrganics.com.au; comshare (at) iinet.com.au; Perth area. Natural foods store. Juice and smoothie bar. Closed on Sunday. They also run the online raw food supply store HealthyValleyOrganics.com.au. +61-8-9371-9903.

All Organic Shop, 341 Elisabeth St., North Hobart, Hobart & South East, Tasmania, 7000 Australia; 03 6234 9090.

All Raw, south of Adelaide, Fleurieu Penninsula; +61 0406-338-212; remedybliss (at) gmail.com

ANU Food Co-op, 7 Kingsley St., Acton, ACT 2601, Australia; anu.foodco-op.com/blog

AussieHealthCoach.com.au; PO Box 4174, Canning Vale East, WA 6155, Australia. Aimee Devlin. Also: RawPear.com

Australian Community Foods, communityfoods.org.au.

Australian Community Gardens Network, communitygarden.org.au.

Australian Farmers' Markets Association, farmersmarkets.org.au. Lists farmers' markets throughout Australia.

Australian Regional Food Guide, australianregionalfoodguide.com.au. Listings of various organic and local food farms, orchards, vineyards, restaurants, and stores. Not all listings are vegetarian.

Katie Barber, Australia raw food fitness trainer, katiebug (at) iprimus.com.au.

The Beanstalk Organic Food, 3 Morgan St., Newcastle East (St. Marks Church) (POB 87, Islington NSW 2293, Australia; beanstalk.org.au.

Bellamy's Organic Orchards, 68-72 Cameron St., Launceston, North East & Midlands, 7250 Tasmania, Australia. Locally-grown organic fruit.

Bellingen Living Foods and Health, Macs Shop, Cahill St., Bellingen, NSW 2454, Australia; bellingenlivingfoodsandhealth.com; denene (at) bellingenlivingfoodsandhealth.com. Denene Williams McArthur.

The Berry Farm, Bessell Rd. (RMB 222), Margaret River, South-West, 6285, WA; 08 9757 5054.

Biological Farmers of Australia, POB 530 – 766 Gympie Rd., Chermside, QLD 4032, Australia; bfa.com.au.

Bliss Organic Garden Café, 7 Compton St., Adelaide, AU; 08-8231-0205. Vegan with raw and gluten-free foods on menu.

Blue Mountains Berries, Berridale, 174-184 Shipley Rd., Blackheath, Sydney, Blue Mtns. & Hawkesbury, 2785 NSW, Australia; 02 4787 5990.

Blue Mountains Food Co-op, Shops 1 & 2 Jones House, Ha'penny Lane, Katoomba NSW 2780, Australia; bluemtnsfood.asn.au.

Bodhi Kitchen, 766 Glenhuntly Rd., Caulfield, South VIC 3162, Australia.

Gay Campbell, Sydney, Australia; GaiasTable.com. Holds raw food events, classes.

Grant Campbell (aka rawaussiealthelete) rawreference.com; rawaussieathlete (at) gmail.com. Ultra marathon runner, 811 lifestyle coach, father, musician, raw retreat organizer.

Canberra Organic Growers Society (COGS), POB 347, Dickson, ACT 2602, Australia; cogs.asn.au

Candelo Bulk Wholefoods Cooperatvie, 34 Church St., Bega, NSW 2550, Australia. Not-for-profit co-op run by volunteers. BYO bags and jars.

Carlisle Health Foods, 238 Carlisle St., Balaclava 3183, Australia

Cedar Creek Orchard, 269 Mulhollands Rd., Thirlmere, South Coast, New South Wales; 02 4681 8457.

Celtic Organic Wholefoods, 19-21 Alicia St., Southport, QLD 4215; Australia; celticorganic.com.au. Market and home delivery. Fresh juices and smoothies.

Cherrydale Orchard, New England Hwy., Teneterfield, Heart of Country (North), 2372, New South Wales; 02 6736 2781. Stone fruit orchard offering pick-your-own.

The Chia Company, POB 105, Leederville, WA 6902, Australia; thechiaco.com.au. Sells raw chia seeds.

Christma Hills Rasperry Farm, 9 Christmas Hills Rd., Elizabeth Town, North Wales 7304, Tasmania, Australia.

City Farm Organic Produce Markets, 1 City Farm Pl., East Perth, Australia; cityfarm.org.au. Saturday 9-noon. Organic produce and nursery.

City Food Growers, cityfoodgrowers.com. Organic gardening organization.

CNR Kitchen, Lake and James St., Northridge, Perth, 6003, Australia. Eclectic menu with everything from gourmet vegan to cooked not vegetarian. Check their FaceBook page.

Community Foods, 74 Shields St., Caims, GLD, 4870, Australia; comfoods.org.au.

Conscious Choice, Sydney; 02-9990-9204. Conscious-Choice.com. Catering and classes by Julie Mitsios, and an on-line store.

The Darrington Brothers, Paul and Ryan, creating a biodynamic permaculture healing center. Email only paul.darrington (at) hotmail.com

The Desert Fruit Company, datesaustralia.com.au. Dave Berrick, owner.

Aimee Devlin, PO Box 4174, Canning Vale East, WA 6155, Australia; RawPear.com; AussieHealthCoach.com.au

Diggers Seeds, POB 300, Dromana, VIC, Australia, 3936; diggers.com.au. Rare and unusual seeds for your garden.

Doonkuna Orchard, Binda Rd., Crookwell 2583, Crookwell, Southern Highlands, 2583, NSW, Australia; 02 4832 1127. Stone fruit and apples.

Down to Earth Organics Market, 1/98 Marine Pde, Kingscliff, Northern Rivers, NSW 2487, Australia; 02 6674 2140.

Dunsborough Home of Health, Shop 28d, 55 Dunn Bay Rd., Dunsborough, WA 6281, Australia; 08-9756-8188.

Earthbound Organics, 1 Soldiers Rd., Roleystone, Australia. Open Wednesday through Sunday 9:30-5.

Earth Garden Magazine, POB 2, Trentham, VIC 3458, Australia; earthgarden.com.au. Magazine for sustainable living

Earth Market & Café, Shop 14, 375 Subiaco Mews, Hay St., Subiaco, WA 6008, Australia; earthmarket.com.au. Closed Sunday and holidays.

Earth to Table, 85 Bronte Rd., Bondi Junction, Sydney, NSW 2022. Vegan, raw, juices, salads, gourmet, organics, etc. Julie Mitsios. Open late 2012.

Eatem Organic Farm, 1333 Lonnavale Rd., Lonnavale, Hobart & South East, Tasmania 7109, Australia. Organic fruits and vegetables.

Eco Directory (EcoShop), ecodirectory.com.au. Information on sustainable living in Australia.

Eden Gate Blueberry Farm, 685 Eden Rd., Youngs Siding, 6331, WA, Australia. You can also pick your own berries here.

Eden Seeds, M.S. 905, Lower Beechmont, QLD 4211, Australia. edenseeds.com.au. Gardening seeds.

Embracing Health, Lisa Wheeler N.D., (mailing address only: Suite 299, 15 Albert Ave., Broadbeach QLD 4218, Australia); embracinghealth.com.au; Info (at) EmbracingHealth.com; EmbracingHealthBlog.com. Raw coach Leisa Wheeler's health transformation education and retreats.

Energetic Greens, Lot 1, Cedar Rd., Wilsons Creek, Northern Rivers, NSW. Organic sprouts and shoots.

Flame Tree Community Co-op, 3.374 Lawrence Hargrave Dr., Thirroul NSW 2515 (POB 178, Thirroul, 2515); flametreecoop.org.au. Opened in 2010.

Flannery's, Bronberg Plaza, Slatyer Ave., Benowa, QLD 4217, Australia; flannerys.com.au. Organic market.

Flannery's, Corner Rode & Webster Roads, Chermside, QLD 4032, Australia; flannerys.com.au. Organic market.

Flannery's, Shop 5/1 Bryants Rd., Loganholme, QLD 4219, Australia; flannerys.com.au. Organic market.

Flannery's, Central One, 45 Plaza Pde., Maroochydore, QLD 4558, Australia; flannerys.com.au. Organic market.

Flannery's, 2184 Gold Coast Hwy., Miami, QLD 4220, Australia; flannerys.com.au. Organic market. Across from Miami High School.

Flannery's, 7, East T Centre, Robina, Gold Coast, QLD 4226; flannerys.com.au. Organic market.

Flannery's, 191 Moggill Rd., Taringa, QLD 4068, Australia; flannerys.com.au. Organic market.

Flannery's, 52 Annerley Rd., Woolloongabba, QLD 4102, Australia; flannerys.com.au. Organic market.

Flannery's, 2021 Wynnum Rd., Wynnum Plaza, QLD 4178, Australia; flannerys.com.au. Organic market.

Food Connect, foodconnect.com.au. Food Connect's aim is to supply local, sustainably produced food to the community in South East Queensland.

Food Forest, Annemarie and Graham Brookman, POB 859, Gawler, SA 5118, Australia; foodforest.com.au.

Food Not Bombs Sydney, sydfoodnotbombs.blogspot.com.

Freshline Organics Delivery, Perth, Australia; fresline.com.au; 9284-6503

Friends of the Earth Food Co-op, 312 Smith St., Collingwood (POB 222, Fitzroy, VIC, 3065, Australia); Melbourne.foe.org.au.

From Earth and Water, Shop 6, 30 James St., Burleigh Heads, QLD 4220, Australia; fromearthandwater.com. Raw and organic food, catering, and classes. At the Northy Street Organic Market. Delivery service available. Also produces raw organic vegan ice cream for sale at local markets. Nicki.

Freelee Fruititionist, TheFruititionist.com.

The Fruit Shack, 55 Dunn Bay Rd., Dunsborough, WA 6281, Australia; fruitandvegshack.com.au.

FruVenu, Sydney, Australia; 02-9636-2268; fruvenu.com.au. Raw food classes. Joy Mozzi.

Gaia's Table, Sydney, Australia; gaiastable.com. Gay (at) gaiastable.com. joymozzi (at) gmail.com. Classes, raw food gatherings, picnics. Gay Campbell and Joy Mozzi.

Garden Organics, Queen Victoria Market, 1 Shed Stalls 71-77, Therry St., Melbourne; gardenorganics.com.au; 03 8618 6976. Also delivers.

Genesis in the Hills Café, Roleystone, Australia. Reservations: (08) 9397 7799; genesisinthehills.com.au. Email: info (at) genesisinthehills.com.au. Vegetarian and vegan food.

Glo Health, 358 Glenhuntly Rd., Elsternwick, VIC 3185, Australia

Gosia O'Reilly, rawgosia.com.au. Mother of two children offering information to build healthier families.

Go Vita, Shop 31 Southlands Blvd., Willetton, WA 6155, Australia.

Go Vita Margate Health Foods, 8b;270 Oxley Ave., Margate Beach, QLD 4019, Australia; (Office warehouse: 3/14 Childs Rd., Chipping, Norton, NSW 2710; Austrralia); govita.com.au.

Granny Smith Natural Food Market, 6 Princes St., Turramurra, NSW 2074, Australia; grannysmith.net.au. Smaller store focused on local foods. Features "food kilometer" (relating to locally-grown and carbon footprint) ratings on the produce signs. Store named after Maria Ann Smith, the English woman who raised her children in Australia, and who grew the first of what became known as Granny Smith Apples, from a seed of an apple from Tasmania.

Green Harvest Organic Gardening Supplies, POB 92, Maleny, QLD, 4552, Australia. greenharvest.com.au.

Green Lizard Vegan, 20/230 William St., Kings Cross, Syndney, Australia. Vegan and raw fusion foods, drinks, smoothies, deserts. Opened 2011.

Green Tucker Store Co-op, Shop 4, 51 Arthur St., Forestville, Sydney, NSW, 2087, Australia; greentucker.org.au.

Happy Bellies UOW Food Co-op, Wollongong Campus.

Healthy Valley Organics, healthyvalleyorganics.com.au.

Hepburn Retreat Centre, 9 Lone Pine Ave., Hepburn Springs, VIC 3461, Austraila; HepburnRetreatCentre.com.au. A vegan retreat amongst hot springs land 100 km west of Melbourne. Zalen Glen, proprietor.

High Vale Bio-Dynamic Farm, 35 Merrivale Rd., Pickerying Brook, Australia; higvale.com. Farm produce.

Hippocrates Australia, POB 1760, Mudgeeraba, 4213 QLD, Australia; Hippocrates.com.au. Health retreat center

It's Up To You, Peter and Linda, POB 421, Manbucca Heads, NSW 2448, Australia; itsuptoyou.com.au. Coaching.

Joe's Organic Markets, 64 Victoria Rd., Northcote 3070 VIC, Australia; joesorganic.com.au. Joe has an interesting and helpful Web site.

Joy Discovery Café, 13 Bent St., Adelaide, SA 5000, Australia; joydiscoverycafe.com.au. Vegetarian café with some raw options, juices, and smoothies.

Jura Books Organic Food Co-op, Parramatta Rd., Petersham, Sydney, Australia (POB N32, Petersham North, NSW 2049, Australia); jura.org.au. Weekly boxes of fruits and veggies.

Ken Little's Fruit and Vegetables, 35 Munster St., Port Mcquarie, Mid North Coast, NSW; 02 6583 5685. Seasonal and locally-grown.

Kings Seeds, POB 2785, Bundaberg, QLD, 4670, Australia; kingsseeds.com.au. Gardening seeds.

Kits Living Foods, POB 818, Coolangatta, QLD 4225, Australia; kitzlivingfoods.com.au.

Kiwi Down Under Organic Farm & Teahouse, 430 Geleniffer Rd., Bellingen, Mid North Coast, 2441, NSW, Australia; 02 6653 4449. Organic fruit and nut farm.

La Diosa, Shop 4/139, Military Rd., Neutral Bay, NSW, 2089; LaDiosa.com.au. They offer some raw food prep classes as well as a variety of "natural health" services.

Le Cru, 137 Victoria Ave, Albert Park, Melbourne, VIC 3206, Australia. 03 9699 1144. lecru.com.au. Carolyn Trewin. Helen and Avril. Opened 2009. Raw restaurant. Vegan, but honey is used in some recipes.

Leo's Fine Foods and Wine, Hartwello, 1 Summerhill Rd., Glen Iris, VIC 3146, Australia

Leo's Fine Foods and Wine, 26 Princess St., Kew 3101, Australia

Life Foods, Australia; Scott Mathias of ScottMathiasRaw.com

The Little Larder Organic Produce Market, Shop 2, 15 Orlando St., Coffs Harbour, Mid North Coast, 2540 NSW, Australia; 02 6651 1088.

Live Food Education, Australia; livefoodeducation.com. Anand (at) livefoodeducation.com. Anand Wells and Runi Burton's site.

Living Foods, 78 Park Ave., Yandoit, VIC 3461, Australia; livingfoods.com.au; livingfoods (at) activ8.net.au; 0432 487 122. Specialises in raw living foods bars.

Living Foods Co-op, Melbourne, Australia; livingfoodcoop (at) gmail.com; facebook.com/profile.php?id=1005695401&ref=ts

Loose Produce, 2 Hobbs Ave., Como, Experience Perth, WA, Australia; looseproduce.com. 08 9474 9100. Closed Sundays.

Casey Lorraine Thomas Raw Food Coach, Australia; caseylorraine.com.

The Lost Seed, POB 321, Sheffield, Tasmania 7306, Australia; thelostseed.com.au. Rare, open-pollinated, heritage, and heirloom seeds that are non-hybrid, non-GMO.

Loving Earth, (Mailing address: 89B Harding St, Coburg, Melbourne, VIC 3058, Australia); 03 9095 6250; 9005 3071; Mobile 0410 910 464; lovingearth.com.au; info (at) lovingearth.net. Raw-Chocolate.net. Online store selling raw foods. Products are available in many health and specialty stores. Scott Fry.

Jessica Loyer, raw gastronome (writes about and researches food). Jessloyer (at) gmail.com. Rawgastronomy.blogspot.com.

Kemi's Raw Kitchen, KemisRawKitchen.com.au. Kemi Nekvapil

Kind Living Café, Brisbane, Australia; KindLivingCafe.com. Opened in Brisbane in 2012.

Lynton Fruit & Veggie Farm, 64 Devlot Rd., Bobigana, North East & Midlands, 7276 Tasmania, Australia.

Macro Wholefoods Market, 31-37 Oxford St., Bondi Junction, NSW 2022, Australia; 029389-7611

Mani Organic Produce, 409 Princes Hwy., Woonana, South Coast, NSW, Australia; 02 4285 9875.

Manly Food Co-operative, 21B Whistler St., Manly NSW 2095, Australia; manlyfoodcoop.org.

Manna Wholefoods, 274 S. Terrace, South Fremantle, Australia.

Maple Street Co-op, 37 Maple Street, Maleny QLD 4552, Australia; maplestreetco-op.com.

Scott Mathias, Australia; ScottMathiasRaw.com and LifeFoods.com

Maya Malamed, changingmaya.com.au. She has organized raw events in Sydney.

Meadow View Orchard, Convent Ln., Borenore, Heart of Country (South), 2800, NSW; 02 6365 2249. Apples, stone fruit, and figs.

Mecca Bros Fruit City, 322 Queens Parade, North Fitzroy 3068 Australia

Miami Markets, Miami High School, Miami, Australia. Corner of Gold Coast Hwy. and Pacific Avenue. Held on Sundays. ROAR foods sells their raw food products here.

Mimsbrook Farm & Café, 65 C Etwell St., East Victoria Park, Australia. Wednesday through Saturday.

Miss Organic, Melbourne, Australia; missorganic.com.au. Organic produce delivery service. Nicci.

Julie Mitsios, Sydney, Australia; conscious-choice.com. Catering and classes by Julie Mitsios, and an on-line store.

Moss-side Berry Farm, 2268 Frankford Rd., Frankford, North East & Midlands, Tasmania 7275, Australia.

Mt. Claremont Farmers' Markets, Mt. Claremont Primary School, Corner of Alfred Road and Davies Road, Mt. Claremont, Australia. Saturday 8-11:30 a.m.

Mt. Lawley Wholefoods & Tempting Thyme Café, Unit 3, 885 Beaufort St., Inglewood Ave., (at Ninth Ave.), Inglewood, WA 6052, Australia; mtlawleywholefoods.com.au. Allen and Marlene Robinson. Closed Sundays.

Mullumbimby Fruit Market, 65 Burringbar St., Mullumbimby, Northern Rivers, 2482, NSW; 02 6684 2169. Fruit and vegetables.

My Heart Garden Café, Shop 5, 225 Hawken Dr., St. Lucia, QLD 4067, Australia. 617 3870 8898.

My Rainbow Dreams, Shop G1B, Dickson Chambers, Dickson Pl., Canberra, Australia; myrainbowdreams.com.au. Vegetarian restaurant with some raw options. Run by students of Sri Chinmoy.

Naked Treaties, nakedtreaties.com.au. Produces truffles and deserts sold at various locations. Jemma (at) nakedtreaties.com.au.

Natural Health Supplies, 78 Ormond Rd., Elwood ,VIC 3184, Australia; naturalhealthelwood.com. Organic produce and supplies. Said to be the oldest natural foods store in Australia. Also, the home of the Vegetarian Society of Australia.

National Association for Sustainable Agriculture Australia (NASAA), Unit 7/3 Mount Barker Rd., Stirling, SA 5152, Australia; nasaa.com.au.

Nimbin Organics Market, 50 A Cullen St., Nimbin, Northern Rivers, NSW 2480, Australia; 02 6689 1445.

Nushies Natural, Level 1, 137 Victoria Ave., Albert Park, Melbourne, 3206 Australia; nushiesnatural.com.au. Maker of raw vegan ice cream, crackers, and granola sold to a growing number of natural food stores. Nushie and Carolyn.

Organic Energy Pure Produce, Shop 8A, Griffith Shops, Barker St., Griffith, Snowy Mountains & ACT, NSW; 02 6295 6700.

Organic Farm Share, Australia; OrganicFarmShare.com. Alf and Marina Orpen.

Organically Grown, 85b St. Bernards Rd., Magill, Adelaide, SA 5087, Australia; 08 83641699. Clinton is the owner, is into raw foods, and seeks out the best he can find in fresh organics. Clinton (at) senet.com.au.

Organic Angels Food Delivery, 8 Andrew St., Blackbourn South, Australia; 1300-792-775; organicangels.com. Organic produce delivery service.

Organic Biodynamic Deliveries, Perth, Australia; Helen 9418-8842

The Organic Collective Delivery, Perth, Australia; theorganiccollective.com.au; 9331-5590.

Organic Farm Share, organicfarmshare.com. Building an organic food community-supported farm for the northern NSW and southern QLD.

Organic Federation of Australia, POB 369, Bellingen, NSW 2454, Australia; ofa.org.au. Site contains information on organic farming certification, and many links to information about toxicity issues of farming chemicals and about organic farming methods, education, and organizations.

Organic Food & Farmers' Markets, Sydney, Australia; organicfoodmarkets.com.au. Site lists organic farmers' markets in Sydney area.

Organic Gertrude, 108 Station St., Fairfield, VIC, 3078, Australia; organicgertrude.com.au. Market.

Organic Larder, 167 Malop St., Geelong, VIC 3220, Australia; organiclarder.com.au. Grocery store.

Organic Markets, organicmarkets.com.au.

Organic n' Green, 5-3 Adalia St., Kallaroo, WA 6025, Australia; organicngreen.com.au. Closed Sundays and holidays.

Organic n' Green Shop & Café, 617 Wanneroo Rd., Manneroo, Australia. Closed Sundays and holidays.

Organic on Charles, Shop 7, 299 Charles St., North Perth, WA 6006, Australia; 9227-7755; organiconcharles.com.au. Closed on Sunday. Loren and Lyndon McMath, proprietors.

Organic Oz, Melbourne, Australia; organicoz.com.au. Home delivery.

Organic Revolutions, Shop 15, 33 Tallebudgera Creek Rd., West Burleigh QLD 4219, Australia. Café and produce. Sells ROAR food products, an Australian raw food company. Next to West Burleigh Post Office.

Organic Valley, 391 Welshpool Rd., East Cannington, WA 6107, Australia; organicvalleywa.com.au. Thursday through Saturday.

Organic Works, 412 Burke Rd., Camberwell, VIC 3124, Australia; organicworks.com. Home delivery.

Passionate Gourmet, Australia; passionategourmet.com.au. Coaching, classes, catering. In Wilson, Como, and Perth.

Passion Foods, 219 Ferrars St., South Melbourne, VIC 3205

Peaches Fresh Food Market, 195 Hampton Rd., South Fremantle, WA 6162, Australia. Seven days 7 a.m. – 7 p.m.

People & Animal Welfare Society, 112-114 Beaufort St., Perth, WA 6000, Australia; paws.org.au. Sells organic produce on Saturdays.

Permaculture Melbourne, POB 3020, Auburn, VIC 3123, Australia; permaculturemelbourne.org.au.

Pick Your Own, pickyourown.org/Australia.htm. On this site you can find farms where you can harvest your own food. You can also add information about self-harvest farms to the site.

Prahan Health Foods, 201 Commercial Rd., South Yarra, VIC 3141, Australia

The Radical Grocery Store, 347 Sydney Rd., Brunswick, VIC 3056, Australia.

Rare Fruit Society of South Australia, rarefruit-sa.org.au.

Raw and Peace, 34 Coral St., Maleny, Queensland, 4552; RawAndPeace.com.au. Raw food café.

Raw Aussie Family, rawaussiefamily.blogspot.com. Eve Zhu is a mother in Australia who keeps this blog about raw food. Formerly it was called Raw Aussie Mom.

Raw Energy (Mullalyup Fruit & Veg), Westland Orchards, Mullalyup, South-West, WA; 08 8764 1514.

Raw Events Australia, RawEventsAustralia.com

Raw Fit, Australia; 0414-646-377; rawfit.com.au. Fitness training and raw food workshops run by Ricardo Riskalla.

The Raw Kitchen, 14 Piazza Arcade, 36 S. Terrace, Fremantle, WA 6160; TheRawKitchen.com.au.

RawPear.com, PO Box 4174, Canning Vale East, WA 6155 Australia; Aimee Devlin. Also: AussieHealthCoach.com.au

Raw Pleasure; Raw-Pleasure.com.au; raw food supplies online; raw chat group; raw events.

Raw Power. Brisbane, Australia; RawPower.com.au. Gourmet raw food classes, events, online education, superfoods, and equipment. Valerie Morkel and Jane Brice bought the company in 2011 from Runi and Anand Wells.

RawReference.com, Grant Campbell

Rawsome, QLD, Australia; rawsome.com.au.

RealFoodFestival.com.au

Raw the Natural Food Store, 118 King St., Hobart, Hobart & South East, Tasmania 7005, Australia. Rawnaturalfoodstore.com.au. Organic produce, honey, wine, coffee, chocolate. Not a vegetarian or all raw store. Many locally-grown foods.

Real Organics, 46 The Parade, Norwood, SA 5067, Australia. Organic produce.

Revive and Replenish, Shop 15, 33 Tallebudgera Creek Rd., West Burleigh, QLD 4219, Australia. Café with some raw food and organic produce.

Roar Food, Burleigh, QLD, Australia; roarfood.com.au. Roarfood (at) me.com. Their prepared raw foods are sold at various locations. Check the website. Brendan Jones and Suki Kasinathan do catering, give lessons in raw food prep, and install culinary gardens. Their raw pizzas are becoming legendary. Jennie Murphy of raw-pleasure.com.au describes ROAR food's pizzas as "phenomenal."

Ruby's Place Performance Café, Bondi Beach, Australia. Has had raw food dinners.

Rusty's Market, 57-89 Grafton St., Cairns, QLD 4870, Australia; rustysmarkets.com.au. Between Shields St. and Spence St. by Gilligan's

Backpackers Hotel & Resort. Market with a stand that sells fresh fruit, including some organic.

Sadhana Kitchen, 76 A Wilford St., Newton, NSW 2042; Australia; SadhanaKitchen.com. In Jivamukti Yoga Centre off Enmore Road. Vegan, mostly raw. Opened 2012.

Sallydale Orchard, 225 Marshalls La, Blayney, Heart of Country (South), NSW 2799, Australia; 02 6368 2550. Organic fruit.

Samadhi Raw Yoga Retreat, North Stradbroke Island, QLD, Australia; samadhiflowyoga.com. Sub-tropical island retreat with yoga, dance, meditation, hikes, surfing, high-fruit raw food. Kath Ford. Kath (at) samadhiflowyoga.com

Samudra, POB 295, Dunsborough 6281, Western Australia; +61 897740110; Samudra.com.au. Runs yoga and surf retreats. Raw food café and organic store, also has raw food chefing classes. Beautiful location. This is the raw place to visit in Australia! Sheridan Hammond.

Santos Natural Food Store, 105 Johnson St., Byron Bay, NSW 2481, Australia; 6685-7071; SantosTrading.com.au. Open 7 days.

Santos Natural Food Store, 51-53 Burringbar St., Mullumbimby, Australia; 6684-3773; SantosTrading.com. Open 7 days

Seed Savers Network Australia, POB 975, Byron Bay, NSW 2481, Australia; seedsavers.net.

Seventh Pillar, Shop 5, Robina Village Shopping Centre, 195 Ron Penhaligon Way, Robina, QLD 4226, Australia; 07 5580 8822; seventhpillar.com.au. Herbs, oils, and health products. Carries Roar Food products.

Slow Food Sydney, slowfoodsydney.com.au. Dedicated to locally-grownn and homegrown foods. Not a vegan organization, but a source of information for a variety of food issues.

Soul Lube City Farms, soulube.com.

Soul Tree Organic Shop & Café, Shop 6, 3 Railway Parade, Glen Forrest, WA 6071, Australia; soultree.com.au. Monday-Sunday 8:30-5.

The Source Real Food Store, Shop 3, Figtree Sq., Strickland St., Denmark, South-West, WA 6333, Australia; 08 9848 1183.

Sprout Organic Wheatgrass, POB 383, Carlton North, VIC 3054, Australia; sprout.net.au. Nathan.

Steenholdt's Organic Products Orchard Farm, 270 Cyngnet Rd., Pethcheys Bay, Cygnet,, Hobard & South East, 7109, Tasmania. 03 6295 0141.

SunBread, Perth, Western Australia; sunbread.com/stockists. Grain-free raw breads sold in markets. Therese De Wolfe

Sun & Earth Organics, 845 Brunswick St., New Farm, QLD 4005, Australia; sunandearth.com.au. Natuaral foods store. Organic juice and smoothie bar.

Sunnybrook Health Store, 553 a North Rd., Ormand, VIC 3204, Australia

Sydney Food Fairness Alliance, GPO Box 1241 Sydney, NSW 2001, Australia; sydneyfoodfairness.org.au. Group working for a more sustainable food system.

Taste Organic Market, Shop 1, 25 Falcon St., Crows Nest, NSW 2065, Australia; tasteorganic.com.au; info (at) tasteorganic.com.au. Not vegetarian, but sells organic fruits and vegetables and raw packaged foods. Has had a raw café held on weekends organized by Maya Melamed of changingmaya.com.au.

Thirty Bananas a Day, 30bananasaday.com. A site for Australian raw foodists. Especially for those into the 80/10/10 high-fruit, low-fat, raw, vegan diet. Freelee Fruititionist, TheFruititionist.com

Casey Lorraine Thomas, Perth, Western Australia; caseylorraine.com; lifestyleraw.blogspot.com. Casey is a raw food coach, has detox programs, and is a colon-hydrotherapist. Has an e-book about the process, including recipes.

Thortas Organic Ginseng Farms, 33 Back Cam Link Rd., Somerset, North West, Tasmania 7322, Australia.

Thoughtful Foods, Roundhouse, University of New South Wales; thoughtfulfoods.org.au. Volunteer-run co-op.

Three Worlds Organic Pizza Cafe, 2558 Gold Coast Hwy., Mermaid Beach, Gold Coast, QLD 4218, Australia; 0401 555 958; myspace.com/thepizzapatch. threeworlds.com.au/life. threeworlds.com.au. Matt Lees and Jason Ure opened Three Worlds Drum Shop and Café in 2001. In 2008 the cafe was operating as a "pay as you feel" raw food café with food Katya of Rawjuvenate helped develop. They have converted an adjoining parking lot into a community activities garden and drum circle area. ROAR foods, a raw food company, also sells their products here.

Totally Organic Plus, Ferry Rd., Shop 8, Centro Shopping Centre, Southport, Queensland 4215, Australia; totallyorganic.com. Market.

Tried, Tasted, Served, TriedTastedServed.com. Email: customerservice triedteastedserved.com

Dr. Sandra Tuszynska, TheRawFacts.BlogSpot.com. She has a PhD in Cell Biology and Detoxification from UNSW, and has studied at Rutgers in the U.S. Author of the book, Fruitful Nutrition.

Tyndale Organic Farm, 2992 Pacific Hwy., Tyndale, Northern Rivers, NSW 2460, Australia; 02 6647 6513. Organic seasonal produce.

The USYD Food Co-op, usydfoodcoop.org.au.

Vegan Online, POB 451, Stirling, South Australia, 5152; veganonline.com.au

Vegan Society NSW, VeganSocietyNSW.com. Site contains information of interest to vegans, including vegan restaurant guide and links to environmental, sustainable living, and animal rights organizations.

The Vegetarian Network, Ste. 6, Kindness House, 288 Brunswick St., Fitzroy, VIC 3065, Australia; vnv.org.au.

Vegetarian Victoria, vegetarianvictoria.org.au. Listing of vegetarian and vegan businesses in the region.

Vegie Bar, 380 Brunswick St., Fitzroy, Melbourne, VIC 3065, Australia; VegieBar.com.au.

The Village Grocer, IGA Supermarket, 19-21 Armsrong St., Middle Park 3206, Australia

Violeta's Garden, Shop 20 Pioneer Village, 2 Southwest Hwy., Armadale WA 6112, Australia; violetasgarden.net.au. Organic market. Not vegan.

Waru Organic Farm, Emu Swamp, Heart of Country (South), NSW, Australia; 02 6365 9269. Organic produce and herbs.

The Wholefood Garden, 46 Pound Crossing Rd., Gresford, Hunter Valley, NSW 2311, Australia; 02 4938 9159. Organic produce.

Wilsons Organics, 57A Gouger St., Adelaide, SA 5000, Australia; 08 8231 5014. Organic and local produce at this market.

Helen and Robin Wolf, Byron Bay; lynne_wolfe (at) hotmail.com. Own an organic fruit and vegetable farm near Byron Bay. Members of WWOOF (Willing Workers on Organic Farms) and can host travelers willing to work on the farm.

Wray Organic, Victoria Ave., Oasis Shopping Centre, Broadbeach, QLD 4218, Australia; wrayorganic.com.au. Market.

Wray Organic, 110 Enoggera Rd., Newmarket, QLD 4051, Australia; wrayorganic.com.au. Market.

Wray Organic, 155, 19th Ave., Palm Beach, QLD 4221, Australia; wrayorganic.com.au. Market.

Wray Organic, 14 Lambert Rd., Indooroopilly, QLD 4068, Australia; wrayorganic.com.au. Market.

WWOOF, Mt. Murrundal Co-op, Buchan VIC 3885, Australia; WWOOF.com.au. Willing Workers On Organic Farms, Australia.

Yamba Organics, POB 224, Northern Rivers, 2464, NSW. Organic fruit and vegetable delivery.

Yong Green Food, 421 Brunswick St., Fitzroy, Melbourne, VIC 3065, Australia. Chef Sunju. Small vegan restaurant with some raw.

Yorktown Organics, 120 Bowen Rd., Yorktown, North East & Midlands, 7270, Tasmania, Australia; 03 6383 4624.

• AUSTRIA

Check MeetUp.com for raw food meetups.

The Heart of Joy, Franz-Josef-Strasse 3, Salzburg, Austria; 43 662 890 773; heartofjoy.at. Vegetarian restaurant with some raw options. Free wireless. Run by students of Sri Chinmoy.

• BALI

Check MeetUp.com for raw food meetups.

Big Tree Farms, No. 36 JI By Pass Ngurah Rai Br. Kertalangu, Desiman, Denspasar Timur, 80237, Bali, Indonisia; bigtreebali.com/story.html. Blair and Ben Ripple. They are the company that has gone to extreme measures to creat truly raw chocolate products. They also have other products.

Juice Ja Café, Dewi Sita Rd., Ubud, Bali. Fresh tropical fruit juices, wheatgrass juice, coconuts, and some food choices.

Kafe, Jln Hanoman 44b, Ubud, Bali; +62-361-7803802; balispirit.com/kafe. Email: kafe (at) balispirit.coom. Some raw foods, smoothies, juices.

Ubud Sari Organic Cafe, 35 JL, Jajeng Ubud, Bali; 62-361-974-393; ubudsari.com. Nila makes raw food. Much of which is freshly picked from their garden.

• BERMUDA

Check MeetUp.com for raw food meetups.

Rock On the Health Store, Butterfield Place, 67 Front St., Hamilton HM 11, Bermuda; 441-295-3468; rockonforhealth.com

• CANADA: ALBERTA

Check MeetUp.com for raw food meetups.

Homegrown Foods Natural Foods Store, #10 – 19 Granite Dr., Stony Plain, Alberta, Canada; 780-963-5305; homegrownfoodanagriproducts.com

Mother Nature's Health Food, 13231 – 20th Ave., Blaimore, Alberta, Canada; 403-562-8684; mothernatureshealthfoods.ca

Planet Organic, 7917 104 St., Edmonton, Alberta, Canada; planetorganic.ca

Sunrise Natural Foods, The Pacific Place, #521 999 36 St. NE, Calgary, Alberta, T2A 7X6, Canada; 403-273-3065

• CANADA: BRITISH COLUMBIA

Check MeetUp.com for raw food meetups.

Body Energy Club, 746 Davie St., Vancouver, BC, V6Z 1B6, Canada; 604-697-0466; 1-877-776-4844. Supplement store with raw foods and supplements hard to find in the city including maca, cacao, Pure Synergy, Vitamineral Green, goji berries, e3live, wheatgrass.

Café Cafe, 556 Pandora Ave., Victoria, BC, V8W 1N7, Canada; 250-590-5733; cafebliss.ca. Organic fresh juices and smoothies including wheatgrass and e3live, salads, and raw crackers.

Capers Market – Whole Foods Market, 2285 W 4th Ave, Vancouver, BC V6K 1N9, Canada; WholeFoodsMarket.com/Capers

Capers Market – Whole Foods Market, 1675 Robson St., Vancouver, BC V6G 1C8, Canada; WholeFoodsMarket.com/Capers

Capers Market – Whole Foods Market, 510 W. 8th Ave., Vancouver, BC V5Z 1C5, Canada; WholeFoodsMarket.com/Capers

Capers Market – Whole Foods Market, 925 Main St., West Vancouver, BC V7T 2Z3, Canada; WholeFoodsMarket.com/Capers

Country Sun Natural Foods, 1377 Johnson Rd., White Rock, British Columbia, V4B 3Z3, Canada; 604-531-1112

Drive Organics, 1045 Commercal Dr., Vancouver, BC, V5L 3X1 Canada; 604-678-9665. Organic grocery store, e3live, wheatgrass trays.

Eternal Abundance/Truffle Café, 1025 Commercial Dr., Vancouver, BC V5L 3X1, Canada; 604-255-8690. Organic produce grocery store with half raw cafe in the back.

Gorilla Food, 101-422 Richards St., Vancouver, British Columbia V5Z 2K6, Canada; 604-722-2504; GorillaFood.com. Aaron Ash, owner.

Kootenay Co-op, 295 Baker St., Nelson, British Columbia V1L 4H4, Canada; 250-354-4077; kootenay.coop

Organic Connections Café, 15622 Marine Dr., White Rock, BC. Vegan and vegetarian and raw menu. Across from Sandpiper Pub.

Organic Lives, 1829 Quebec St., Vancouver, BC V5T 2Z3, Canada; 778-588-7777; organiclives.org. Raw food cafe/superfood store. Also sells food and supplements online. Store carries variety of foods, nuts, and seeds, e3live, etc. Some entrees, including raw pizza, lasagna, nori rolls, and wraps. Wide selection of cakes and pies.

Planet Organic Market, 10-2755 Lougheed Hwy., Port Coquitlam, BC, V3B 5Y9, Canada; PlanetOrganic.ca.

Radha Yoga and Eatery, 728 Main Street, Vancouver, BC , V6A 2V7, Canada; 604-605-0011; radhavancouver.org. All vegan with daily raw specials.

Raw BC, POB 19020, 4th Ave. RPO, Vancouver, BC V6K 4R8; rawbc.org. Vancouver, British Columbia, Canada. A non profit raw food organization promoting the raw lifestyle. Brings in speakers to talk about raw foods.

Raw Food Meetup, Vancouver, British Columbia, Canada; rawfood.meetup.com/372; Raw food potluck and other raw events meetup group based in Vancouver, BC.

Raw Foundation Culinary Arts Institute, 1333 W. Georgia St., Vancouver St., Vancouver, BC; RawFoodFoundation.org

Rawk the Planet Raw Vegan Café, 240-12240 2nd Ave., Richmond, BC V7E 3L8.

Rawmbas, 101 572 Stewart Ave., Nanalmo, British Columbia, CA V9S 5T5; Rawmbus.ca. Has a Facebook page.

Rawsome Living Foods, 854 Long Harbour Rd., Salt Spring Island, BC, V8K 2L8, Canada; RawsomeLivingFoods.ca.

Rawsta Flora Organics, Vancouver, British Columbia, Canada; rawstafloraorganics.com. Produces raw packaged raw food products sold in various stores throughout Canada. Chantale Roy is the owner and is a graduate of the Living Light Culinary Institute. In 2010 she developed and taught a course in raw food cuisine for the University of British Columbia.

Rawthentic Eatery, 744 A Memorial Ave., Box 233, Qualicum Beach, BC V9K 1SB, Canada; rawthenticeatery.com; rawthenticeatery (at) shaw.ca. In strip mall with Pharmasave. Annette, Pam, and Amy Hadikin.

Roots Natural Organic Foods, 22254 Dewdney Trunk Rd., Maple Ridge, British Columbia, V2X 3H9, Canada; 604-467-1822; rootsnatural.ca.

Chantale Roy, Vancouver, BC, Canada; ChantaleRoy.ca. Gourmet raw food chef.

SeJuiced, 1958 West 4th, Vancouver, BC V6J 1M5, Canada; 604-730-9906. Vegetarian/Vegan. Some raw food. Organic juices.

Sunfruit Organics, 1041 B Ridgeway Ave., Coquitlam, British Columbia, V3J 1S6, Canada; 604-936-3405

Sunny Raw Kitchen, BC, Canada; thesunnyrawkitchen.blogspot.com. Carmella's blog is popular.

Sprouts at UBC, 66 Lower Level SUB; Vancouver, British Columbia, Canada; 604-822-9124; ams.ubc.ca/clubs/nfc. Student-run. Has café, and store. Weekly vegan lunch.

Truffles Café at Eternal Abundance, 1025 Commercial Dr., BC, V5L 3X1, Canada; 604-255-8690.

Whole Foods Market, 925 Main Street, West Vancouver, Canada; 604-678-0500; wholefoodsmarket.com/stores/westvancouver. Organic grocery, great selection of bulk foods plus produce.

Zen Zero 407B 5th St., Courtenay BC V9N 1J7, Canada; 250-338-0571; ZenZero.ca.

• CANADA: MANITOBA

Check MeetUp.com for raw food meetups.

Aviva Market, 1224 St. James St., Winnipeg, MB, R3H 0L1, Canada; aviva.ca. Sells a variety of products of interest to raw foodists.

• CANADA: NOVA SCOTIA

Check MeetUp.com for raw food meetups.

Ellora Natural & Organic Foods Buying Club, 3772 Highway 331, Lahave, Nova Scotia B0R 1C0, Canada; 902-688-2541; ellora.ca.

Satisfaction Feast, 3559 Robie St., Halifax, NS B3K 4S7, Canada; 902-422-3540; satisfaction-feast.com. Vegetarian restaurant with some raw options. Run by students of Sri Chinmoy.

• CANADA: ONTARIO

Check MeetUp.com for raw food meetups.

Annapurna, 1085 Bathurst St., Toronto, ON, Canada; annapurna.ca. Vegetarian café with some raw options, juices, and smoothies. Run by students of Sri Chinmoy.

Belmonte Raw, belmonteraw.com. Classes and catering.

The Best Food Ever, US Address: 3909 Witmer Rd., #574, Niagra Falls, NY 14305; thebestfoodever.com. Distributor of products. Packaged and bottled things, nuts, powders, and things marketed as "superfoods."

The Big Carrot Natural Food Market, 348 Danforth Ave., Toronto, Ontario M4K 1N8, Canada; 416-466-2129; thebigcarrot.ca. Large co-op.

Booster Juice, Canada; boosterjuice.com. Some raw items on manu, including wheatgrass juice. Various locations.

The Fairy's Tonic Kombucha, Toronto, Canada; thefairystonic.com.

Forever Healthy, online store, 1 Yorkville Ave., Ste. 1, Toronto, Ontario M4W 1L1, Canada

The Green Smoothie Bar, 236 James St. North, Hamilton, ON, Canada; TheGreenSmoothieBar.com

Harmony Whole Foods Market, 163 First St., Orangeville, Ontario, L9W 3J8; Canada; 519-941-8961; harmonymarket.com

In the Raw, Toronto, ON, Canada; intheraw.ca. Lindsay (at) intheraw.ca, and Erin (at) intheraw.ca sell their products at The Big Carrot, Noah's, Organics on Bloor, and Sweet Potato.

Jugo Juice Bars, jugojuice.com. Has some raw items, including wheatgrass juice. Various locations throughout Canada.

Karma Co-op, 739 Palmerston Avenue, Toronto, ON, M6G 2R3, Canada; 416-534-1470; KarmaCoop.org

Live Organic Food Bar, 264 Dupont St., Toronto M5R 1V7, Canada; 416-515-2002; LiveFoodBar.com. Also has packaged food available at the Big Carrot Natural Food Market.

The Living Centre, 5871 Bells Rd., London, ON N6P 1P3, Canada; thelivingcentre.com. Classes, seminars, speakers, retreats.

Lotus Heart Blossom, 185 Syndenham St., Kingston, Otario K7K 3M1, Canada; lotus-heart-blossom.com. Vegetarian restaurant with some raw options. Run by students of Sri Chinmoy.

The Naked Sprout, 4040 Palladium Way, Unit 11, Burlington, Ontario, L7M 0C2, Canada; TheNakedSprout.com.

Nature's Emporium, 16655 Yonge St., Unit 25, New Market, Ontario L3X 1V6, Canada; 905-898-1693; naturesemporium.ca.

Noah's Natural Foods, 667 Yonge St., Toronto, Ontario, M4Y 1Z9 Canada; noahsnaturalfoods.ca.

Noah's Natural Foods, 2395 Yonge St., Toronto, Ontario, M4Y 1Z9, Canada; noahsnaturalfoods.ca.

Noah's Natural Foods, 322 Bloor St. West, Toronto, Ontario, M5S 1W5, Canada; noahsnaturalfoods.ca.

Naoah's Natural Foods, 9121 Weston Rd., Vaughan, Ontario, L4H 0L4, Canada; noahsnaturalfoods.ca.

Nujima Living Foods, 588 Bloor St. West, Toronto, Ontario, M6G 1K4, Canada; info (at) nujima.com; nujima.com

Organics on Bloor, 468 Bloor St. W., Toronto, Ontario, M5X 1S9, Canada; 416-538-1333; organicsonbloor.com. One block east of Bathurst.

Peace Garden, 47 Clarence St., Ottawa, Ontario, Canada; 613-562-2434. Vegetarian restaurant with some raw options. Run by students of Sri Chinmoy.

Perfection-Satisfaction-Promise, 167 Laurier Ave., E. Ottawa, Ontario K1N 7R9, Canada; 613-234-7299. Vegetarian restaurant with some raw options. Run by students of Sri Chinmoy.

Power of Raw, Erika Wolff, powerofraw.com. Classes, retreats, seminars, recipes.

Raw Aura, 94 Lakeshore Rd. E., Mississauga, Ontario, L5G 1E3, Canada; raw-aura.com. Raw organic cuisine. Also serving juices, smoothies, and teas. Opened 2009.

Raw Elements Inc., RR #2, Acton, Ontario, L7J 2L8, Canada; 519-853-8729; rawelements.ca. Raw products company. Mail order.

Rawlicious, 3092 Dundas St. W., Toronto, ON, M6P 1Z8, Canada; 416-519-7150; rawlicious.ca

Ruth's Hemp Foods, ruthsfoods.com. Makes hemp seed nutrition products, including some that are raw. Distributed internationally.

S.E.E.D Culture, Kensington Market, 64 Oxford St., Toronto, Canada; 647-801-0833. Organic seeds and sprouting supplies.

Simply Raw Express, 989 Wellington Street West, Ottawa, Ontario, K1Y 2Y1; Canada; SimplyRaw.ca. Author Natasha Kyssa opened her raw food café in 2012.

Taloola Café, 396 Devonshire Rd., Windsor, Ontario, N8Y 2L4, Canada. Cooked vegetarian and vegan options with raw deserts, organic teas. A Bohemian type of café in an historic building. Linda Zagaglioni.

TerraTree, Toronto, Ontario, M6M 5G3, Canada; terratree.com. info (at) terratree.com. One of the oldest raw companies in Canada. They produce raw organic crackers, snacks, and deserts.

Toronto Sprouts, Mississauga, Toronto, Ontario, M5S 2R4, Canada; 416-977-8929; 416-535-3111; TorontoSprouts.com; Marie Larsson and Benjamin Stone

Toronto Vegetarian Association, veg.ca.

Upaya Naturals, Toronto, Ontario, Canada; 416-617-3096; upayanaturals.com.

WOW Wild Organic Café 22 Carden St., Guelph, Ontario, N1H 3A2, Canada; 519-766-1707

• CANADA: QUEBEC

Check MeetUp.com for raw food meetups.

Crudessence Service Traiteur, 5333 rue Casgrain, Suite. 801, Montreal, Quebec H2T 1X3, Canada; 514-271-0333.

Crudessence Pignon sur Rue, 105 rue Rachel Quest, Montreal, Quebec H2T 1X3, Canada; Crudessence.com. Raw food menu, classes, speakers, delivery.

Ecollegey – The Real Green Grocer, 4627 Wilson, Montreal, Quebec, H4A 2V5, Canada; 514-486-2247; ecollegey.com

Le KirlianCafé, 1337 de la Sapinière #3

Val-David, QC, J0T 2N0 Canada; gabriellesamson.com

Raw In Montreal, RawInMontreal.com. A Web site featuring information about raw events and things in Montreal. Info (at) RawInMontreal.com. Ildikó Brunner is from Budapest.

Tau, 4238 rue Saint-Denis, Montreal, Quebec, H2J 2K8, Canada (at Rachel); 514-843-4420; marchestau.com. Organic fruits and vegetables, bulk section.

Tau, 7373 Langelier Boul, St. Leonard, Quebec, H1S 1V7; 514-787-0077; marchestau.com. Organic fruits and vegetables, bulk section.

Tau, 3188 St. Bartin West Boul., Laval, Quebec H7T 1A1; 450-978-5533; marchestau.com. Organic fruits and vegetables, bulk section.

Tau, 6845 Tachereau Boul., Brossard, Quebec J4Z 1A7; 450-443-9922; marchestau.com. Organic fruits and vegetables, bulk section.

• CANADA: SASKATCHEWAN

Check MeetUp.com for raw food meetups.

Eat Healthy Foods Organic Grocery Store, 3030 12th Ave., Regina, Saskatchewan, S4T 1J6, Canada; 306-522-4167; eathealthyfoods.ca

• CARIBBEAN

Check MeetUp.com for raw food meetups.

Rest' O Cru, Galeries de Houelbourg, Z.I. de Jarry, 97122 Baie-Mahault, Guadeloupe - F.W.I.; restocru.com

• CENTRAL AMERICA: COSTA RICA

Check MeetUp.com for raw food meetups.

Finca de Vida (Food of Life); SW Costa Rica near San Isidro and Playa Dominical; fincadevida.com; 011-506-8-373-3261; info (at) fincadevida.com; Brian and Jody Calvi

Raw in Costa Rica, RawInCostaRica.com

• CENTRAL AMERICA: PANAMA

Check MeetUp.com for raw food meetups.

Tanglewood Wellness Center, Costa Rica;; tanglewoodwellnesscenter.com. Has promoted their supervised fasting and healing programs. Although Tanglewood is included in this book because people are interested in it, I would like to encourage anyone considering a visit to Tanglewood to research the background of the founder, and question the therapeutic techniques promoted there, such as long-term, supervised fasting. I do not advise people to go on long-term water fasts. According to the Quackwatch.org site in 2010, Loren Eric Lockman, who founded Tanglewood, has an interesting history with The Maryland Board of Physicians, which issued cease-and-desist orders against Lockman and Timothy Trader for practicing medicine without a license – after a woman with diabetes died after going through Lockman's guided fast. There is also information you can find out about Loren Lockman by doing a simple Google search for his name. Research before paying money or booking a flight.

• **CHINA**

Check MeetUp.com for raw food meetups.

Rawthentic Food, POB 224, Sai Kung Post Office, Hong Kong; RawThenticFood.com.

• **ENGLAND**

Check MeetUp.com for raw food meetups.

Aconbury Sprouts, aconbury.co.uk; info (at) aconbury.co.uk. Produces sprouts, wheatgrass, and other products.

Alchemy The Centre, Unit 101, Stables Market, Chalk Farm Rd., London NW1 8AH, England; 020 7267 6188; alchemythecentre.co.uk. Café with juice bar, smoothies, seed milks, elixirs. Yoga, workshops, events.

Alexandra Palace Farmers Market, Wood Green, N22. Sunday 9-3. Takeaway foods.

The Better Food Company, Proving House, Sevier St., St. Werburghs, Bristol, BS2 9QSEngland, BetterFood.co.uk. Organic supermarket and café.

Blackheath Farmers' Market, Blackheath Rail Station Car Park. Sunday 10-2. Near Greenwhich park.

Bonnington Cafe, 11 Vauxhall Grove, Vauxhall, SW8 1TD, London; bonningtoncafe.co.uk. Vegetarian and vegan café that has raw food. Check site.

Brixton Whole Foods, 59 Atlantic Rd., Brixton, SW9 8PU, London; 020 7737 2210. Organic produce.

Broadbery's, London, England; broadberys.co.uk. Makes and sells packaged raw food items, including flax crackers. Dustin Broadbery. Formerly associated with Dragonfly.

Bumblebee, 30, 32, 33 Brecknock Rd., N7 ODD; 020 7607 1936. Organic produce, nuts, seeds, herbs, spices.

China Town, London. Some shops in China Town sell durian, coconuts, mangosteen, and some other tropical fruits. See Woo 18-20 Lisle St.; New Loon Moon, 9 Gerard St.; Loon Fung, 42-44 Gerrard St.; Golden Gate, 100 Shaftesbury Ave.

Choice Organics, Units 3 & 4, Enterprice Way, Osiers Rd., Wandsworth, London, SW18 1EJ, UK; Wandsworth, choice-organics.com. Organic produce available here.

Conscious Events, consciousevents.co.uk. Kyle Vialli.

Country Life, London, England; countrylife-restaurant.co.uk. In 2009 they were closed.

Detox Your World, detoxyourworld.com

Earth Natural Foods, 200 Kentish Town Rd., London NW5 2AE; EarthNaturalFoods.co.uk

Fareshares Food Co-op, 56 Crampton St., Walworth, SE17 3AE; fairshares.org.uk. Some organic produce and dried whole foods. Thursday 2-8; Friday 3-7; Saturday 3-5.

Festival of Life, FestivalOfLife.net. 0207277 6882. Yearly festival

42˚Raw, 6 Burlington Gardens, Wistminster, London, W1S; 42Raw.co.uk. Royal Academy of Arts. Salads, smoothies, juices. Jesper Rydahl

Fresh Network, fresh-network.com

Friends Organic, 83 Roman Rd., E2 0GQ; 020 8980 1843. Organic produce.

Funky Raw Magazine, FunkyRaw.com. A quarterly magazine and a company that is a resource of information, and sells various products of interest to raw foodies.

Global Tribe Café, 18 Swan St., Leeds, L5I 6LG; GlobalTribeCafe.co.uk; Vegetarian, vegan and some raw. Has a Facebook page.

Happy Apple GreenGrocer, 60 High St., Totnes, Devon, TQ9 5SQ, England. Organic produce available.

Health Etcetera, Winchester, England; healthetcetera.com. A residential living foods centre.

Hornbeam, 458 Hoe St., Walthamstow, London E17 9AH, England; hornbeam.org.uk. Center for community involvement. Some raw food in café and in fruit and veg market stall.

InSpiral Lounge, 250 Camden High St., London NW1 8QS, England; 020 7428 5875; inspiralled.net

Itadaki Zen, 139 King's Cross Rd., WCIX 98J. Vegan, organic with some raw.

Karuna, 26 Bossel Rd., Buckfastleigh, Devon, TQ11 0DD, England; +44 (0) 8456-341-466; karunadetox.com; info (at) karunaretreates.com. Detox, fasting, yoga, and juicing retreats.

Kitchen Buddy, (mailing address: Theresa Webb, Kitchen Buddy, 49 South Park Crescent, Catford, London SE6 1JJ, England); kitchenbuddy.eu. Purechocolate.kitchenbuddy.eu. Workshops (at) kitchenbuddy.eu. Theresa holds raw food chef classes.

Langridge Organic, langridgeorganic.com. Delivers organic produce. Not a vegan company.

London Farmers' Markets, lfm.org.uk; 020 7833 0338. Markets are located in Acton, Blackheath, Clapham, Ealing, Islington, Marylebone, Notting Hill, Peckham, Pimlico Road, Queens Park, South Kensington, Swiss Cottage, Twickenham, Walthamstow, and Wimbledon Park.

Luscious Organic, 240 Kinsington High St., W8 6NE; 020 7371 6987; lusciousorganic.co.uk. Market with some organic produce.

Kate Magic, RawLiving.eu

The Manna House, themannahouse.com

Manna, 24 Coombe Rd., Brighton, BN2 4EA, England. Live food and cooked vegan café. Kyle Hayden Vialli.

Marylebone Farmers' Market, Cramer Street Car Park, off Marylebone, High Street, W1. London. Sunday 10-2.

Nama Artisan Raw Foods, 19 Lonsdale Rd., London, NW6 6RA, England; NamaFoods (at) hotmail.com. Opened December 2012.

Nectar, 16 Onley St., Norwich, NR2 2EB; TheNectarCave.co.uk. Mostly raw café with juices and smoothies. Opened 2011.

New Covent Garden Market, Covent House, London, SWB 5NDX England; newcoventgardenmarket.com

Notting Hill Farmers' Market, Car park behind Waterstones. Saturday 9-1.

Ocean Wave Vibrations, OceanWaveVibrations.com. Raw foods.

Oliver's WholeFoods and Natural Remedies, 5 Station Approach, Kew Gardens, Richmond, Surry TW9 3QB; oliverswholefoods.co.uk; info (at) oliverswholefoods.co.uk.

Organic Republic, A7 Eldon Way, Park Royal, London, NW10 7QY UK; organicrepublic.com. Organic produce delivery.

Purely Raw, PurelyRaw.com.

Rainforest Creations, Hammersmith Lyric Square, Kind Street, W6, London. Thursdays 9-3. rainforestcreations.co.uk.

Rainforests Creations, Chelsea Market, Duke of York Square, Kings Rd. SW3, London. rainforestcreations.co.uk. Saturdays 9-3.

Rainforest Creations, Old Spitalfields Market, Brushfield St., E1, London; rainforestcreations.co.uk.

Rainforest Creations at Urban Bliss, North Kensington, 333 Portobello Rd., North Kensington, London; rainforestcreations.co.uk.

Raw Alchemy, RawAlchemy.org.uk

The Raw Chocolate Company, Unit E 3, Blacklands Farm, Wheatsheaf Road, Henfield, East Sussex BN5 9AT; therawchocolatecompany.com

Raw Fairies, RawFairies.com. 07879 246 501. Raw food delivery daily.

Raw Living, rawliving.co.uk

RawLoveUK.com. Malachi's site. Info, education, and events in England.

Rawseedsrambles.blogspot.com, England. Blog of a sister who calls herself Cosmic.

Saf Restaurant, 152-154 Curtain Rd., Shoreditch, London EC2A 3AT; +44 (0) 20 76130 007; SafRestaurant.com. safrestaurant.co.uk. Chad Sarno's restaurant

Saf, Whole Foods Market, The Barkers Building, Kensington High Street, London, W8 5SE, England; safrestaurant.co.uk. Opened 2010 at the Whole Foods Market.

Second Nature, 78 Wood St., Walthamstow, E17 3HX; 020 8520 7995. Organic produce.

The Shop On The Hill market 7b Harefield Rd., Brockley, London SE4 1LW England; 0208 6922175; theshoponthehill (at) hotmail.com. Tiny market

Spirited Palace, 105 Church Road, Crystal Palace, London, SE19 2PR, England; 020-8771 5557 or 07939 474 507; thespiritedpalace.com. Vegan Caribbean food.

Sun Chlorella, sunchlorella.co.uk.

Susu Organic, susuorganic.co.uk. Directory of organic companies.

Sweet Senstions, sweetsensations.uk.com. liz (at) sweetsensations.uk.com. Lizbygrave (at) gmail.com. Liz Bygrave teaches vegan and mostly raw food chefing classes.

Jill Swyers, jillswyers.com; info (at) jillswyers.com. Workshops in raw food in London, England, and Algarve, Portugal.

Tony's Hemp Store, 10 Caledonian Rd., London N1 9DU, England; 7837 5223. Vegetarian and vegan menu with some raw.

Total Raw Food, POB 129, Brighton, BN51 9BW; 01273 248 697; TotalRawFood.com

222 Veggie Vegan Restaurant, 222 North End Rd., West Kensington, London W14 9NU, England; 222veggievegan.com. Some raw options on menu, including juices.

Unicorn Co-op Market, 89 Albany Rd., Chorlton, Manchester, M21 0BN, England; unicorn-grocery.co.uk. Organic groceries. Also owns a farm in Glazebury.

Vantra, West End, 22-13 Soho St., W1D 3DJ. Raw options. London, England; Vantra.co.uk. Opened late 2010.

Vegan London, veganlondon.co.uk

Vegan Runners, veganrunnersmakessense.co.uk.

Vegan Society, vegansociety.com

Vgango, 39 Webbs Rd., Battersea, London; Vgango.co.uk. Vegan café. Opened 2012

VitaO, 74 Wardour St., London W1F 8TE, England; VitaO.CO.uk. Extensive raw and juice menu. Formerly known as VitaOrganic. Changed in 2010.

Whole Foods Market, The Barkers Building, 63-98 Kensington High St., W8 5SE, London; 020 7368 4500; wholefoodsmarket.com. Large store, small raw foods section. Some organic produce. Likely all overpriced, like the American Whole Foods Market. Better to support mom and pop, independent stores, and to go to fruit wholesalers to purchase by the case and save money.

Wild Food Café, first floor, 14 Neal's Yard, Covent Garden, WC2H 9DP; wildfoodcafe.com. Opened 2011. Mostly raw. Some cooked.

• EUROPE: BELGIUM

Check MeetUp.com for raw food meetups.

Raw Creations, RawCreations.be. Serge Lenssense-Wynen

• EUROPE: CROATIA

Jesse Bogdanovich, Island of Vis, Croatia, TheWholeLifestyle.com/retreat/. Runs a raw vegan retreat in Croatia by the Adriatic beaches. With Jesse's mother, Dr. Ruza Bogdanovich of The Cure Is In The Cause Foundation and author of a book by the same name (Access: TheCureIsInTheCause.com). Jesse Boganovich is also on FaceBook.com.

• EUROPE: CZECH REPUBLIC

Check MeetUp.com for raw food meetups.

Life Food, lifefood.cz

•EUROPE: FINLAND

Check MeetUp.com for raw food meetups.

Antonia keeps a blog about fruits and vegetables: nutrition-facts-in-fruits-and-vegetables.com

• EUROPE: FRANCE

Check MeetUp.com for raw food meetups.

Biocoop Grenelle, 44 Boulevard de Grenelle, Paris, 75015, France; 0145777014. Organic market.

Bob's Juice Bar, 15, Rue Lucien Sampaix, Paris, 75010, France; 0682637274; bobsjuicebar.com. Metro: Jacques Bonsergent. Small place that has some juices, salads, and vegan food.

Ero Dom Cameroun, 28 Bd Jules Carteret, 69348 Lyon Credex 07, Lyon. Fresh tropical fruit.

Grand Appetit, 9, Rue La Cerisale, Paris, 75004, France; 0140270495. Metro: Bastille. Some vegan food and wine.

Green Garden, 20, Rue Nationale, Paris, 75013, France. Metro: Porte d'Ivry. Café with some vegan options. Natural foods store next door.

Le Pas-Sage Oblige, 29 rue du Bourg-Tibourg, 75004, Paris, France; lepassageoblige.com. Vegetarian restaurant with some raw options.

La Paradis du Fruit, Paris; LeParadisdufruit.fr. Vegetarian restaurant with juices and smoothies.

Le Potager du Marais, 22, Rue Rambuteah, Paris, 75003, France; 0142742466. Metro: Rambuteau. Vegetarian restaurant with some vegan food.

La Vie en Fruit, 116 Boulevard St. Germain, Paris. Juice bar with smoothies and salads.

Les Nouveaux Robinson – Pont de Neuilly, 16 Rue des Graviers, Paris, 73400; 0147479280. Organic market.

Rainbow Juice, 1 Rue Marauerin, Paris; Restaurant with fresh juices and smoothies.

Soupie Fruitie, 1 Rue Alexandra Parodi, Paris. Juice and smoothie bar.

Tripti-Kulai, 20, rue Jacques Coeur, 3400 Montpellier, France; Tripti-Kulai,com. Vegetarian with some raw options. Also has a snack shop at 3, rue Massillian, 3400 Montpellier, France. Store at 22, rue Bernard Delicieux, 3400 Montpellier, France.

Torce Viviers En Charnie, Pays de Loire France; dawncampbellholistichealth.eu. Welcomes guests interested in natural alternative lifestyle and vegetarian, vegan, raw and natural hygiene diet. English host, Dawn Campbell. master coach, living foods practitioner, chef, teacher, author and offers reiki, thought field therapy, massage and yoga.

Wanna Juice, 65 rue Saint-Andre des Arts, 75006 Paris; WannaJuice.com

• EUROPE: GERMANY

Check MeetUp.com for raw food meetups.

Aphrohdisia, aphrohdisia.com. MelanieMaria (at) aphrohdisia.de. Melanie Holzheimber is a gradudate of the Living Light Culinary Institute.

Bio-Corner Naturkost Health Food Store, Fiedelerstrasse 23, Hannover, Germany; +49-511-836037

BistROH, Café, RohKöstlich Messe & Verlag GmbH, Nelly & Volker Reinle-Carayon, Birkenweg 2, 67346 Speyer, Germany; Rohkoestich.com; rhovolution.de. Café, BistROH. School, KulinaROH. Shop.

Effulgence Waves, Kurfurstenanlage 9, 69115 Heidelberg, Germany; das-grune-restaurant.de. Vegetarian restaurant with raw options. Run by students of Sri Chinmoy.

German Goes Raw, germanygoesraw.de. Site contains information on where to get raw cuisine in Germany.

Lebensfroh Café, Görlitzerstr 38, D-10997 Kreuzberg, Berlin, Germany; lebensfroh.org. Mandy und Metin.

La Mano Verde, Wesbadener Str. 79-D, 12161, Berlin, Germany; 030 827 031 20; lamanoverde.de/english/index.html. Vegan restaurant with some raw foods.

Raw Meister, rawmeister.jimbo.com

RohVolution (rawvolution), Berlin, Germany; rohvolution.de. Nelly & Volker Reinle-Carayon

• Europe: Hungary

Check MeetUp.com for raw food meetups.

Mannaturel Etelmanufactura – Manna Restaurant, Garibaldi UTCA 5; Pincehelyseg BAL, olbali, Budapest, Hungary, 1054; Mannatural.hu. Patrick Hliva, proprietor.

• Europe: Italy

Check MeetUp.com for raw food meetups.

Nudo Crudo; NudoCrudo.net. Chef Vito Cortese.

Ristorante Bliss, Via Teodosia, 9 R, 16129 Genoa, Italy; blissblissbliss.com. Vegetarian restauran with some raw options. Run by students of Sri Chinmoy.

• Europe: Lithuania

Check MeetUp.com for raw food meetups.

Raw42, Rudninu G. 12, LT-01135, Viluius, Lithuania. Juice and smoothie bar. Jesper Rydahl is proprietor. Has locations in London and Copenhagen.

• Europe: Netherlands

Check MeetUp.com for raw food meetups.

42˙Raw, Pilestraede 32, 1112 Copenhagen, Denmark; 42Raw.co.uk. Smoothie and juice bar. Jesper Rydahl is proprietor. Locations in London and Lithuania.

Mastercare, cafe/shop, and Chocolate Club, mastercare.nl. Bastiaan Swager

Rock It Raw, weekly raw event in Amsterdam; RockItRaw.nl

Raw Supoerfoods, Raw food supply company in Amsterdam.

Raw Food Café, Chocolate Club, Spuistraat 239, 1012 VP Amsterdam, The Netherlands; rawfoodcafe.nl

Simple Raw, Oehlenschlaegersgade 12, Kobenhavn V, Kobenhavn 1663 (Copenhagen), Denmark; SimpleRaw.com. Vegan and vegetarian.

Unlimited Health, van Ostadestraat 234 A+B, 1073 TV Amsterdam; unlimitedhealth.nl; info (at) unlimitedhealth.nl. Yoga and raw food center.

• EUROPE: NORWAY

Check MeetUp.com for raw food meetups.

The Fragrance of the Heart, Fr. Nansens plass 2, 0160 Oslo; 47 22 33 23 10; fragrance.no. Vegetarian restauran with some raw options. Run by students of Sri Chinmoy.

Helt Rå, Elias Smiths vei 7, 1337 Sandvika. In Sandvika, outside of Oslo.

• EUROPE: PORTUGAL

Check MeetUp.com for raw food meetups.

Jill Swyers, jillswyers.com; info (at) jillswyers.com. Workshops in raw food in London, England, and Algarve, Portugal.

Tacao Viva e Sustentavel, alimentacaoviva.blogspot.com

• EUROPE: ROMANIA

Check MeetUp.com for raw food meetups.

Torturi Raw Vegan (raw vegan cakes); Tablariei, 2200 Brasov, Romania. Andrei Andi, proprietor. Has a Facebook page.

• EUROPE: SPAIN

Check MeetUp.com for raw food meetups.

811-friendly.net. Stephanie.

Crua Gourmet Cuisine, Barcelona, 08037, Spain; CruaGourmetCuisine.com. Christine Mayr.

Crucina, Calle del Divino Pastor 30, 28004 Madrid, Spain. Malasana Neighborhood. Crucina.com. Opened 2011. Menu and staff training done by Raw Chef Dan of Quintessence, a raw restaurant, New York City.

Eco Forest, EcoForest.org. An intentional community of raw foodists living together.

Organic, C. de la Junta de Comera 11, Barcelona, Spain 08001; 001 34 93 301 0902

• EUROPE: SWEDEN

Check MeetUp.com for raw food meetups.

Blueberry Lifestyle, Stockholm, SE; blueberrylifestyle.se. Several stores selling organic produce and various for raw food items. Not all vegan products. Ulrika Holm, owner.

Sanna Ehdin, SannaEhdin.com. Sanna wrote a book about raw smoothies titled, Sanna's Smoothies for the Self-healing Human.

Fresh Food Festival, FreshFoodFestival.com

Gryningen Halsobod, Folkungargatan 68; 08-641- 27 12. Shop sells a variety of vegan items.

Erica Palmcrantz Aziz, Goterborg, Sweden; pzi.se. info (at) pzi.se. Raw food chef.

Levende Foda, LevandeFoda.se

Organic Green, Rehnsgatan 24; 08-612 74 84. Vegetarian café with some vegan food, including some raw.

Sunfood Yoga, SunfoodYoga.com

Vegan Stockholm, veganstockholm.se. Site lists restaurants and shops that sell vegan.

• Europe: Switzerland

Check MeetUp.com for raw food meetups.

Bergidylle Gourmet-Cru, Schwarzsee; rohvolution.ch. Edeltraut Preissard

BioSamara, biosamara.ch

Christie is a contact for raw food information in Switzerland, chrebe (at) peacemail.com

Genève Raw & Living Food, Geneva; rawfood.meetup.com/461. David Newbery

Hier und Jetzt Café, Bubenbergplatz 10, 3011, Bern, Switzerland; 41 31 311 7271. Vegetarian café with some raw options, juices, and smoothies. Run by students of Sri Chinmoy.

Hiltl, Zurich, Switzerland; hiltl.ch. Said to be the oldest vegetarian restaurant in Europe.

Keimling, keimling.ch

Naturlich Leben, Silvia Dörig; NatuerlichLeben.ch

Orkos, de.orkos.com/default.aspx?tabid=53

Passion for Fruit, passion4fruit.com

Raw Vegan Geneva, rawvegangeneva.com. Site contains a list of raw sources, juice bars, organic food shops, etc. in Geneva.

Rohkost Treffen Schweiz, Zurich; rawfood.meetup.com/349. Ilanta Sa and Rafael Järmann

Tropenkost, tropenkost.de

• Iceland

Check MeetUp.com for raw food meetups.

Ecstacy's Heart Garden, Klapparstigur 37, Reykjav; 354 56 12345. Vegetarian restaurant with some raw options. Run by students of Sri Chinmoy.

Kaffi Hljomalind Co-op, Laugavegur 21; Reykjavik, Iceland; 5171980; kaffihljomalind.org. Organic fair trade co-op coffee house with some raw organic foods. Music store, activist center, community information boards.

Solla, Himnesk Hollusta, Sundaborg 5, 104, Reykjavík; 554 7273; himneskt.is

• India

Check MeetUp.com for raw food meetups.

Energy Home, 35-A, Chetty St, Pondicherry, India; EnergyHome.in. EnergyHome.in. Vegan restaurant near Mother's Ashram.

• Ireland

Check MeetUp.com for raw food meetups.

Bernadette Bohan, 34 Sonesta, Malahide, Dublin; changesimply.com; b (at) changesimply.com. Author and raw foods teacher.

Castelruddery Organic Farm, Donard, Wicklow, Ireland; casorg (at) eircom.net.

Dublin Food Co-op, 12 Newmarket, Dublin 6; dublinfood.coop.

The Happy Pear, Church Rd., Greystones, Wicklow, Ireland; thehappypear.ie.

Healthy Habits Café and Store, Quarantine Hill, Wicklow Town, Co. Wicklow, Ireland; healthyhabis.com; veronicasol (at) eircom.net.

Irish Living Foods, irishlivingfoods.com.

The Irish School of Natural Healing, The Old Rectory, 25 Coote Street, Portlaoise, County Laois, Ireland; +353 (0)57 8682567; herbeire.ie/School/About.html. Focus is on "cleansing the body and mind using organic vegan and living food programmes, herbal medicines, bodywork and environmental and lifestyle awareness."

The Irish School of Herbal Medicine, The Old Rectory, 25 Coote St., Portlaoise, County Laois, Ireland; herbeire.ie.

Living Green, Moma Lynn, Ballinclea, Donard, Wicklow, Ireland; livinggreen.ie; info (at) livinggreen.ie. Source for sprouting supplies and information.

Loop de Loop Eco Shop Healthfood Store, Bank Place, Castletownbere, Ireland; 00353 27 70770

Natasha's Living Foods, Unit B3, Space Enterprise Centre, North King St., Stoneybatter, Dublin 7, Ireland; natashaslivingfoods.ie; Natasha (at) natashaslivingfood.ie.

The Natural Food Market, St. Andrews, Pearse St., Dublin 2; supernatural.ie. Has a raw food café.

Organico Café and Natural Foods Store, No. 2 Glengarriff Rd., Bantry, County Cork, Ireland; 02751391; organico.ie

Select Stores, 36 Tubbermore Rd., Dalkey, Dublin, Ireland. 01 2859611.

• Israel

Check MeetUp.com for raw food meetups.

Israel Gone Raw, IsraelGoneRaw.com

• Jamaica

Check MeetUp.com for raw food meetups.

Ashanti Foods Monthly Brunch, Yvonne Hope; 876-944-3316

Earl's Juice Garden, 16 Derrymore Rd., Kingston 10, Jamaica; 876-906-4287; 876 920-7009

Earl's Juice Garden #2, Shop #6, 6 Red Hills Rd., Kingston 10, Jamaica, 876-754-2425

• Japan

Check MeetUp.com for raw food meetups.

RawFood-KenTei.com

Raw Café by Cacao Magic, 41-1 Ishibashi-cho, Jyodoji, Sakyo-ku, Kyoto, Japan, 606-8406; cacaomagic.com. Sumire Matsuda

• Mexico

Check MeetUp.com for raw food meetups.

The Green Corner, Mexico City; TheGreenCorner.org. Organic shops and restaurants in a building aiming to be sustainable.

• New Zealand

Check MeetUp.com for raw food meetups.

Alpha & Omega, Asian and Organic Market, 39 Queen St., Blenheim, New Zealand; 03-579-5684

Rene Archner, Warkworth, New Zealand; ReneArchner.com. Raw food chef and educator.

Blueberry Farm, 1229 Akatarawa Rd., Upper Hutt, New Zealand; 04-526-6788; blueberryfarm.co.nz. Harvest your own blueberries and dive in the swimming hole.

The Blue Bird, 299 Dominion Rd., Mt. Eden, Aukland; thebluebird.co.nz. Vegetarian café with some raw options, juices, and smoothies.

Brydone Growers Farm Shop, 469 Alma-Maheno, Main South Rd., Oamaru, New Zealand; 03-434-6744

Ceres Organics, 121 Carbine Rd. Mt Wellington, Auckland, New Zealand; 09-920-2500

Ceres Wholefoods Store, 181 Ladies Mile Ellerslie, Auckland, New Zealand; 09-579-7126

Chantal Organic Wholesalers, Organic Vege Boxes, 13 Northe St., Napier, Hawke's Bay 4001, New Zealand; +64 6 835 7898; +64 6 835 8784; chantal.co.nz; orders (at) chantal.co.nz. Delivery.

Christchurch Vegetarian Center, Rm 121, 141 Hereford St., Christchurch, New Zealand; vegetarianchristchurch.org.nz.

City Markets, 2 Owens Pl, Bayfair, Tauranga, New Zealand; citymarkets.co.nz. Open 7 days.

Commonsense Organics, 260 Wakefield St., Wellington 6011, New Zealand; commonsenseorganics.co.nz. Market.

Commonsense Organics, 37 Waterloo Rd., Lower Hutt 5010, New Zealand; commonsenseorganics.co.nz. Market.

Commonsense Organics, Tenancy 4, New Tenancy Bldg., Coastlands, Paraparaumu 5032, New Zealand; commonsenseorganics.co.nz. Market.

Commonsense Organics, 7 Bay Rd., Kilbirnie, Willington 6022, New Zealand; commonsenseorganics.co.nz. Market.

Cornucopia The Organics Shop, 221 Heretaunga St., East Hastings, New Zealand; 06-876-6248. Market.

Down to Earth Market, 268 Devon St. West, New Plymouth, New Zealand; 06-758-3700; downtoearthorganics.co.nz. Organic fruits and vegetables. A full-range natural store: not all vegetarian.

Driving Creek Café and Organics, 180 Driving Creek Rd., Coromandel, New Zealand; 07 866 7066; drivingcreekcafe.com. Vegetarian with vegan and raw options, juices, and smoothies.

East West Organics, 273G West Coast Rd., Glen Eden, Auckland, New Zealand; eastwestorganics.co.nz. Market.

Eternal Delight, Central Christchurch, New Zealand; 021 703 345. Raw food catering. Offers classes. Paul and Patricia Granswind. Patricia also has her site:.

Golden Bay Organics, 47 Commercial St., Takaka 7110, New Zealand. A vegetarian store.

The Good Earth, 5 Merivale Rd., Merivale, Tauranga, New Zealand. Organic fruits and vegetables, wheatgrass, and used and new juicers.

Harvest Wholefoods, 405 Richmond Rd., Grey Lynn, Auckland, New Zealand; huckleberryfarms.co.nz. Full line natural foods store.

Hot Yoga of New Zealand, 20 Nile Street West, Nelson 7010, New Zealand; hotyoganz.com. Yoga studio with some raw snacks.

Hot Yoga of New Zealand, 250 Wakefield St., Wellington 6011, New Zealand; hotyoganz.com. Yoga studio with some raw snacks.

Huckleberry Farms Glen Innes, 150 Aprirana Ave., Glen Innes, Auckland, New Zealand; huckleberryfarms.co.nz. Full line natural foods store.

Huckleberry Farms Greenlane Market, 240 Greenlane Rd., Epsom, Auckland, New Zealand; huckleberryfarms.co.nz. Full line natural foods store.

IE Produce Ltd. Natural Food Store, No. 1 Barry's Point Rd., Takapuna, New Zealand; +64 9 488 0211; ieproduce.com. Large selection of organic fruits and vegetables.

Imago Organic Orchard, 50 Arapaepae Rd., Levin, New Zealand; 06-368-3858

Kerikeri Organic, 1188 State Hwy. 10, Kerikeri 0470, New Zealand; kerikeriorganic.co.nz. Market. Organic fruits, vegetables, nuts, and seeds. Many of which they grow and harvest.

The Lotus Heart Cafe, 595 Columbo Street, Christchurch 8011, New Zealand; thelotusheart.co.na. Vegetarian with some raw options, juices, and smoothies.

The Lotus Heart Restaurant, Second location: Level 1, Orginal Chief Post Office Building, 15-31 Cathedral Square, Christchurch, New Zealand; thelotusheart.co.nz. Vegetarian restaurant with some raw options, juices, and smoothies.

Lyttel Piko WholeFoods Co-opperative, 12 London St., Lyttelton; pikowholefoods.co.nz.

Mahamudra Retreat Centre, RD4 Colville, Coromandel, New Zealand; mahamudra.org.nz. Budhist-run retreat center.

Michelle's Health and Nutrition, 28 Boon St., Whakatane, New Zealand. Organic fruits, vegetables, nuts, seeds, and bulk itmes.

Monk Street Market, 1 Monk St., Whitianga Coromandel; 07-866-4500. Organic fruits and vegetables.

Naturally Organic, Rosedale Plaza, 215 Rosedale Rd., Albany, New Zealand; naturallyorganic.co.nz.

The New Zealand Vegetarian Society, POB 26664, Aukland, New Zealand; vegetarian.org.nz.

Oetpoti Urban Organics, urbanorganics.org.nz. Information about home gardening in New Zealand.

Opawa Organic Grocer, Shop 6, 124 Opawa Rd., Opawa, Christchurch, New Zealand; 03-982-3749

Organic Co-op Thames, 736 Pollen St., Thames, New Zealand; 07-868-8797

Organic Explorer, organicexplorer.co.nz. Site that lists a variety of businesses in New Zealand, including natural foods stores and restaurants.

Organic Green Grocer, 40 Tasman St., Nelson, New Zealand; 64 3 548 3650; organicgreengrocer.co.nz.

Organic Living Healthfoods, Broadtop Shopping Centre, 336 Broadway Ave., Palmerston North, New Zealand; organic-living.co.nz. Market with full range of products.

Organic Matters, Shop 9, Richmond Centre, Egmont St., New Plymouth, New Zealand. Market.

Organic New Zealand Magazine, organicnz.org

Organic World, 181 Point Chevalier Rd., Point Chevalier, Auckland, New Zealand; organicworld.co.nz. Market for fresh produce, and full store items. Also sells organic seedlings for home culinary gardens.

Papatuanuku Alternative Health Market, 209 Pora St., Te Kuiti, New Zealand. Market that also makes fresh fruit and vegetable juices.

Parito Coastal Yoga Retreat, 1574 Whaanga Rd., RD2 Ruapuke, Raglan, New Zealand; parito.co.nz. A vegetarian yoga retreat center.

Permaculture in New Zealand, permaculture.org.nz.

Phoenix Organics Distribution, 17 Fatima St., Redwood, Christchurch, New Zealand; 03-352-3464

Piko Wholefoods, 12 London St., Lyttelton, New Zealand; pikowholefoods.co.nz. This store opened in 2007.

Piko Wholefoods, 229 Kilmore St., Christchurch, New Zealand; pikowholefoods.co.nz. Opened in 1977.

Pure Wellbeing, 1/12 Menin Rd., Raumati South, Kapiti Coast 5032, New Zealand; alxo, 3 Shearwater Rise, Paraparaumu Beach, Kapiti Coast, 5032, New Zealand; purewellbeing.com. Raw food classes, retreats, events, juice bar. Michael Hayman and Jules Barber.

Putiputi Ra Organic Traders, 79 Walton St., Whangarei, New Zealand; putiputira.co.nz

Real n' Raw, 48 Rukutai St., Mission Bay, Auckland 0630, New Zealand. Produced a film about raw foods.

Riley's Market, 5 Chambers St., Kakanui, Maheno, New Zealand; 03-439-5453

Riverslea Retreat, 733 Otaki Gorge Rd., RD2 Otaki, New Zealand; riversleаretreat.co.nz. Vegetarian yoga retreat center.

Riverton Organic Food Co-op, 154 Palmerston St., Riverton, New Zealand.

Seed Coastal Organics, 67 Carthew Street, Okato, Taranaki, New Zealand, 4335; seedcoastalorganics.jimdo.co

Soulfood Organic Store and Cafe, 74 Ardmore St., Wanaka, New Zealand; 03-443-7885

SuJu; fromgreytogreen.co.nz; Fromgreytogreen (at) home.org.nz. Renata Holicova is a graduate of Cherie Soria's Living Light Culinary Institute in Fort Bragg, California.

Sunset Coast Organics, 1510 Waiuku Rd, RD1, Waiuku, Pukekohe, New Zealand, 09-235-7835

Taste Nature, 131 High St., Central City, Dunedin 9016, New Zealand. Market with organic fruits and vegetables and bulk supply.

Taste Nature, 7 Moray Pl., Dunedin, New Zealand

Thames Organic Shop, 736 Pollen St., Thames, New Zealand. Market with a good amount of organic fruits and vegetables.

The Vegan Society of New Zealand, vegansociety.co.nz.

Village Organics, 245 Commerce St., Frankton Village Shopping Centre, Hamilton, New Zealand; villageorganics.co.nz. Market with some organic fruits and veggies.

Waiheke Organic Food, 20 Tahi Rd., Waiheke Island, Auckland, New Zealand; 09-372-8708

Waihi Beach Natural Health, 31B Wilson Rd. Waihi Beach, New Zealand. Market.

Wellness Grocer Deli and Café, 581 Beach Rd., Rothesayn Bay, Auckland, New Zealand; 09-476-6154

Whymore Organic Orchard, 879 Downs Rd., West Eyreton Cust, New Zealand; 03-312-5177

Wild Gypsy Raw, wildgypsyraw.com.

• PANAMA

Check MeetUp.com for raw food meetups.

Aris Latham, sunfired.com/site

• PERU

Check MeetUp.com for raw food meetups.

Shaman Vegan Raw Restaurant, Santa Catalina Ancha 366-B, Cuzco, Cusco, Peru 08484; ShamanVegan.com. Open late 2012. Mallku Aribalo, proprietor.

• RUSSIA

Check MeetUp.com for raw food meetups.

Svobodnie Ludi (translated as People of Freedom) Raw Club-Cafe, Saint-Petersburg, Russia. Sergey Martynov is on FaceBook. This had closed down, but Sergey is hopeing to have another café in the future.

• SCOTLAND

Check MeetUp.com for raw food meetups.

Fruit Market, Blochairn Road, Glasgow, Lanarkshire, G21 2EP

Grassroots Shop and Deli, 20 Woodlands Rd., Charing Cross, Glasgow, G3 6UR, Scotland; 0141-353-3278; grassrootsorganic.com. Not a vegan business. Offers some products of interest to raw foodists.

Orb Café, Shining Light, 246 Morrison Street, Edinburgh, EH3 8DT, Scotland; OrbCafe.com.

Real Foods, 37 Broughton St., Edinburgh, EH1 3JU; RealFoods.co.uk; info (at) realfoods.co.uk.

Real Foods, 8 Brougham St., Edinburgh, E3H 9JH; RealFoods.co.uk

Scottish School of Herbal Medicine, Alexander Stephen House, Suites 20-22, 91 Holmfauld Rd., Gladgow. G51 4RV. Scotland; herbalmedicine.org.uk. Keith and Maureen Robertson, owners. Not a raw food company, but offers information, products, and services of interest to those interested in natural health.

• SINGAPORE

Check MeetUp.com for raw food meetups.

BalancedLivingAsia.com

Raw Food Centre, rawfoodcentre.com. Sunita Vira is a certified, Gourmet Raw Food Chef from the Living Light Culinary Institute in California.

• South America: Argentina

Check MeetUp.com for raw food meetups.

Verde Llama - Life Food / Comida con Vida, Jorge Newbery 3623, Buenos Aires (near Charlone y Roseti, Colegiales); 4554-7467, Suite B, Federico Lacroze/39, 65, 93 bus; Chacarita (Neighborhood). Organic vegetarian creations, colorful, relaxed café. Diego Castro opened this café and juice bar in early 2007. Café also sells organic produce (when they have extra), wheatgrass, granola bars.

• South America: Brazil

Check MeetUp.com for raw food meetups.

Universo Orgânico Produtos Orgânicos e Alimentação Com Vida, Rua Conde de Bernadote nº 26 / Lojas 105 e 106 Leblon - Rio de Janeiro – RJ; 3874-0186/2274-8983; contato (at) universoorganico.com; universoorganico.com.

• South America: Columbia

Check MeetUp.com for raw food meetups.

Raw Kowabunga Juice Bar, CRA 8 #127-82 Bella Suiza, Bogota, Columbia. Smoothies, juices, salads.

• South America: Ecuador

Check MeetUp.com for raw food meetups.

Vida, Centro de Transformacion, 5-56 Avenida Loja y Remigio Crespo, Cuenca, Ecuador; 094160419; 092961570; blovins (at) hotmail.com

• South America: Peru

Check MeetUp.com for raw food meetups.

Maca Punch, Gomez del Carpio 140 C, Lima, Peru; 511-4462162; macapunch.com. Supplier of natural products, including maca, Yacon, camu camu, lucama, purple corn, and other natural products from various regions.

• Spain

Check MeetUp.com for raw food meetups.

Antonia Organic Kitchen, Carrer de la Junta de Comera 11, Barcelona, 08001, Spain; AntoniaOrganicKitchen.com. Veggie restaurant. Indian and Spanish influence. Salad bar. Full moon raw gatherings. Frank and Giselle.

• Thailand

Check MeetUp.com for raw food meetups.

Ariya Organic Café, 2nd flr., MBK Center, Bangkok, Thailand; 02-6260188. ariyaorganic.com. Vegan, raw and cooked foods, juice bar, smoothies, deserts, take-out. In Siam Square.

Rasayana Raw Food Café, 57 Soi Sukhumvit 39 (Prom-mitr), Sukhumvit Rd., Klongton-Nua Wattana 10110; Bangkok, Thailand, 66-2662-4803-5; 0-2662-4803-5; rasayanaretreat.com

• Turkey

Check MeetUp.com for raw food meetups.

Max Green, Akmerkez Food Court (Nispetiye Cad.), Istanbul, 34335, Turkey. MaxGreen.co. Mehmet Ozderici, proprietor.

• RAW FOOD BUSINESS 101

A message for those conducting business in the raw food industry

BECAUSE I've written some books, I get mail and email from all over the planet. Unfortunately, some of it has to do with people being ripped-off, or having a far from ideal experience, in some business venture when they have dealt with certain people, such as so-called "raw gurus," and also companies trying to cash in on the raw food craze.

Some of these unfortunate experiences have resulted in people losing thousands of dollars and/or being left in deep debt.

Many small companies are servicing the demand for raw food. Some have jumped at opportunities they thought were going to dramatically improve their business, only to find out too late that they were not going to get paid for their product or service.

The point of including this section in the book isn't about identifying which companies and people have been involved in these unfortunate business situations. It is simply to encourage people to be wise I their business practices.

To prove their cases that they have been treated unfairly, certain people and companies have gone to the extent of sending me paperwork showing which people and companies have been dishonest with them. They see certain people and/or companies listed in my global raw food guide, *Sunfood Traveler*, and they want me to know that certain people are not trustworthy.

There is really nothing I can do to correct any of these situations. But I can include information in this book to advise people involved in business to beware, to use critical thinking, and to do business smartly. Also, don't buy anything that you don't need.

In 2010, I was told of a situation in which one person dealing with another person in a raw food business deal ended up losing tens of thousands of dollars with one using legal maneuverings to avoid payment. While I believe there was some dishonesty involved, I think the chief component of that mess was simply unwise business practices, including not having a defined business plan, not keeping records, and one person being too impressed with and trusting the other who has a bit of that "raw celebrity' aspect going on.

Another unfortunate business situation involved one person who has a raw food business losing money when a well-known person living in a different country skipped out on paying a bill that was in the thousands of dollars.

Some people hearing about such dishonest business practices state the knee-jerk reaction of, "File a lawsuit!" But, taking on the expense and time of an international lawsuit is out-of-the-question for a small businessperson – especially when the legal fees and and other costs would greatly exceed the debt involved. So there is another case of a person who had to try to forget about that and move on – and, is probably cringing every time they see the person on a Web site or hear about them spoken of as if they are good and righteous and inspirational.

Every type of business, community, and culture seems to have a side that is not so wonderful, and has its rotten apples. The raw food world is like that. There are some really wonderful people, and then there are some others. I tell myself that, becaust the raw veganism offers a lot of healing it attracts people who need that, and a few here and there come from very damaged backgrounds. Like children, some need more loving than others, some need nurturing and guidance, and some need tough love. And some need to learn to be more honest with and respectable to their brothers and sisters, and with themselves.

Over the years I've been told a lot of stuff about various people in the raw food world, but I try not to believe in rumors. And I'd rather not hear the gossip and lies, or hear about the ugly behavior as a form of entertainment by some storyteller who feeds off of drama and/or feels validated because they know the latest nonsense and how to spew it in a way that triggers desired reactions.

I'm including this little bit of information in this book because there have been too many cases of people getting ripped-off in business deals of some sort when dealing with others that position themselves as some sort of righteous raw food authorities (if you dig into their past, you can find some interesting psychological aspects as to why people work to display themselves as celebrities, why they behave the way they do, and what the roots are of their unfavorable issues).

When the various incidents are taken into account, this really isn't about one person, but about a number of people. And it is not about certain people in one country, but is about a variety of people in many countries. It also isn't limited to those selling food products, but is about those selling other products and providing other services not related to food products (such as seminars canceling events and not refunding money).

If you are someone who is dealing with buying and selling things, or providing services within the raw food industry (and that is what it has turned into: a global raw food industry in which hundreds of millions of dollars are being exchanged for products and services, including books, seminars, chef training, retreats, equipment, food products, reselling, product design, packaging, shipping, Web services, accounting, staff services, etc.) DO NOT automatically trust someone because you view the person as well-known. "Well-known" does not translate to "honest" or "trustworthy."

Just because someone is considered well-known, or they have a really cool Web site, or they know how to promote themselves, or they have fancy promotional materials, or they smile pretty, or they have taken on a trendy nic-name, or they are related to someone, or they have a number of YouTube videos in which they say really cool stuff, or they have written books, or they give seminars attended by hundreds of people, or they know how to say big words, or they are married to so-and-so, or they stayed at your house, or you like the way they dress... does not mean that you should automatically trust them when doing business.

I know specifically that some of these people use the list of raw food companies, retreats, Web sites, and restaurants in my book, *Sunfood Traveler*, to contact others and do their business. While I meant for my book to make it easier to know about the raw food world, I didn't mean for it to be a manual for deceptive people searching for the gullible.

While there are very many good people doing business in the raw food industry, there are certainly some who have not been so honest or good. Included are those who are selling products they know are not of the quality or origin they are claiming. And there are those who have blatantly taken advantage of others, are creating a long history of doing so, and appear to show no signs of changing their ways.

My point in writing this is this: if you are going to do business, no matter if it is with a recognizable raw food person, or with your neighborhood repair person, be smart about it.

Just because some recognizable person in the raw food industry says something is good and holds some ideal value does not necessarily mean their claims hold truth. They are a businessperson. Their main point may be this: to get money from your pocket into theirs. Their charm, cheer, positioning, and presentation may have to do with one thing: getting money.

Just because a packaged product says "raw vegan" on the label doesn't necessarily mean it is your idea of raw or vegan, nor does it automatically mean that the product is good for you, or that the ingredients are sourced from where you may think, or that the ingredients are grown under established organic standards, of that the product isn't GMO. There is no government entity that certifies products as raw or vegan. You have to do your own research to find out which products fit your standards.

I know firsthand that certain people working in the raw food industry lack honor, which is truly dishonoring the person they see in the mirror. I also know some well-known people who have been ripped off or have otherwise been taken advantage of by others in the raw food industry who have either been dishonest, misleading, or at least behaved in ways that are not reflective of a person with high business ethics.

It's up to you. You can keep believing in the razzle dazzle and publicity of these people selling overpriced products of unknown origin and/or providing services of questionable value, you can keep eating up their nonsense, and you can keep throwing your money at them every time they spew a claim that you favor. Or, you can be wise with your resources.

If you really want raw food, grow a garden, nurture wild edible plants, research and plant native fruiting trees and berry bushes, and support your local organic farmers. When you go to the market, skip the shelves of packaged so-called "raw foods" with their Mylar and plastic and weak endorsements and questionable "superfood" claims. Instead, proceed to the produce section. Also, find the organic fruit and vegetable wholesalers in your region that will sell cases directly to consumers.

If you are going to start a raw food business, or already own one, read at least several books about how to run a small business. Be professional about it. Avoid getting ripped-off.

Be your own guru.

• Raw Web Sites

CHEFS, AUTHORS, CLASSES, HEALTH COACHES, FOOD COMPANIES

INCLUSION in this list does not imply that the author of this book, John McCabe, endorses the company or organization, its products, its owners, teachers, or founders, or any other aspect of the business, organization, owners, founders, teachers, products, services, facilities, or concepts.

Businesses, organizations, and persons often relocate or change the focus of their offerings. Before doing business or using the services or purchasing the products of any person, company, or organization on this list, do your own research to find out if you are getting what would be beneficial to you.

Sue Aberle, MS, RD, CD, Vancouver, WA; health.aberle.net. Sue is a dietitian who follows a plant-based diet.

AJ, chooserawnotwar.blogspot.com.

Alive Foods, AliveFoods.com. Author Paul Benhaim, Australia. Info (at) AliveFoods.com. Also runs: NotTheCookingShow.com

Diana M. Allen, MS, CNS, Montague Integrative Health, 432 Greenfield Road, Montague, MA 01351, USA; Eat2Evolve.com.

All Raw Directory, AllRawDirectory.com

Matt Amsden: RawVolution.com. Proprietor of Euphoria Loves Rawvolution café, Santa Monica, California. Author of *RawVolution.*

Anabrese, rawlifestyle.co.uk

Angels Healthfood Institute, POB 858, Gold Hill, OR 97525; angelshealthfoodinstitute.com; Farm address: 9394 Blackwell Rd., Central Point, OR 97502; 541-855-1846; angels-visions.com

The Art of Living Well, Florida, USA; ArtOfLivingWell.com

AussieHealthCoach.com.au; Aimee Devlin

Australia Raw Food Community: Raw-Pleasure.com.au

Back to Basics Naturally, Mary Lou Sackett, D.C., 2806 W Carleton Rd., Hillsdale, MI 49242; backtobasicsnaturally.com

Jesse Bogdanovich, Island of Vis, Croatia, TheWholeLifestyle.com/retreat/. Runs a raw vegan retreat in Croatia by the Adriatic beaches. With Jesse's mother, Dr. Ruza Bogdanovich of The Cure Is In The Cause Foundation and author of a book by the same name (Access: TheCureIsInTheCause.com). Jesse Boganovich is also on FaceBook.com.

Ruza Bogdanovich, TheCureIsInTheCause.com. Author and lecturer.

Heather Baker, theorganicacorn.com. Raw foodist with a hemp and organic clothing and household goods company in Santa Barbara, California.

Bar-Yochi Carob Fudge, Los Angeles, CA; baryochaifudge.blogspot.com

Thor Bazler, ThorBazler.com. Author and owner of Raw Power nutritional supplement company in Idaho, USA.

Paul Benhaim, AliveFoods.com. Chef, chocolateier, and entrepreneur in Australia.

Don Bennett, Health101.org

The Bliss Bar, Los Angeles, 310-909-6612; theblissbar.org; email: activate (at) theblissbar.org. Traveling raw food café available for events.

Boutenko Family: RawFamily.com. Authors and chefs who have traveled the world teaching about raw food. Victoria lives in Ashland, Oregon. Igor lives in Russia. Of their three children, Sergei and Valya are active in raw food education, including through their recipes books.

Sergei Boutenko, Harmony Hikes, HarmonyHikes.com. SergeiBoutenko.com. Chef and author Sergei Boutenko of RawFamily.com in southern Oregon conducts adventurous wild food foraging hikes.

Valya Boutenko, valyaboutenko.com. Artist, author, filmmaker, educator, and daughter of Victoria and Igor Boutenko.

Brad's Raw Chips, BradsRawChips.com. Brad Gruno.

Bright Earth Foods, 9391 Wagner Creek Rd., Talent, OR 97540; brightearthfoods.com. A raw foods supply company selling bulk items.

Sapoty Brook. eco-eating.com. Australian inventor of the KaPNak chart.

Café Gratitude, CafeGratitude.com. San Francisco restaurant and store, 5 locations (1 in San Francisco, and one each in Berkeley, San Rafael, Oakland, and Healdsburg). Mostly raw. Matthew and Terces Englehart are authors of recipe books. They also own an organic farm and a vegan Mexican restaurant with some raw on menu.

Karyn Callabrese, Chicago, IL, USA; KarynRaw.com.

Cardinal House, TheCardinalHouse.com. Carissa.

Helen Castillo, New York; TheRawPalate.com

Steve Charter. 5 Hoathly Hill, West Hoathly, West Sussex, RH19 4SJ, UK; Permaculture-steve.net

Chocolate Superfoods, 1595 West SR 89A, Sedona, AZ 86336; chocolatesuperfoods.com

Katherine Clark, kcclark.biz. Has been director of Hippocrates Health Institute's Health Practitioner's Academy and lecturer with Viktoras Kulvinskas.

Brenda Cobb. LivingFoodsInstitute.com. Author and owner of this New Age healing center offering raw food prep classes in Atlanta, Georgia. Brenda healed herself from cancer with the help of raw food and healthful thought.

Coconut Bliss, POB 288, Eugene, OR 97440; coconutbliss.com. Luna and Larry are makers of raw ice cream.

Comfortably Raw, ComfortablyRaw.com

Conscious Chocolate, ConsciousChocolate.co.uk.. Emma Jackman's chocolate company in England.

Conscious Events, consciousevents.co.uk. Kyle Vialli.

Cora Cacao Confections; coracaoconfections.com. Daniel Korson and Mitthew Rogers. Raw chocolate company.

The Daily Raw Café, Terilynn, TheDailyRawCafe.com.

Dave The Raw Food Trucker, Dave Conrardy/The Raw Food Trucker, POB 544, Auburn Washington 98071. He dropped over 200 pounds by following a raw food diet. Vidoes on YoutTube.

Date People, California; 760-359-3211. They grow and sell organic dates.

Brenda Davis RD, 1094 Lambeth Crt., Kelowna, BC V1V 1N2, Canada. BrendaDavisRD.com. She is the co-author of Cherie Soria's book, The Raw Revolution Diet.

Jim Dee, creator of AllRawDirectory.com.

Aimee Devlin, Australia; RawPear.com; AussieHealthCoach.com.au

Rick and Karin Dina, Santa Rosa, CA; RawFoodEducation.com

Draw, Jason Andrew Wrobel, Los Angeles, CA, USA; 310-383-0445; jasonwrobel.com/jw. Jason Andrew Wrobel. Raw chef, catering, instruction, events.

Discount Juicers, Rhonert Park, CA., DiscountJuicers.com; John Kohler

Earth Foods TV, Minnesota, USA; EarthFoods.TV. Ryan. Source for scientifically / evidence-backed nutrition information on fruits, vegetables, sprouts, superfoods, sea vegetables, herbs, seeds, and the like. Sharing juicing recipes, smoothie recipes, testimonials, and videos. Also, EarthFoods on FaceBook.

EarthKitchen.co.uk

Earth Shift Products, earthshiftproducts.com. Sells packaged dry raw foods, nuts, seeds, sea vegetables, nutrition bars, books, and other products.

EatRaw Corporation, 140 58th St., Ste. 6E, Brooklyn, NY 11220; 718-210-0048; eatraw.com

Eco Forest, Apdo 29, Coin 29100, Malaga, Spain; EcoForest.org

Elizabeth Howard: RawRawGirls.com. Eugene, OR, USA. Chef, life coach, runs seminars.

Angelina Elliott, CA; She-ZenCuisine.com. Author of *Alive in 5.*

Empress Organics, empressorganics.vpweb.com. Jennifer makes raw baby food.

Euphoric Organics, EuphoricOrganics.com. Author and chef Renee Loux Gordon of Maui, Hawaii.

Everything Raw, Essential Living Foods, 922 Colorado Ave., Santa Monica, CA 90401, USA; EverythingRaw.com; EssentialLivingFoods.com.

Fat Uncle Farms, funclefarms.globspot.com; funclefarms (at) gmail.com. Raw almonds.

Festival of Life, FestivalOfLife.net. England

Finca De Vida, Fincadevida.com (Farm of Life, Costa Rica). Brian and Jody Calvi, raw food health coaches

Forever Healthy, ForeverHealthy.net. Canadian raw food supply company.

Laura Fox, VisionaryCulture.com; BestOfRaw.net; RawInspirations.com; DivineMeditations.net; RawAlliance.org

Fresh Food Festival, Denmark; FreshFoodFestival.com

Fruitarian Worldwide Network, fruitnet.org. Dave Klein. Also runs Vibrance Magazine, (formerly Living Nutrition): LivingNutrition.com.

Fortina Chocolate, San Diego, CA, USA. FortinaChocolate.com. Raw chocolate company. Vince and Jinelle Wendling, and Jeff Botticelli

Freelee Fruititionist, TheFruititionist.com

Funkey Forest, FunkeyForest.com. Australian yoga and fasting retreat center in mountains near Byron Bay. Erik Adams, founder.

I am careful about listing "fasting retreats" in this book. While short fasts can be beneficial, I do not advise anyone to go on long-term water fasts of more than a few days. Even if the fasts are supervised by people who say they have experience with the process.

Funky Raw Magazine, London, Endland; FunkyRaw.com; funkyraw.com/shop. Email: magazine (at) funkyraw.com. Rob Hull, publisher.

Joanne Gero, N.D., VibeAlive.ca.

Frank Giglio's Raw for All, rawforall.com. Raw recipe collection. Frank Giglio is a classically trained chef with The New England Culinary Institute, VT and the Institute for Integrative Nutrition in NYC.

Gnosis Chocolate, New York; gnosischocolate.com.

Go Raw Chicago, GoRawHaveFun.com. Lenette Nakauchi

Gourmet Vegan Chef, Patricia Granswind of Eternal Delight restaurant in New Zealand is originally from Germany. EternalDelight.net. GourmetVeganChef.com.

Adam Graham, livefoodexperience.com

Greenivore, Greenivore.net

Green Smoothie Revolution, greensmoothierevolution.com

Green Smoothies Rock, greensmoothiesrock.ning.com

Santiago Guido, Maryland, U.S.; TheRawFoodMuscle.com.

Roger Haeske, Hawaii; RogerHaeske.com; LightningSpeedFit.com; PushUpBlaster.com; InstantEnergyExercises.com

Rob Ocean Hall, icaneatraw.com. Traveling raw chef who teaches classes and caters events.

Happy Healthy Human, Florida; happyhealthyhuman.com. Jason gathers people for raw food classes. He has opened a café.

Healthy Living Show, Los Angeles, CA; thehealthylivingshow.com. Cathy Silvers, formerly an actress on the TV show, Happy Days, she is an author and has a raw foods store.

Hemp: What The World Needs Now, HempNowBook.com. John McCabe's book about hemp, and why the laws prohibiting industrial hemp farming need to end.

Brenda Hinton, St. Helena, California; rawsomecreations.com. Brenda is a chef certified by the Living Light Colinary Institute.

Renata Holicova, New Zealand; fromgreytogreen.co.nz; Fromgreytogreen (at) home.org.nz. Teaches classes in gourmet raw food. She is a graduate of the Living Light Culinary Institute in Fort Bragg, California.

Harmony Hikes, HarmonyHikes.com. Chef and author Sergei Boutenko of RawFamily.com in southern Oregon conducts adventurous wild food foraging hikes.

Woody Harrelson, VoiceYourself.com

Healing Journeys, HealingJourneys.info. Ninaya Laub of Santa Barbara, California. Mom, massage therapist, yoga teacher, watsu giver, hydrotherapist, and raw food instructor. Her husband, Daniel, is involved in permaculture, helps run an organic farm, keeps an amazing culinary garden, and installs food gardens.

Jon Hinds, Monkey Bar Gym, 600 Williamson St., Ste. K2. Madison, WI 53703; 608.663.7511 MonkeyBarGym.com. Wisconsin yoga, calisthenics, and fitness course gym founded by Hinds, a personal fitness coach to many professional athletes.

Bruce Horowitz, thesunkitchen.com. Raw chef classes and catering. LongevityChef.com. RawPermaculture.com.

How 2 Eat Raw, How2EatRaw.com. Sheri Rivera.

Hunab Ku Portal, HunabKu.biz

Igniting Your Life, IgnitingYourLife.com. John McCabe's site for his book of the same name.

Jaffe Bros Natural Foods, Valley Center, CA, USA; OrganicFruitsAndNuts.com

Joel's Food, USA; JoelsFood.com. Joel Oohner.

Juice Feasting, JuiceFeasting.com

Nwenna Kai, Taste of the Goddess author. Nwenna (at) hotmail.com. Nwenna Kai. Formerly had a restaurant in Hollywood.

Chris Kendall, the-raw-advantage.com; Nutritionist, yoga practitioner, professional skateboarder.

David Klein, Living Nutrition, LivingNutrition.com.

Dr. Rosa Kincaid, Kincaid Medical Associates, P.C., 3016 Locust St., Ste. 104, St. Louis, MO 63103, USA; DrRosaKincaid.com; Medical doctor, teacher, raw food chef, professional dancer, mother, wife, grandmother.

Karen Knowler, England; TheRawFoodCoach.com.

John Kohler, California, GrowingYourGreens.com, and DiscountJuicers.Com
Kori Runs Dogs, nieko.com/korirunsdogs. Vegan blog.
JacQui Lalita, DanceOfTheDivine.org.
Mari Larsson, Toronto Sprouts, Toronto M5S 2R4; 416-977-8929; 416-535-3111; TorontoSprouts.com
Ninaya Laub, HealingJourneys.info. Mom, yoga teacher, watsu giver, hydrotherapist, chef, and raw food instructor in Santa Barbara, California.
Brenda Lee, overthemoonrawfoods.com; overthemoonrawfoods (at) gmail.com.
Levande Foda, Sweden; LevandeFoda.se
LifeFoods.com. Australia. Scott Mathias of ScottMathiasRaw.com.
Live Food Experience, LiveFoodExperience.com. Raw food chefiing and training by Adam Graham.
Living Earth Beauty, 93 S. Jackson St. #17775, Seattle, WA 98104, USA; LivingEarthBeauty.com. Jed and Jill sell raw, vegan, organic skincare products.
Ellen Livingston, LivingYogaNow.com.
Living Tree Community, LivingTreeCommunity.com. Living Tree Community Foods. Raw food products, including nut butters, oils, dried fruit, sprouting seeds, mesquite, carob, and North American wild rice.
Living Source, LivingSource.co.uk
Andrea Livingtson, phytofoods.blogspot.com. Andrea is a graduate of the Living Light Culinary Institute. She was the garden manager at Bastyr University in Kenmore, Washington, and is very knowledgeable about organic gardening.
Living Yoga, Ellen Livingston, Ann Arbor, MI; LivingYogaNow.com.
Lizby Grave, LizbyGrave.co.uk
Renee Loux, EuphoricOrganics.com. Chef, author, and TV personality who lives in Maui, Hawaii.
Elaina Love, PureJoyAcademy.com; PureJoyPlanet.com
Jillian Love, JillianLove.com; RawYogaRetreats.com; RawYogaJedi.com. Sanoma, CA.
Love Raw, LoveRaw.com
Love Snax, lovesnaxinc.com. Raw organic chocolate.
Jessica Loyer, raw gastronome (writes about and researches food). Jessloyer (at) gmail.com. Rawgastronomy.blogspot.com. Australia.
Brian Lucas, 310-460-9253; ChefBeLive.com; BeLiveLight.com. Known as "Chef BeLive." Lives in Los Angeles. Has written an ebook of his recipes. Co-creator of L.A. Raw Bazaar with Baruch Inbar and Maya Kriheli: LARawBazaar.com.
Lulu's Chocolate, Oregon; luluschocolate.com
Kate Magic, RawLiving.eu
Maine Sea Coast. 1-207-565-2907. Company that sells a variety of raw seaweed.
Mango the Fruitarian, MangoDurian.blogspot.com. Australia.
Anna Marcon, TheRawLife.co.uk
Bridgitte Mars, Boulder, Colorado, USA; BrigitteMars.com. Chef and author.

Rainbeau Mars, Santa Monica, CA; RainbeauMars.com. Daughter of Bridgette. Yoga teacher.

Scott Matthias, Australia; ScottMatthiasRaw.com. Also, LifeFoods.com.

John McCabe, C/O Carmania Books, POB 1272, Santa Monica, CA 90406-1272; SunfoodLiving.com. IgnitingYourLife.com. SunfoodTraveler.com. Author, ghostwriter, artist, environmental activist.

Dan McDonald & Krista Peterson, POB 722, Sultan, WA 98294; youtube.com/liferegenerator.

Andrea McNinch, How2EatRaw.com.

Mediterranean Goes Raw, MediterraneanGoesRaw.com. Mrs. Flora Papadopoulou, author of book *Mediterranean Goes Raw*

Vesanto Melina, MS, RD, 20543 96th Ave., #34, Langley, B.C. V1M 3W3, Melina; NutriSpeak.com. Co-author of Cherie Soria's book, The Raw Revolution Diet.

Dalila Miranda, radiantcuisine.com. Chef in Los Angeles who gives private classes.

Monkey Bar Gym, Wisconsin; MonkeyBarGym.com. Jon Hinds, personal trainer to many professional athletes.

Mike Mullen, raw chef, deserts, catering. 415-283-7045. OmMikeOm (at) gmail.com

Nature Raw, POB 870, 257 S Moapa Blvd., Overton, NV 89040; NatureRaw.com. Raw products company.

Eloise Nelson, PhD, thepowerofchow.com. Author of *14 Day Gourmet.*

Noyo Food Forest, POB 974, Fort Bragg, CA 95437; NoyoFoodForest.org. Impressive organic learning farm. Susan Lightfoot, Executive Director. They use the compost from Cherie Soria's Living Light Culinary Institute.

Nude Food, NudeFood.com

Ocean Wave Vibrations, 33 Punchards Down, Follaton, Totnes, TQ9 5FD; OceanWaveVibrations.com

Joel Odhner, RawLifeLine.com. Chef.

Joyce Oliveto, Health Horizons, 963 Peaceful Ct., Brighton, MI 48114, USA; naturalagelessliving.com. Email: Rejoyce (at) comcast.net. Organized the Midwest Living Foods Healthy Living EcoFestival.

Optimum Health Institute, OptimumHealth.org. Cedar Creek, Texas, and Lemon Grove, California.

Rene Oswald, reneoswald.com. rawfoodrene.com. Instructional chef. Author of *Transitioning to Living Cuisine.*

Over The Moon Raw Foods, Charlotte, NC; overthemoonrawfoods.com; overthemoonrawfoods (at) gmail.com. Catering. Brenda Lee Gambill.

Cath Parker, CathParker.WordPress.com

Andrew Perlot, Connecticut; Raw-Food-Health.net.

Plant Powered Living, Encinitas, CA; PlantPoweredLiving.com

Susan Powers, POB 184, Crystal Bay, MN 55323; RawMazing.com. Recipes and blog.

Premier Organics, 2342 Shattuck Ave., #342, Berkeley, CA 94704; 510-875-2146; premierorganics.org. Produces Artisana nut butters, coconut spreads, and other raw foods.

Pure Joy, Elaina Love's companies, PureJoyPlanet.com; PureJoyAcademy.com

Purely Raw, PurelyRaw.com

Pure Raw Lifestyle, PureRawLifestyle.com. Founded by Amy Rachelle of AmyRachelle.com

Qito, Qito.co.uk. Blog of Suki in England

Quantum Chocolate. Justin Ligeri's raw, organic, and vegan chocolate company. Jligeri2005@yahoo.com.

Amy Rachelle, AmyRachelle.com. Conducts seminars. PureRawLifestyle.com

Radiant Cuisine, RadiantCuisine.com. Site for chef Dalila Miranda in Los Angeles

Karen Ranzi, Ramsey, New Jersey; SuperHealthyChildren.com. Karen coordinates the New Jersey Raw Food Support Network. Karen (at) SuperHealthyChildren.com

Raw and Vegan, rawandvegan.com. The blog of Kate Quinn of Australia.

Raw Beauty Calendar, RawBeautyCalander.com. Tanya Wood.

The Raw Body Twins, POB 26311, Shawnee Mission, KS 66225-6311; TheRawBodyTwins.com. Susan and Stacey.

The Raw Chef Blog, U.K.; TheRawChefBlog.com. James Russell.

Raw Chef Dan, RawChefDan.com. Dan of Quintessence restaurant in New York City: Raw-Q.com.

The Raw Chocolate Company, Unit E 3, Blacklands Farm, Wheatsheaf Rd., Henfield, East Sussex BN5 9AT, England; TheRawChocolateCompany.com.

Raw Denver, RawDenver.com. Info (at) rawdenver.com.

Raw Divas, 2710 Thomes Ave., Ste 246, Cheyenne, WY 82001, USA; 2620 Frontenac, Unit 1, Montreal, QC H2K 3A1, Canada; TheRawDivas.com. Tera Warner.

Raw Dog Rory, USA; RawDawgRory.com

Raw Done Tastefully, Marina del Rey, CA; RawDoneTastefully.com. Raquel Smith teaches raw food courses.

Raw Edge Productions, RawEdgeProductions.com. Steven Prussack.

Raw Elements, Ontario, CA; RawElements.ca. Dawn (at) RawElements.ca. Raw products company.

Raw Epicurean, rawepicurean.net. The site of Ingrid Weithers-Barati.

Raw Family, Ashland, OR, USA; RawFamily.com. The Boutenko family of chefs and authors.

Raw Food Blogs, for a list of bloggers on raw food, access: rawfoodrightnow.blogspot.com/2007/07/ultimate-list-of-raw-food-blogs.html

Raw Food Central, POB 1537, Sebastopol, CA 95437; RawFoodSebastopol.com. Kathryn Ackland. Classes, meetings, events.

Raw Food Chef, Fort Bragg, CA; RawFoodChef.com. Site for author and chef Cherie Soria's chef training school, Living Light Culinary Institute. Facility includes a raw café, and retail store. She also hosts an annual Chef Showcase: Hot Chefs, Cool Kitchen! An event highlighting some of the best raw food chefs on the planet – streamed live over the Internet. She owns and operates an eco-friendly inn. She is the author of *Raw Food Revolution Diet.*

Subscribe to her free enewsletter by accessing the Web site and entering your email address into the enewesletter subscription box.

Raw Food Coach, Karen Knowler, U.K.; TheRawFoodCoach.com

Raw Food Health, Connecticut; raw-food-health.net. Andrew Perlot is a journalist and promotes the raw food lifestyle.

Raw Food Ideas, Jeff, England; RawFoodIdeas.com.

Raw Food Info, Rhio, New York; RawFoodInfo.Com.

Raw Food Media, Christopher Ciabarra, Los Angeles, CA; rawfoodmedia.ning.com.

Raw Food Network, Aaardvaaark P. O. Box 522 Bakersville NC 28705; RawFoodNetwork.com

Raw Food Planet, RawFoodPlanet.com

Raw Food Rehab, RawFoodRehab.ning.com

The Raw Food Muscle, TheRawFoodMuscle.com. Santiago Guido.

Raw Foods Bible, RawFoodsBible.com. rawfoodsbible (at) rawfoods.com. Author Craig B. Sommers N.D., C.N.

Raw-Foods-Diet-Center.com, USA. Hugh Cruickshank

Raw Foods News Magazine, RawFoodsNewsMagazine.com

Raw Foods On A Budget, rawfoodsonabudget.com. Brandi Rollins

Raw For 30 Days, Raw for Thirty, LLC, 156 Chestnut Ridge Rd., Bethel, CT 06801, USA; RawFor30Days.com. April (at) SimplyRawMovie.com. Site for documentary about diabetic patients who got off their medication by going raw under the supervision of Gabriel Cousens in Arizona.

Raw From The Farm, Oakland, CA, US; rawfromthefarm.com

RawFullyTempting.com. Hillborough, NJ. "Online café."

Raw Games, Attn: PMB 8696, 15-2662 Pahoa Village Rd., Pahoa, HI 96778; RawGames.org; contactus (at) rawgames.org. Paul Speros, founder, speros (at) rawgames.org.

The Raw Greek, TheRawGreek.com. Gina Panayi, England

Raw Intent, RawIntent.co.uk. England raw food online store.

RawKinRaw, rawenergyandlife.com. Erinn Williams began making chocolate brownies and distributing them to stores in the Los Angeles area. She is also a songwriter: erinnwilliams.com.

Raw Kosmickreations, Genevieve, POB 653, Culver City, CA 90232; RawKosmickreations.com; rawkosmickreations (at) gmail.com.

The Raw Life, Anna Marcon; TheRawLife.co.uk; anna (at) therawlife.co.uk

Raw Lifeline, Joel Odhner, RawLifeLine.com. Chef.

Raw Living, rawliving.eu. Kate Magic. Author of *Eat Smart, Eat Raw.*

RawLivingLove.com, North Carolina, USA. Brian Yonce lost over 100 pounds on the raw food diet starting in spring 2010.

RawLoveUK.com. Malachi's site about raw food info, education, and events in England.

Raw Matt, USA; rawmatt.com.

RawMazing, Susan Powers, POB 184, Crystal Bay, MN 55323; RawMazing.com. Recipes and blog.

Raw Mom, rawmom.com. Shannon 'Shakaya Breeze' LeoneTera Warner.

Raw Natural Hygiene, rawnaturalhygiene.ning.com

Raw n Delish, David Klein, Ph.D., Manager, POB 256 Sebastopol, CA 95473 USA; rawndelish.us.

Raw Network of Washington, Monika Kinsman, 9805 NE 116th St., PMB 7127, Kirkland, WA 98034; RawWashington.org. Monika also has opened Thrive Restaurant in Seattle.

Raw Nirvana, Sedona Media Company, POB 1194 Sedona, AZ 86351; RawNirvana.tv. Ron James and Kim McDermitt.

Raw Pear, Australia; RawPear.com. Aimee Devlin

Raw People, Carlsbad, CA; RawPeople.com.

Raw-Pleasure, Jennie Murphy, Raw Pleasures Australia, POB 2627 Nerang DC, Nerang, Queensland, 4211, Australia; Raw-Pleasure.com.au. Orders (at) raw-pleasure.com.au. Raw food forum, store, and seminars.

Raw Power, Thor Bazler, Idaho, USA; RawPower.com. Company that makes raw nutritional supplements. Formerly known as Steven Adler.

Raw Princess Studio, 1511 SW Market Street, Portland, OR 97201; rawprincess.org. Cindy Cummins. Makes and sells raw food items. Conducts juicing gatherings. Has a MeetUp group. Site has blod with recipes.

Raw Quest, Denmark; RawQuest.dk; Freshfoodfestival.com.

Raw Sacramento, RawSacramento.net

Raw Sangha, RawSangha.com. RawSangha (at) gmail.com. Brother Echo. A news and information site about raw issues and events in California.

Raw School, rawschool.com. Nora Lenz.

Raw Spirit Fest, RawSpirit.com. Raw Spirit Festival was first held in Arizona. A version was held in California in 2009, but attendance was weak. Contact Happy Oasis: Heavenly (at) RawSpirit.com.

Raw Superfoods, RawSuperfoods.com. Raw food supply company in Amsterdam.

Raw Vegan Radio, RawVeganRadio.com. Steven Prussack.

Raw Vegan Source, Tom Armstrong & Susan Park, 22336 NE 85th St., Redmond, WA 98053, USA; RawVeganSource.com

Raw Vortex, Kara Maia Spencer, OR, USA; rawvortex.squarespace.com. Inspiration and recipes.

RawVolution, Matt and Janabai Amsde, Santa Monica, CA; RawVolution.com. Matt is the author of the recipe book, RawVolution. He and Janabai own ELR Café (Euphoria Loves Rawvolution).

Raw Washington, Monika Kinsman; RawWashington.org. Monika opened Thrive restaurant in Seattle.

Raw Way, Bethany Herr-Hatfield, Michigan; rawwaylife.com; rawwaylife (at) gmail.com. Raw food products.

RawYogaRetreats.com; RawYogaJedi.com; Jillian Love, JillianLove.com. Sanoma, CA.

Rejuvenative, Rejuvenative.com. Site for the raw foods product company Rejuvinative Foods, POB 8464, Santa Cruz, CA 95061; 800-805-7975; 831-427-2196; mail (at) rejuvenate.com

Rhio's Raw Energy, New York; RawFoodInfo.com. Author and chef Rhio.

Erik Rivkin, VivaLaRaw.com. ERivkin (at) mindspring.com; chef.

Ginger Robinson, therawpath.com

Rock It Raw, RockItRaw.nl. Weekly raw event in Amsterdam

Rod Rotundi, Rod Rotundi, Marina del Rey, CA, USA; rodrotondi.com; LeafCuisine.com. Formerly owned a restaurant in Culver City that closed in 2010. Rotundi, who remains active in other projects. He is also the author of a book on green living and making raw foods. Rod (at) LeafOrganics.com.

Running Raw, Tim Van Orden; RunningRaw.com. Orden is a raw athlete.

Seeds Green Printing and Design, Pittsburgh, PA; seedsgreenprinting.com. Formerly printnetinc.com. Jeffrey Shaw. A printing company that uses 100% recycled paper. Also, other eco-friendly printing options available, such as biodegradable labels. They printed John McCabe's book, *Sunfood Living.*

Self Healing, Eric Karlsson; Self-Healing.se/naturecure.htm. Sweden and Australia.

Selina Naturally, 4 Celtic Dr., Arden, NC 28704, USA; CelticSeaSalt.com. Markets unheated salts.

Shaman Shack, Dean Thomas, Santa Monica, CA, USA; ShamanShack.info. Chinese tonic herbal products and mushrooms.

Shazzie, England; Shazzie.com. Co-author of *Naked Chocolate.*

She-ZenCuisine.com, CA. Angelina Elliott, author of *Alive in 5.*

Cathy Silvers, Los Angeles, CA; thehealthylivingshow.com. Formerly an actress on the TV show, "Happy Days," she now is an author and has a raw foods store.

Simply Raw, Natasha Kyssa; Ottawa, Canada; SimplyRaw.ca. Raw company that also has a yearly raw festival.

Sara Siso, Arizona; 480-760-3387; chefsara.com; chefsarasignaturecreations (at) gmail.com. Raw chef. Graduate of Tree of Life.

Chad Sarno, rawchef.com. Info (at) rawchef.com.

Sirova, Ames, Iowa, USA; Sirova.com. Raw food supplies. Kori Radke and Joanna Steven. Sirova is the Czech word for raw.

Jim Sloman, mayyoubehappy.com

Smart Monkey Foods, SmartMonkeyFoods.com. Company started by recipe book author Ani Phyo that produces raw nutritional bars.

Jonathan Snell, Johnny's Hot Sauce, Vital Heat, Venice, CA; VitalHotSauce.com. Organic raw hot sauce made my hand.

Cherie Soria, Fort Bragg, CA, USA; RawFoodChef.com. Author, chef, and owner of Living Light Culinary Institute. Also has café and eco-friendly inn. Subscribe to her free enewsletter by accessing the Web site and entering your email address into the subcription box.

SplendorInTheRaw.com. Tina Jo.

SproutHouse.com. Rita.

SproutPeople.com

Terry Stiers, chef in Missouri; RawFoodBasics.com, rawfoodbasics (at) yahoo.com

Straight From The Garden, POB 420921, San Diego, CA 92142; straightfromthegarden.com

Shawna Stursa, Columbus, OH; rawshawna.com. Also has a Raw Columbus group on MeetUp.com.

Sunfood Living, SunfoodLiving.com. Site for John McCabe's book, *Sunfood Living: Resource Guide for Global Health.*

Sunfood Traveler, SunfoodTraveler.com. John McCabe's site.

The Sun Kitchen, Bruce Horowitz; thesunkitchen.com. Catering and chef classes.

Super Hero Snacks, Chad Johnson, Santa Cruz, CA, USA; superherosnacks.com.

Sura Detox, Ham Farm, Dolton, Nr. Winkleigh, Devon, EX19 8QT, U.K.; SuraDetox.com.

Synergy Chef, 1825 Del Paso Blvd. Ste. 2, Sacramento, CA 95815, USA; SynergyChef.com; TheArtOfFood.org.

Dean Thomas, Santa Monica, CA, USA; ShamanShack.info. Chinese tonic herbal products and mushrooms.

Thor Bazler, Idaho, USA; ThorBazler.com. Makes the Raw Power raw food nutritional supplements sold in many stores.

Lawrence Todd, Formerly owned Earthsong Living Cuisine in Hermosa Beach, CA. Closed in 2011. Chefraw.com. 16.lawrence (at) gmail.com

Tyler Tolman, 1271 Oakridge Rd South, Park City UT 84098, USA; tylertolman.com

Toronto Sprouts, Marie Larsson, Toronto M5S 2R4, Canada; 416-977-8929; 416-535-3111; TorontoSprouts.com.

Total Raw Food, Brighton, England; TotalRawFood.com.

Tree of Life Rejuvenation Center, Arizona, Dr. Gabriel Cousens, TreeOfLife.nu. A health retreat and learning center.

U.B.Raw Inc., 380 Bannock St., Mesquite, NV 89027; 702-346-5029; UBRaw.com; Email: info (at) UBRaw.com. Not a restaurant. Ronnie and Minh provide raw food training and restaurant consulting.

UNFI – United Natural Foods, Inc. 1-800-679-6733. This is a food distribution company with offices throughout the US, including Hawaii.

Vegan Body Building, Robert Cheeke, veganbodybuilding.com. Robert (at) veganbodybuilding.com.

Vegan Girl blog, vegangirl.com

Vermont Fiddle Heads, Linda Wooliever, Raw Vermond, 18 Worcester Village Rd., Worcester, VT 05682-9684, USA; vt-fiddle.com

Kyle Vialli, galaxyofvitality.com, consciousevents.co.uk.

VibeAlive.ca, site of Joanne Gero, N.D.

Vibrance Magazine, (formerly Living Nutrition); LivingNutrition.com. Raw food magazine. Dave Klein. Also runs Fruitarian Worldwide Network: fruitnet.org.

Vibrancy Homestead, Dr. Gina Shaw, England; Vibrancy.Homestead.com.

Viva La Raw, Erik Rivkin, VivaLaRaw.com. Founded Viva La Raw Project to educate people on raw foods and healthy planet ventures.

Vivapura, 320 Smelter Ave., POB 431, Patagonia, AZ 85624-0431; 877-787-6457; Vivapura.net. Not a restaurant. Company produces and distributes raw food products.

WE Juice for Joy Experience, TheWEConference.com. Kaci Christian, founder of The WE Conference, leads quarterly 10-day juice fasting and teleclass with Chef Xian. The WE Conference is a women's empowerment organization base on compassionate principles that promotes health, wellness, compassion, love and peace via plant-based nutrition.

Wilderness Family Naturals, 99 Edison, Silver Bay, MN 55614; wildernessfamilynaturals. Food supplies.

Women Go Raw, womengoraw.com

Jason Andrew Wrobel, Draw, Los Angeles, CA, USA; jasonwroble.com; 310-383-0445; Jason (at) jasonwroble.com. Raw chef, catering, instruction, events

Maris Yeager, Ukiah, CA, USA; icaneatraw.com. Raw chef graduate of Cherie Soria's Living Light Culinary Institute.

Yoga In The Raw, YogaInTheRaw.com. Michael Stein and Angela Starks of New Paltz, New York. Yoga studio, raw food and green living seminars.

Zenergy, Santa Monica, CA 90403, USA; 310-866-0820; zenergysuperfoods.com.

• Raw Chef Training

MANY raw food restaurants offer raw food preparation courses. If you live near a raw food restaurant, check to see if they offer classes in food preparation. Or see below for information about **Cherie Soria's Living Light Culinary Institute** in Fort Bragg, California. Access: rawfoodchef.com.

If you are considering attending a raw chef school, and especially if it is for professional reaons, such as you want to work at restaurants, resorts, or do private chefing, please consider Living Light Culinary Institute. Compare it to other so-called chef training programs. Consider the cost per hour, and you will likely find that Living Light is the best choice, especially when considering that it is fully licensed in the state of California, and, upon completion of their program, you will be a graduate.

It may be fun to take classes from other chefs, and at raw food restaurants, but attending a fully state-licensed chef school is what will look good on your resume, and will give you the hands-on teaching that will benefit your skills. Other places and people teaching raw chef classes are more demonstrative, less hands-on, and charge much more per hour than Living Light. Their qualifications and teachings are not of the quality that you will receive at Living Light.

Also to consider when attending a so-called raw chef school is that, they may be operating outside of the law and misrepresenting the value and quality of training that you will receive. So, do your research before paying anyone for classes. And, do not be romanced or charmed into paying for raw chef classes, including from authors or so-called raw food celebrities.

As raw culture spreads across the world, more retreat centers and raw food restaurants are offering food prep classes. These may be one-day, multiple-day, or multiple-weekend classes.

In Australia, there is **Samudra**, the yoga and surf school that also has a raw food café. They offer multiple-day courses in raw food preparation. Contact samudra.com.au.

Author and chef Matthew Kenney has built **105 Degrees,** an upscale raw cafe, culinary academy and retail shop at Classen Curve in Oklahoma City, OK; matthewkenneylifestyle.com/105-degrees. In 2012, he opened a chef school and restaurant in Santa Monica, California.

There are also chefs who teach private raw prep classes, such as

Aris Latham, sunfired.com/site

Lenore Baum of **Lenore's Natural Cuisine**, 164 Ox Creek Rd., Weaverville, NC 28787; lenoresnatural.com. Lenore teaches raw organic vegan classes near Asheville.

Sergei and Valya Boutenko, in Ashland, Oregon, rawfamily.com

Rachel Carr and Kristan Andrews of **Cru Silverlake,** this restaurant in Los Angeles offers chef classes. CruSilverlake.com. 1521 Griffith Park Blvd., Los Angeles, CA 90026. They also have a Good Karma Truck that drives around to various events serving vegan food.

Patricia Granswind of **EternalDelight.net** in New Zealand. She is part Italian, is from Germany, and has lived in Vancouver, BC and Santa Monica, California. GourmetVeganChef.com. GourmetVeganChef (at) gmail.com.

Brenda Hinton of rawsomecreations.com in St. Helena, California. She is certified as a chef from Living Light Culinary Institute.

Brian Lucas, Los Angeles; ChefBeLive.com; BeLiveLight.com. Co-creator of L.A. Raw Bazaar with Baruch Inbar and Maya Kriheli: LARawBazaar.com.

Alicia Parnell of Que Se Raw Se Raw restaurant in Burlingame, California has a kitchen angel internship program in which volunteers learn to make raw food by working in the restaurant. 1160 Capuchino Ave., Burlingame, CA 94010; QueSeRawSeRaw.com.

Raquel Smith, Raw Done Tastefully, Marina del Rey, CA; RawDoneTastefully.com. Raquel Smith teaches raw food courses.

Raw Foundation Culinary Arts Institute, 1333 W. Georgia St., Vancouver St., Vancouver, BC; RawFoodFoundation.org

Rod Rotundi, formerly had the Leaf Cuisine restaurants in Culver City, Sherman Oaks, and Redondo Beach, California. Rod (at) LeafOrganics.com.

Angela Starks and Michael Stein, YogaInTheRaw.com. Upstate New York

Linda Szarkowsky of **Green Spirit** in Chicago is a graduate of Living Light Culinary Institute. Linda (at) GreenSpiritLiving.com.

Sabina Torrieri of **La Vie En Raw Café** in Coral Gables, Florida, lavieenrawcafe.com.

Theresa Webb of **Kitchen Buddy** in England. Theresa (at) KitchenBuddy.eu.

A person can also learn a lot by using the popular raw food recipe books. Many of them are available in public libraries, are sold at the raw restaurants, and are available through traditional book stores and Web sites. Many raw recipe book authors also teach raw food or sunfood preparation classes.

Brenda Cobb's Living Foods Institute is a New Age healing center offering classes in raw food preparation. After being told that she was going to die, Brenda healed herself from cancer with the help of raw food and healthful thought. 1530 Dekalb Ave., NE, Ste. E, Atlanta, Georgia, 30307; 404-524-4488; LivingFoodsInstitute.com.

Alissa Cohen former owner of Grezzo restaurants in Boston and author of a popular recipe book. She has a chef training program. AlissaCohen.com.

Cousins Incredible Vitality, hold regular culinary arts classes. 3038 W. Irving Park Rd., Chicago, IL 60618; 773-478-6868; CousinsIV.com

Glaser Organic Farms, offers "raw food cuisine culinary arts classes" taught by chef Tracy Fleming. 19100 SE 137th Ave., Miami, FL 33177; 305-238-7747; GlaserOrganicFarms.com. They also have a weekly raw street market, Green Market, on Saturday.

Angels Healthfood Institute, POB 858, Gold Hill, OR 97525; angelshealthfoodinstitute.com; Farm address: 9394 Blackwell Rd., Central Point, OR 97502; 541-855-1846; angels-visions.com. Offers raw food prep classes and retreats.

For those wishing to experience professional raw chef training, consider Cherie Soria's **Living Light Culinary Institute**, 301-B North Main St., Fort Bragg, California 95437; 800-816-2319; 707-964-2420; RawFoodChef.com.

WITH the **Living Light Culinary Institute**, Cherie Soria has raised the bar on the standards of gourmet raw vegan foods. She has taken over nearly half of an historic two-story building in this small town on the Northern California coast, and has transformed it into a fully-staffed teaching facility with top-of-the-line equipment.

As Soria's Web site states, "In the comprehensive 19-day chef and instructor training program students learn all aspects of creating raw living foods – from appetizers to desserts, breads to confectioneries. Attendees range from Parisian executive chefs to novices." As a bonus for those who complete the full program, the Institute has a chef referral service designed to help connect graduates to potential employers.

Living Light Culinary Institute also holds workshops and seminars for those who can't commit to the full-length program, and for those who simply wish to learn how to make truly healthful food that tastes amazing. Additionally, the Institute offers an entire nutritional science program, including a nutrition educators' certification course.

Soria runs a raw food café and retail store in the same structure that holds her Institute. She has also restored a nearby mansion into an eco-friendly inn serving students and travelers.

Check out Cherie's wonderful book: *Raw Food Revolution Diet: Feast, Lose Weight, Gain Energy, Feel Younger.* It is not only a recipe book, it contains a tremendous amount of information that substantiates the benefits of a raw food diet – proving that the raw food diet not only meets, but exceeds our dietary needs. It is co-authored by dietitians, Vesanto Melina, and Brenda Davis using peer-reviewed studies.

Sign-up for the Living Light enewsletter by accessing RawFoodChef.com and entering your email address in the subscription box.

• Sunfoodist Retreats Inside U.S.

BEFORE traveling to attend any retreat, raw food or otherwise, do research on the Internet and ask around to find out if the retreat is offering what you would like to experience. Don't simply and only rely on promotional material provided by the retreat.

There are a variety of raw food retreats that offer different styles and share their own philosophies. One may focus more on detoxing and fasting, while another may focus on yoga and learning to make healthful food. Some may focus on success theory and inspiration. Or, they may be a mix of all of those things. They may be held in hotels; bed and breakfast hotels; retreat centers, or at resorts. Others are held in more of a rugged surrounding, such as at a hot springs center where you stay in a tent. Select a retreat based on your comfort level and needs.

I have been careful about listing "fasting retreats" in this book. While short fasts can be beneficial, I do not advise anyone to go on long-term water fasts of more than a few days. Even if the fasts are supervised by people who say they have experience with the process.

Also, some intentional communities host and/or function as retreat centers. To find a list of raw food intentional communities, access: RawCommunities.com. The site contains a growing list of raw food intentional communities around the world.

• Arizona Retreats

Eden Hot Springs, AZ. Various raw food retreats have been held at this hot springs center. Retreats are organized by various authors and teachers. Before visiting, do some research to find out what it is that is being offered, and if it is what you would like to experience.

Tree Of Life Rejuvenation Center, 686 Harshaw Rd., POB 778, Patagonia, AZ 85624; 520-394-2520; healing (at) treeoflife.nu; TreeOfLife.nu; Dr. Gabriel Cousens' center.

• California Retreats

Living Light Culinary Institute, 301-B North Main St., Fort Bragg, California 95437; 800-816-2319; 707-964-2420; RawFoodChef.com; info (at) rawfoodchef.com.. This is Cherie Soria's raw food chef school. It also has a café and retail store. Check schedule for raw food seminars and her annual chef showcase. Cherie owns and runs an eco-friendly inn serving students and other travelers in Fort Bragg. She is the author of *Raw Food Revolution Diet: Feast, Lose Weight, Gain Energy, Feel Younger.*

Sign-up for the Living Light enewsletter by accessing the Web site, RawFoodChef.com, and entering your email address in the subscription box.

Optimum Health Institute, 6970 Central Ave., Lemon Grove, CA 91945; 619-464-3346; OptimumHealth.org.

• FLORIDA RETREAT

Hippocrates Health Institute, 1443 Palmdale Court, West Palm Beach, FL 33411; 800-842-2125; hippocratesinst.com

• GEORGIA RETREATS

Living Foods Institute, Atlanta, GA; LivingFoodsInstitute.com.

Enota Mountain Retreat, Hiawassee, GA; Enota.com. This isn't a vegan venue, but they have many events throughout the year of interest.

• HAWAII RETREATS

Banyan Tree Santuary, 73-4464 Kohanaiki Rd., Kaulua Kona, Big Island, HI 96740; banyantreesanctuary.com. Healing sanctuary run by raw vegans. 3.3 acres, 200 fruit trees, organic carden, yoga, medication, workshops, massage. Contact: Raybo: iamrg51 (at) gmail.com.

Vacation Inn Paradise, 593 Poipu Dr., Honolulu, Oahu, HI 96825; 808-239-2030; toll free 877-398-6220; vacationinnparadise.com; Email: HealingWithNature (at) hawaii.rr.com. Near Hanauma Bay. 20 Minutes from Waikiki. Raw food vacation packages offer massage, acupuncture, lymphatic drainage. Inn has infrared sauna, chlorine-free ozonated pool, gardens, fruit trees,

Kalani, Big Island, near Pahoa, Hawaii. Kalani.com. This is a yoga retreat center that is like summer camp for adults with a large pool, massage, and a special watsu pool. Rooms are simple with screens instead of windows. There is also a camping field for those with tents. Communal dining is mostly vegetarian or vegan. They will accommodate the raw food diet upon request.

Yoga Oasis, POB 1935, Pahoa, HI 96778; 808-965-8460; YogaOasis.org. info (at) yogaoasis.org. On Big Island. Check schedule.

• MICHIGAN RETREAT

The Assembly of Yahweh Wellness Center, 7881 Columbia Hwy., Eaton Rapids, MI 48827; 517-663-1637; Hiawatha Cromer

Creative Health Institute, 112 West Union City Rd., Union City, MI 49094; 517-278-6260; CreativeHealthInstitute.us. CreativeHealthInstitute.com.

• NEW MEXICO RETREAT

Ann Wigmore Foundation, POB 399, San Sidel, New Mexico 87049; 505-552-0595

• NEW YORK RETREAT

Turquoise Barn, 8052 Country Hwy. 18, Bloomville, NY 13739; turquoisebarn.com. Michelle Premura and Michael Milton. Bed and breakfast, art gallery, event venue, retreat, vacation rental, and camping space. Organic, vegetarian, vegan, and raw food. Check site for information about events. Area is popular with athelete bikers. Next to the Catskills Scenic Trail. Access: catskillscenictrail.com.

• OREGON RETREATS

Boutenko Family, POB 172, Ashland, OR 97520; RawFamily.com; HarmonyHikes.com. The Boutenko family are authors, chefs, and wild food foragers who have traveled the world teaching about raw food. They offer various types of raw food seminars, gatherings, and hiking/camping adventures. Check with them for schedule and location of events.

• TEXAS RETREATS

Optimum Health Institute, Rural Route 1, Box 339-J, Cedar Creek, TX 98612; 512-303-4817; OptimumHealth.org.

Oxygen Life Spa and Raw Superfood Store, 609 N. Locust, Denton, TX 76201; 944-384-7946; OxygenLifeSpa.com. Asha Cobb

Rest Or Your Life Health Retreat, POB 102, Barksdale, TX 78828; 830-234-3488; vvvhaag (at) swtexas.net; Gregory and Tosca Haag.

• WASHINGTON RETREAT

Thrive Wellness Center - Cedar Springs Renewal Center, 31459 Barben Rd., Sedro Woolley, Washington 98284; 360-826-3599; mohappy (at) cedarsprings.org. In connection with Thrive raw restaurant in Seattle. 43 Acres in the foothills of the Cascade mountins, 90 minute drive from Seattle.

• PUERTO RICO RETREAT

Ann Wigmore Institute, POB 429, Rincon, Puerto Rico 00677, USA; 787-868-6307; Wigmore (at) coqui.net; annwigmore.org

• SUNFOODIST RETREATS OUTSIDE U.S.

THERE are a variety of raw food retreats that have different styles. One may focus more on detoxing and fasting, while another may focus on yoga and learning to make healthful food. They may be held in hotels; bed and breakfast hotels; retreat centers, or at resorts. Others are held in more of a rugged surrounding, such as at a hot springs center where you stay in a tent. Select a retreat based on your comfort level and needs.

Also, some intentional communities host and/or function as retreat centers. To find a list of raw food intentional communities, access: RawCommunities.com. The site contains a growing list of raw food intentional communities around the world.

• AUSTRALIA RETREATS

Embracing Health, Lisa Wheeler Retreats, embracinghealth.com.au/retreat

Funkey Forest, 1321 Main Arm Rd., Mullumbimby, NSW 2482, AU; 02-66845279; FunkeyForest.com. Surrounded by wildlife sanctuary in mountains 30 minutes from Byron Bay. Not a resort. Has dorms, camping, meditation/yoga rooms, massage, kitchen facilities, broad deck, hiking excursions. Various yoga, fasting, detox retreats. Erik Adams.

Hippocrates Health Center of Australia, Elaine Ave., Mudgeeraba 4213, Gold Coast Queensland, Australia; 07-5530-2860; Hippocrates.com.au

Raw Power, Brisbane, Australia; RawPower.com.au. Valerie Morkel and Jane Brice bought the company in 2011 from Runi and Anand Wells.

Samadhi Raw Yoga Retreat, North Stradbroke Island, QLD, Australia; samadhiflowyoga.com. Sub-tropical island retreat with yoga, dance, meditation, hikes, surfing, high-fruit raw food. Kath Ford. Kath (at)

samadhiflowyoga.com

Samudra, POB 295, Dunsborough 6281, Western Australia; +61 897740110; Samudra.com.au. Runs yoga and surf retreats with raw food. Raw food café and organic store opened 2008. Beautiful location. Sheridan Hammond.

• Belize Retreat

Vida Clara, 011-501-668-8866; vidaclara.com. Email: heal (at) vidaclara.com.

• Brazil Retreat

Pid Rama, Nova Friburgo – RJ, Brazil; pindorama.org.br/en. Conducts raw vegan retreats, as well as a number of other educational seminars.

• Canada Retreats

Hollyhock, POB 127, Manson's Landing, Cortes Island, BC V0P 1K0, Canada; hollyhock.ca/cms. 100 miles north of Vancouver on Cortes Island. There are some retreats held here of interest to raw foodists.

New Life Retreat, RR4, 453 Dobbie Rd., Lanark, Ontario, K0G 1K0, Canada; 613-259-3337; healing (at) newliferetreat.com; newliferetreat.com. Chas and Madeline Dietrich

Nonpareil Natural Health Retreat, RR#3, Stirling, Ontario, K0K 3E0, Canada; 613-395-6332; nonpareil (at) sympatico.ca; David Gouveia and Ms. Mano McNabb. 173 acre country estate.

• Costa Rica Retreats

Cascada Verde, Costa Rica, cascadaverdelodge.com. cascadaverde (at) hotmail.com

Finca de Vida (Farm of Life), wellness center and eco-adventure, foods from organic farm. Wellness Program teaches the principals of optimal health. Private accommodations; yoga; communal center for facilitating small retreats, workshops and personal gatherings. Opening Fall 2009. Located in SW Costa Rica, near San Isidro and Playa Dominical; fincadevida.com; 011-506-8-373-3261; info (at) fincadevida.com;

Spirit of the Earth, 5871 Bells Rd, London, Ontario, N6P 1P3, Canada; 519-652-9109; Walter and Lorenna. Canadian address, but retreats are held in Costa Rica.

Pacha Mama, 506-289-7081; pacha-mama.org. Intentional community on the West coast of Costa Rica. Holds many gatherings and has massage therapists, yoga teachers, and other healers and instructors present.

Waterfalls Villas AKA Cascadas Farallas, Costa Rica; waterfallvillas.com. Fateh and Franco Bolivar, Near Dominical Beach. "Raw Foodist Heaven - Retreat with private waterfalls in an amazing natural setting perfect for rejuvenation, detox, honeymoons and weddings." – Fateh.

• Croatia Retreat

Jesse Bogdanovich, Island of Vis, Croatia, TheWholeLifestyle.com/retreat/. Runs a raw vegan retreat in Croatia by the Adriatic beaches. With Jesse's mother, Dr. Ruza Bogdanovich of The Cure Is In The Cause Foundation and author of a book by the same name (Access: TheCureIsInTheCause.com). Jesse Boganovich is also on FaceBook.com.

• England Retreats

Health Etcetera, Enland, healthetcetera.com
Heart Spring, England, HeartSpring.co.uk
Karuna Detox, karunadetox.com
The Raw Food Retreat, therawfoodretreat.co.uk
Shambhala, England, Shambhala.co.uk
Shekin Ashram, England, ShekinAshram.org
Sura Detox, England, SuraDetox.com

• France Retreat

Retreat Biarritz, retreat-biarritz.com

Torce Viviers En Charnie, Pays de Loire France; dawncampbellholistichealth.eu. Welcomes guests interested in natural alternative lifestyle and vegetarian, vegan, raw and natural hygiene diet. English host, Dawn Campbell. master coach, living foods practitioner, chef, teacher, author and offers reiki, thought field therapy, massage and yoga.

• Honduras Retreat

La Casa Verde; wendygreenyoga.com. Wendy Green's yoga and relaxation retreat.

• Ireland Retreat

The Irish School of Natural Healing, The Old Rectory, 25 Coote Street, Portlaoise, County Laois, Ireland; +353 (0)57 8682567; herbeire.ie/School/About.html. Focus is on "cleansing the body and mind using organic vegan and living food programmes, herbal medicines, bodywork and environmental and lifestyle awareness."

• Mexico Retreats

Casa Axis Mundi, Valladolid, Yucatan, Mexico; CasaAxisMundi.com. Raw vegan retreat and bed & breakfast. Opened 2012.

Rancho La Puerta, Tacate, Baja, California, Mexico; RachoLaPuerta.com

Rio Caliente Spa and Nature Resort, Primavera, Mexico; 1-800-200-2927; RioCaliente.com/index.html. Although not all vegetarian or raw food, this "nature ranch" in a pine forest provides raw food, fresh juices, and is in a setting of gardens, natural hot spring-fed pools, and offers common spa treatments, including massage, mud baths, steam baths, hiking, and yoga. The spa grows much of its own food. Located 45 minutes from Guadalajara. Group rates are offered.

Sanoviv Medical Institute of Baja California, Mexico; 2602-C Transportation Ave., National City, CA 91950; 800-SANOVIV (726-6848); sanoviv.com

• New Zealand Retreat

Innourish, 82 Mtakana Valley Rd., Matakana, New Zealand; innourish.net; adyama86 (at) yahoo.com; innourish (at) xtra.co.nz

• Panama Retreat

Aris Latham, sunfired.com/site

Tanglewood Wellness Center, Correos Bejuco, Entrenza General, Rep. de Panama;; tanglewoodwellnesscenter.com. Has promoted their supervised fasting and healing programs. Anyone going on a fast or to a health retreat in another country should do their research to know that they are going to be in a situation in which they feel it is best for them. Do an internet search for Tanglewood and see if they are a place that fits your standards.

• PHILIPPINES RETREAT

The Farm at San Benito, Hippocrates Health Resort of Asia, The Farm at San Benito, Isle of Luzon, Philippines; Manila Office, Azalea Room Mezzanine Floor, Mandarin Oriental Hotel, Makati Avenue, Makati City; 632-751 3498; 632-750 8888 loc. 72428; info (at) thefarm.com.ph; thefarm.com.ph; A raw-food resort.

• SPAIN RETREATS

Communidad de Alimentacion Cruda Internacional, Finca Cruda, Revista Naturaleza Cruda, Arroyo del Viejo-Alpujata, 29110 Monda, Malaga, Costa del Sol, Spain; 952 119929, 619 78 85 70; Contact: Balta, Baltacrudo (at) yahoo.es

The Living Raw Retreat, thelivingrawretreat.com

The Retreat Option, Southern Spain, retreatoption.wordpress.com

• THAILAND RETREATS

Atsumi Healing Center, 34/18 Soi Pattana, Saiyuan Rd., Rawai, Phuket Island, Thailand, 83130; English in Thailand: 08 1272 0571; overseas +66-8-1272-0571; Thai enquirees 08-1970-1753; overseas +66-8-1970-1753; atsumihealing.com

ProCynergy, 120/51 Palm Springs Place, Ciang Mai, 500000, Thailand; 053 241 249; Julia (at) juliajus.com; juliajus.com

The Sanctuary, Thailand ;thesanctuarythailand.com/resort-spa-home.htm. Yoga, massage, cleansing, ocean kayaking, beachside hammocks. Not a raw resort, but easy to follow a raw diet here in a remote location. The food is vegetarian, but with some fish on the menu.

• RANDOM RECIPES FOR A RAW KITCHEN

For more recipes, access:
living-foods.com/recipes
goneraw.com/recipes
rawmazing.com/rawmazing-recipes

It is good to eat simply. Instead of always working to make every meal into a gourmet feast, make some meals into monomeals. By that, I mean eating only one thing during a meal: such as eating a melon, or eating several tangerines, or eating a few mangoes, or a big bowl of strawberries, including the leaves.

Get into making green smoothies. These are made by blending water, some fruit, and some green leafy vegetables. Don't guzzle green smoothies, drink massive amounts of them, or rely on them too heavily. Rather, drink slowly, savoring their flavor and allowing the digestive juices of your moth to begin the conversion process. Salads rich in variety are a better choice.

Learn to make salads from scratch, including the dressings – especially from foods you grow in a home garden. Doing so will be more healthful, and save money.

For variety, go for it, and make some of your favorite gourmet raw foods, pimped-out salads, and luscious raw desserts.

There are a growing number of raw recipe books. One is a low fat recipe book by Veronica Grace Patenaude. If you are on the Internet, see Dara Dubinet's YouTube channel. Dara demonstrates low fat raw or mostly raw recipes. I suggest to people that they follow a low-fat diet.

One excellent book about raw food nutrition is *Becoming Raw: The Essential Guide to Raw Vegan Diets*, by Davis, Melina, and Berry.

I wouldn't advise using the nama shoyu that some of the recipes in the book contain. Instead, I advise using coconut aminos, which are becoming more common in healthfood stores.

Replace carob for the chocolate in the recipes.

Use dates, coconut bud sap, coconut sugar, or maple syrup instead of agave. Agave is NOT a healthfood. Raw honey would be a lesser choice, and only for those who use honey.

Cut the oil in recipes in half, or a fourth, or maybe, depending on the recipe, delete the oil altogether.

Brenda Davis and Vesanto Melina are also the co-authors with Cherie Soria of *Raw Food Revolution Diet.* Davis and Melina got into raw foods while researching and helping Cherie Soria write *Raw Food Revolution*, then they wrote the book, *Becoming Raw.*

For athletic performance, read *Thrive Fitness: Mental and Physical Strength for Life*, by Brendan Brazier. He also wrote the *Thrive Diet.* Also, consider Douglas Graham's book, *The 80/10/10 Diet.*

• Simple Salad

In a large bowl, combine:
Half a head of **Romain lettuce or one-half bunch kale**, finely chopped
Juice of one-half **lemon**
One half of a ripe **avocado**, pitted, skinned, and finely cut into cubes
Several raw **pine nuts or fractured raw walnuts**

Optional:
Several **grape tomatoes**
Spoonfull **black currants**
Two pinches **salt** (optional)
One diced **pear or peach**
Ground **black pepper**
Freshly chopped herbs: **oregonao or basil**

• Kale Salad for Four

In a large bowl, combine:
Two bunches of finely chopped **kale**
Two diced **Roma tomatoes**
Several fractured **walnuts**
Eight raw **green olives**, diced
One-fourth of a **red onion**, diced
One-forth of a **red bell pepper**, diced
Two cored, unpeeled **apples**, diced
One-fourth cup **raisins**
Two tablespoons **nutritional yeast** (not brewer's yeast)
One tablespoon **millet** (not heated)
One tablespoon **sesame seeds**
Two tablespoons fractured **hemp seeds**

Dressing:
In food processor, combine:
Three or four **dates**
Juice from one half **lemon**
Tablespoon prepared **mustard** (such as Dijon)
Teaspoon **hemp seed oil** (or no oil)
Teaspoon **dill**
Teaspoon **thyme**
Half a teaspoon **chili powder** (or none)
Two tablespoons **water**

Optional:
Half a teaspoon vegan **probiotic powder**
Dash of **cayenne** powder
Dash of **salt** (optional)
One diced **peach**
Several diced **strawberries**
Handfull **blueberries**

• EINSTEIN SALAD

This salad is a rather involved salad that is particularly rich in brain and bone nutrients. It's a great salad for bringing to dinner parties.

All ingredients raw, unheated, and organically grown.

Presoak the following greens
In one-half cup lemon juice and one-half teaspoon salt for a half day, or overnight, in a covered bowl in the refrigerator. To get the leaves coated with the lemon juice and salt, mix them with your hands. Some people purposely squish the leaves as they do this, and this is why you may hear people describe this is a "massaged salad":
One-half cup finely chopped **chard or kale**
One-half cup finely chopped **broccoli**
One-half cup finely chopped **celery**
One-half cup finely chopped **dandelion greens**
One-half cup finely chopped **Italian parsley**
One-half cup finely chopped **collard greens**

(You can also use spinach, beet greens, or other greens)

After soaking, put in strainer and lightly rinse with water. Spin dry in salad spinner. If you don't have a spinner, spread the rinsed greens on a clean towel, and gently roll to absorb the majority of water.

Soak:
One tablespoon **mustard seeds** in water for about half a day
One-fourth cup **sunflower seeds** in water for 4 to 8 hours

Put into big bowl: the salad mix above with:
One-fourth cup chopped **raw walnuts**
One-fourth cup raw **sunflower seeds** (soaked)
One chopped **apple**
One finely chopped red or **yellow bell pepper**
One-fourth cup fresh **pomegranate seeds or raisins** with seeds
One cubed **avocado** (pitted and peeled)

Dressing: blend together:
One tablespoon **mustard seeds** (soaked)
One clove **garlic**, minced

Six raw **olives**, pitted, chopped
Nine raw, fresh **cranberries, or** about 15 **fresh blueberries**
One-fourth cup **hemp oil** or cold-pressed grapeseed oil, or olive oil
One teaspoon minced fresh **ginger root**
Tiny pinch of **red pepper**
One tablespoon **nutritional yeast** (optional)
One teaspoon **spirulina**
One-fourth teaspoon pink or sea **salt** (optional)
One tablespoon freshly ground **flax seeds** (use coffee grinder)
Juice from half an **orange**, or three to four tablespoons apple juice

Optional:
One to two tablespoons of raw **honey or maple syrup**

Toss the salad and dressing together. Chill.

• MUSHROOM WRAP FILLER

Combine in Cuisinart:
One portobello **mushroom**, chopped
One **carrot,** chopped
Five **walnuts**
One-fourth of a **brown onion**, chopped
Five raw, pitted **green olives**
One tablespoon (or less) **hemp oil**
One tablespoon **thyme**
Dash of **cayenne powder**
One half teaspoon pink or sea **salt** (optional)

After combining the above ingredients in Cuisinart, place in bowl and stir in one-half of a finely cubed **avocado**.

Use as filler for a **collard green** wrap by putting a scoop full on a collard leaf and wrapping it up.

• CORN SALAD

In a bowl, combine:
Kernels cut from one unheated cob of **corn**
Squeeze of one-forth **lemon**
Handful of fractured **cashews or macadamia nuts**
Heaping tablespoon raw **shredded coconut** meat
One **green onion**, diced
Palmfull of diced **cilantro**
One pinch **curry** powder

Optional:
Pinch of **salt**

• Sliver Salad

Key to this salad is to use a mandoline, or a food processor with the shreading blade. The last option would be to slice all very fine with a sharp chef's knife.

Shread:
One large or two medium-sized **carrots**
One 2" slice of a **daikon radish**
One **parsnip**
One **red bell pepper**
One **turnip**

Put all shreaded veggies into a large salad bowl.

Stir in:
One finely chopped **shallot**
Two finely chopped **scalions**
One palmful finely chopped **Italian parsley**
One cup chopped **lettuce** of your choice
One cup finely sliced **black kale**
One finely chopped rib of **celery**
One cup finely chopped **cucumber**
Handful of fresh **sunflower sprouts**

Toss in:
One tablespoon **dulse** flakes or powder
One tablespoon **millet**
Half a teaspoon **black pepper**
One-fourth cup **shreaded almonds**
Fresh squeezed juice of half a **lemon** (or one lime)
One tablespoon **hemp seed oil** (or no oil)

Serve chilled.

Optional:
If you prefer it to be sweet, add a couple of tablespoon of raw **honey**. Or, finely chip three or four **dates**, soak them in half a cup of water, then add these to the salad with a little bit of the soak water. Garnish with organically grown **edible flower**.

• Cucumber Salad

With a fork:
Take four medium-sized **cucumbers** and score them lengthwise with the fork, creating grooves. Some people like to peel the cucumbers. Some don't.

With a chef knife:

Cut cucumbers in halve lengthwise, then slice very thinly

Dice:
One peeled small to medium **red onion**
One-half cup **fresh dill**. If unable to obtain fresh dill, use about one-fourth cup dried dill.

Blend:
One-fourth cup **olive oil** (or less)
Juice from one **lemon**
One-fourth cup **apple vinegar**
Three peeled cloves of **garlic**
One teaspoon pink or **sea salt** (optional)

Place all together in a bowl, stir, chill.

Optional:
Top with a few cut olives and/or grapes.

• Avocado Peach Salad

From Houston's Rawfully Organic Co-op. RawfullyOrganic.com. KristinaBucaram.com; Kristina (at) RawFullyOrganic.com; FullyRaw.com.

Combine in a big bowl:
A variety of fresh greens, such as **romaine lettuce, kale, or swiss chard**, chopped
A small bunch of **spinach**, chopped
One-third to one-half of a ripe **avocado**, cut up
Cherry tomatoes or a cut up beefsteak tomato
One **orange**, pealed and cut up using sharp knife.
Herb of choice, such as **basil, Italian parsley, or cilantro**
Dressing:
In a blender, combine:
Three to four **peaches**
One-third to half of an **avocado**

Optional dressing ingredients:
One-third of a **bell pepper** and half a **mango**.

Pour the dressing onto the salad. Stir and serve.

• Stuffed Red Bell Peppers

From Anand Wells and Runi Burton of Australia's LiveFoodEducation.com

Soak in salty water for eight hours:
Four cups **pecans**

Soak in water for two hours:

One cup **sundried tomatoes**

Put in a food processor and pulse until consistency is not too smooth, but not too lumpy:
The two cups of soaked **pecans**
The one cup of dried **tomatoes**
One medium **carrot**, chopped into small pieces for easy processing
One medium **zucchini**, chopped into small pieces for easy processing
Two **dates**, pitted
One-half teaspoon celtic **salt** (optional)
Two tablespoons **chia seeds**
One tablespoon **lemon juice**
One clove of **garlic**

Optional:
One **chilli**

Slice in half (either through the middle or top to bottom) and scrape out the seeds:
Six red bell peppers (in Australia they are called *capsicums*)
Fill the bell peppers with the mixture from the food processor. You can eat them straight away or dehydrate them at 115 degrees Fahrenheit for four hours.

Serves six.

• Creamy Salad Dressing

In high-speed blender, combine:
One-fourth cup (or less) **pine nuts**
Three tablespoons **apple vinegar**
Juice from one-half **lemon**
Three-fourths cup **hemp seed oil** (or no oil)
Three peeled cloves **garlic**
Palm full of fresh **basil**, or slightly smaller amount of dry basil
Sprig of fresh **oregano**, or one teaspoon dry oregano
One teaspoon pink or sea **salt** (optional)

Chill.

This is nice over a salad of **spinach**, **grape tomatoes**, thin slices of **cucumber**, and some diced bits of **dandelion greens**. Garnish with a sprinkle **dill**, a dash of **nutritional yeast**, and some shredded **carrot**.

• Simple Dressing

From Julie Tolentino, a private chef in California. Julestolen (at) yahoo.com

This recipe can be made any time with just a few ingredients. No blender or food processor necessary.

In a bowl, whisk together:
One-fourth cup **lemon juice**
One-teaspoon **date paste or raw honey**
Pinch of sea **salt** (or no salt)
One-fourth cup (or less) of **olive oil** (or no oil, and use water)

Optional:
One teaspoon **balsamic vinegar**

The best thing about this dressing is you don't even have to measure out the ingredients after you have made it once. Simply add ingredients to a big bowl of mixed greens as you go. Amounts of each ingredient can vary depending on your taste buds. Simple enough to use on just about any green salad variation.

• Alfredo Salad Dressing

Soak in water for half a day:
One and a half cups raw **sunflower seeds**
One and a half cups **pine nuts** (pignolis)

When the seeds and nuts are done soaking, pour into a screen strainer or colander to strain them and then mildkly rinse under water.

Put the seeds and nuts into a blender, and combine with:
Juice of one large or two small **lemons**
Three or four cloves of **garlic**
Half a teaspoon of **black pepper**
Pinch of **kelp powder**
Enough **water** to get the consitency of thick salad dressing.
When done blending, pour into bowl and taste. If **salt** is desired, add salt and stir until desired taste is accomplished. Chill.

Optional:
Some people add a tablespoon of **nutritional yeast** to this mix.

• Sunfood Burgers

In a coffee grinder, grind together:
One cup raw, dehulled **sunflower seeds** (may have to do one-half cup first)
and a sprinkle of raw **pumpkin seeds**

Chop fine:
One **Roma tomato**, or other medium tomato
One handful of **broccoli**

One brown **onion**
Optional:
A palm full of chopped **red bell pepper** and/or **crimini mushrooms**
Blend until the consistency of breadcrumbs:
One-palm full of **walnuts or Brazil nuts**

Shred:
One **carrot**
Two **zucchini**
Stir the above together with:
One tablespoon **cumin**
One teaspoon **coriander**
One teaspoon **thyme**
One teaspoon **turmeric**
One-half teaspoon **wakame or dulse seaweed powder**
Optional:
You might also add a little **pink salt**, **cayenne pepper** [if you like hot spice], and **black pepper**.

Make palm-sized burgers. Place in dehydrator for 8 to 15 hours (depending on how firm you like the burgers).

While the burgers are dehydrating, make the topping.

Topping: in a small processor, blend all of these together:
One cup **pine nuts**
Three tablespoons **nutritional yeast**
One-half teaspoon **dill**
The juice from one half of a **lemon**
One-fourth teaspoon **pink salt** or a combination of salt and **dulse powder**. (or don't use either)

Chill the topping.

When the burgers are ready, spread the topping on top, and add a slice of **tomato**, some diced **avocado**, and wrap in a **collard green** with some **sprouts**.

Collard greens: Some people like to soften them by heating some water, then pouring the hot water over the collard green as it sits in a bowl. I prefer my collards full strength.

Nice to serve these with a salad.

• VEGGIE LOAF WITH GRAVY

Soak:
Three-fourths cup dehulled raw **sunflower seeds**

Three-fourths cup raw **walnuts**
Three-fourths cup raw **Brazil nuts or almonds**

Lightly grind in coffee grinder:
One fresh sprig, or one teaspoon dried **rosemary**
One tablespoon **thyme**
One teaspoon **sage**

Combine in Cuisinart the following into a crumb-like consistency:
The nuts and herb mix with:
One-fourth cup (or less) **olive oil or hemp oil** (or don't use oil and use water instead)
One-half teaspoon **dulse powder**
One teaspoon pink or sea **salt** (optional)
One-half teaspoon **black pepper**

Mince:
Two ribs of **celery**
One half **red bell pepper**
One fistful **Italian parsley**
One-half inch **ginger root**
Three cloves of **garlic**
Four **crimini mushrooms** (optional)

In a large bowl, hand mix together:
The nut/herb combination with the minced vegetables.

Form into two loafs on a platter. Serve chilled, OR place in dehydrator at 118 degrees for ten to fifteen hours.

Can also be served with:

• **GRAVY**

In a Cuisinart, combine:
One **burdock root**, chopped fine
One thumb-sized piece of a **brown onion**
One pitted **date**
Four tablespoons raw **tahini**
Three tablespoons (or less) either **olive, flax, or hemp oil**
A pinch of **dulse powder**
One-fourth teaspoon pink or sea **salt** (optional)
One-fourth teaspoon **black pepper**
A little **water** to make the gravy the consistency you desire

Optional:
One-third cup **dried shiitake mushroom powder**: made by putting shiitake mushroom in a coffee grinder or a high-speed blender.

• CauliRice

One half a head of a **cauliflower** (cut into bits)
One **tomato** (cut into fourths)
One half **red bell pepper** (cut into bits)
One cup fresh **parsley** (cut up)
One forth cup fresh **chives**
Place in food processor and process until the texture of couscous or brown rice. Can be served with grave and burger recipe above. Or wrap a scoop full in a Romain lettuce with slices of tomato and avocado.
Optional:
One or more of the following can be added: crumbled palm-full of raw **walnuts**; one tablespoon of **chili powder**; **currants**; diced **olives**: one-fourth cup diced **red onion**; tablespoon of raw **hemp seed oil** or palm full of fractured raw **hemp seeds**.

• Mashed Not Potatoes

Soak in water for half an hour:
One a a half cup **cashews**

Rinse the cashews.

Drain the cashews, and combine in a high-speed blender with:
One chopped **cauliflower**
One-fourth cup chopped **parsnips**
Two tablespoons **flaxseed or olive oil** (or no oil)
Juice of one **lemon**
One-fourth teaspoon **salt** (or dulse powder, of neither)

Use the blender tamper to keep tamping down the mixture until it is smooth.

If you don't have a high-speed blender, the ingredients can be put through a Champion juicer using the blank plate, then further blended in a standard kitchen blender or in a food processor until smooth.

Pur into serving bowl. Garnish with diced Italian parsley. Serve at room temperature, or chill.

Optional:
These may also be blended in:
One **crimini mushroom**
One thumb-sized slice of **brown onion**

• Marinated Mushrooms

This recipe can be made a day in advance.

In a bowl, mix together:
One-fourth cup (or less) **hemp seed oil or olive oil**

One tablespoon **coconut aminoes or ortganic wheat-free tamari** (or vinegar)
The juice from one half of a **lemon**
One-fourth cup minced Italian **parsley**
One minced **green onion**
One or two minced **garlic** cloves
One-half teaspoon **salt** (or dulse powder, or no salt)
One pinch **white pepper** powder
One pinch **kelp** powder

Using a spoon, scrape out the gills of:
Six **portobello mushrooms** with stems removed
Then cut each mushroom cap in half and thinly slice.

Put the slices of mushroom in the bowl of the marinara mixture. Mix so the mushroom slices are coated. Allow to marinate at room temperature for one to two hours. Then, cover and keep refrigerated.
Serve at room temperature.

These can be served inside a kale leave along with guacamole and wrapped. Also good with caulirice recipe below.

• MARINARA

In the morning, put three-fourths cup of chopped **sundried tomatoes** in water, and let them soak all day.

Combine in food processor until still slightly chunky:
The soaked **sundred tomatoes** (with water strained out)
Two ripe **tomatos**
One-half **red bell pepper**
One clove minced fresh **garlic**
One palm full of chopped fresh **basil**, or one tablespoon dried
One small palm full of chopped fresh **oregono**, or one teaspoon dried
Two or three pinches **black pepper**
One or two pinches **cayenne powder** (or more, depending on if you like spicey)
One-fourth teaspoon of either **salt or dulse powder**, depending on your taste. Or a little of both, or neither of either.
Two to three tablespoons (or less) organic, cold-pressed **olive oil or hemp seed oil** (or no oil)

Chill and serve over shredded **zucchini** (cut with a spiralizer) **or raw kelp noodles**

Note: Because of the herb taste opening up, this marinara may taste better on the second day: keep in fridge.

Optional:
Add one or two pitted, diced **olives** as the sauce is blending; three or four crubled **walnuts**; several **pine nuts** that have been soaked in water for one to ten hours. Also, while it is blending, add one-fourth teaspoon of one of these: **cumin, sage, or dill**. When it is ladeled over shredded zucchini, sprinkle some **nutritional yeast** and/or **sesame seeds** on top.

• No Bean Hummus

By Matt Amsden of RawVolution.
Access: rawvolution.com

In high-speed blender, combine until thick and smooth:
Two **zucchini**, peeled and chopped
Three-fourths cup raw **tahini**
One-half cup fresh **lemon juice**
One-fourth cup **olive oil**
Four cloves **garlic**, peeled
Two and a half teaspoons **sea salt** (optional)
One half tablespoon ground **cumin**

Chill.

You can use this hummus in the following recipe:

• Voona Salad

This is a good salad to bring to dinner parties.

In a big bowl, toss in:
Palm full of **sunflower seeds**
Palm full of fractured **cashews**
Palm full of fractured **walnuts**
One bunch of **chard**, chopped fine
One bunch of **spinach**, chopped fine
Two ribs of **celery**, chopped fine
One small **red bell pepper**, chopped fine
One small **orange bell pepper**, chopped fine
One half **red onion**, diced
One or two **Roma tomatoes**, chopped fine
One ripe **avocado**, cut into small cubes
Handful of **cranberries**
Dash of **black pepper**
One teaspoon (or less) of pink or sea **salt** (optional)
One tablespoon **thyme**
Dash or three of **cayenne pepper**
One-half teaspoon **dulse powder**
One teaspoon **dill**

Sprinkle of uncooked, raw **millet**
Two or three teaspoons of **grape seed oil or olive oil** (or no oil)
One-half cup (or a little more) of **raw hummus** from previous recipe.

After tossing together, chill before serving.

• Kale Salad

Toss in a big salad bowl:
Two bunches of **kale**, finely chopped
Two **Roma tomatoes**, sliced to bits
Several raw **walnuts**, fractured
Eight **green olives**, diced
One-fourth to one-half **red onion**, diced
One-fourth to one-half **red bell pepper**, diced
Two **apples**, diced (black Arkansas or apples of your choice)
A palm-full of **raisins or cranberries or black currants**
One-half cup of **nutritional yeast** (optional)
A tablespoon or two of raw, unheated **millet** seeds
A tablespoon or two of raw **sesame seeds**
A tablespoon or two of raw **hemp seeds**
One teaspoon **probiotic powder**
One tablespoon **thyme**
One teaspoon **dill**
A couple of dashes of **cayenne powder**
Two tablespoons **spirulina powder**

Dressing:
In a Cuisinart, combine:
Four **dates**
Two or three tablespoons of **stone ground or Dijon** mustard
Juice of one-half **lemon** (or more)
Two tablespoons **vinegar**
Two tablespoons (or less) **hemp oil or flax oil** (or no oil)
One tablespoon **water**

Toss together. Chill.

Optional: Blueberries. **Mandarin orance** slices. Diced **pear**. Shreded **beet**. Diced **mango**. Diced **parsley**. Diced **cilantro**. Tablespoon of raw **fennel**. Palm full of raw **pumpkin seeds**. Palm full of **hemp seeds**.

• Hemp Seed Tabouli

In a large bowl, stir together:
Three bunches Italian **parsley**, finely chopped
One-third cup **hemp seeds**
Several cherry or **grape tomatoes** cut n half

One-fourth cup **brown onion**, finely chopped
Two or three (or less) tablespoons **hemp seed oil** (or no oil)
Juice of one **lemon**
One-fourth teaspoon pink or **sea salt** (optional)

Optional:
One teaspoon dill. One tablespoon unheated, raw millet. Diced red bell pepper.

Chill.

• RAW CURRY FALAFEL

From Xam Devesh of the Xammin' UnBakery. Xammin.blogspot.com

In large bowl, stir together:
One and a half cups **flax seeds**
One and a half cups **sunflower seeds**
One and a half tablespoon **turmeric root powder**
One teaspoon whole **cumin seeds**
Two teaspoons **paprika**
One tablespoon **red pepper flakes**
One teaspoon **cayenne powder**
Two teaspoons **tarragon leaves**
Two teaspoons ground **mustard seed**

Then add wet ingredients, and stir all together:
Two tablespoons **tamari** (Ohsawa brand ortganic unpasteurized wheat-free tamari)
Two tablespoons cold-pressed **olive oil**
One-half cup **water**

Patt into six falafels. Place on **dehydrator** trays. Dehydrate for three hours about 105 degrees F. Then flip, and dehydrate another three hours.

• XAM'S HUMMUS

In Cuisinart, grind togther:
One and a half cups **sunflower seeds**
One and a half cups **cashews**

Put ground sunflower seeds/cashew mix into high-speed blender, and add:
Two tablespoons **tamari** (Ohsawa brand ortganic unpasteurized wheat-free tamari)
One tablespoon **turmeric root powder**
One teaspoon **cayenne**
Two tablespoons **nutritional yeast** (optional)

One teaspoon **terragon**
One teaspoon **cumin seeds**
One crushed clove of **garlic**
One tablespoon cold pressed **olive oil**
About one cup **water** (and maybe a little more while blending).

Blend until consistency is smooth.

Top falafels with hummus. Serve on plante with side of more hummus along with slices of **cucumbers** and **carrots** and a salad.

• Cabbage Pumpkin Seed Paté

Soak for 2 hours, and then drain:
One cup **pumpkin seeds**

In food processor, mix the pumpkin seeds with all of the following:
One-fourth chopped head of **cabbage**
One-half cup **water**
One tablespoon **herbs de province**
One teaspoon **marjoram**
One-half teaspoon **cumin**
One-half teaspoon **paprika**
One stalk fresh **rosemary** (or 1 tablespoon dried)
One-half teaspoon **lemon thyme**
One-eighth teaspoon **cayenne**
Pinch of **sea salt**
Place all ingredients in food processor with s-blade attached. Process until smooth. Serve with **flax crackers** and/or **cucumber sticks.**

• Zucchini Chips

Slice zucchini thinly. Placein a dehydrator set to about 105 degrees until dry. Use with dips, paté, and guacamole.

The same can be done with carrots, summer squash, pears, and apples.

• Vegetable Paté

One-third cup **pumpkin seeds**
Seven **walnuts**
One small **zucchini**, chopped
One-fourth cup **brown onion**, chopped
One-third of a **red bell pepper**, chopped
Juice of one **lemon**
Two or three **garlic** cloves
Two tablespoons **dulse powder**
One tablespoon **kelp powder**

Three to four tablespoons **nutritional yeast**
Cherry-sized piece of **ginger root**, diced
One medium **carrot**, chopped
One-fourth teaspoon **black pepper**
Dash of **dark vinegar**

Combine all ingredients in Cuisinart. Use as spread on dehydrated veggie pulp or seed crackers.

Optional:
Some people use a couple tablespoons of Nama Shoyu in this recipe. I don't. You can add coconut aminoes, which is a healthier alternative.

• Mexican Paté

Combine all in a Cuisinart:
Juice from half a **lemon**
One-fourth cup freshly ground (in coffee grinder) **pumpkin seeds**
One-fourth cup freshly ground (in coffee grinder) **flax seeds**
One **carrot**, chopped
One-fourth **tomato**
One-fourth of a **green pepper**, chopped
Three cloves **garlic**, crushed and diced
6 raw **walnuts**
6 raw **Brazil nuts** (or 6 more walnuts)
Two tablespoons (or less) **hemp oil** (or no oil)
One-fourth teaspoon **black pepper**
One-half teaspoon **salt** (optional)
Four tablespoons **cumin**
Two tablespoons **chili pepper powder**
Serve chilled.

For rawduerves, serve on slices of **tomato** or raw **seed crackers**. Top with **avocado** and a bit of **sprouts**.

Optional:
Two tablespoons **carob powder**
If you like cilantro, instead of using a carrot, use an entire bunch of **cilantro**, including the stems. You might also add four pitted green **olives**, a dash of **vinegar**, and a small piece of a **carrot**.

• Pumpkin Soup

From Maya Melamed of Taste Organic raw café in Sydney, Australia. ChangingMaya.com.au.

In a high-speed blender, combine:
Two cups fresh cubed **kabocha pumpkin**

One-half cup of warm **water**
One cup **water of young Thai coconut**
One-fourth cup **flesh of young Thai coconut**
Theree tablespoons of chopped fresh **cilantro** (leaves only)
One-fouth teaspoon dried **ginger**
Cayenne pepper to taste

After blending:
Pour into bowls and sprinkle with **cinnamon**.

Optional:
Sea salt to taste.

• Catch A Healthy Habit Spinach Soup

By Glen Colello and Lisa Storch of Catch A Healthy Habit restaurant in Fairfield, Connecticut; CatchAHealthyHabit.com

Serves three or four.

In a high-speed blender, combine:
One cup fresh **spinach**
One-half to one whole **cucumber** depending on the size
One to two **tomatoes** depending on the size
One-fourth cup pure "flouride free" **water**
One **avacodo**, peeled and pitted
Two tablespoons **coconut aminos**
Pince of **cayenne pepper**
One tablespoon fresh **lemon juice**
One tablespoon cold-pressed, raw olive oil

Chill and enjoy.

• Chilled Tomato Soup with Avocado Salsa

From Helen Castillo of TheRawPalate.com

With garden-fresh tomatoes in season, this quick and easy-to-make chilled soup with only five main ingredients is as comforting as Mom's, but made robust and lively with its garnish of avocado salsa that packs a punch of flavor in this savory dish.

In food processor, pulse the following until a puree:
Six large, juicy **tomatoes**, stemmed, seeded and cut into large chunks
Three Tablespoons **olive oil**
Two Tablespoons **shallot**, finely diced
Three Tablespoons fresh **lime juice**
Three-fourths teaspoon **Celtic sea salt** (optional)

In a serving bowl, toss until well combined:

One-half ripe, firm **Haas avocado**, peeled, pitted and diced
Two teaspoons finely diced **shallot**
Two teaspoons chopped fresh **cilantro**
Two teaspoons **olive oil**
Two Tablespoons fresh **lime juice**
Himalayan salt to taste (optional)

Transfer the soup from the food processor to salad bowls. Top with garnish.

Serves Two.

• Tomato Soup

In high-speed blender, combine:
Three cups **tomatoes**
Two or three stalks **celery**
One-half of a peeled **lemon**
One minced clove of **garlic**
One-half bunch of chopped **cilantro**

Chill and serve in bowls. Sprinkle with diced fresh **cilantro** or **dill** leaf. This could go well with some of the crackers in the following recipe.

Optional:
If you like your soup sweet, have it as it is. For a spicier soup, while it is blending, add half a diced fresh **hot peper**. You can also add some **chili powder**. If you don't stay away from salt, add some pinches of **salt**, or powdered **dulse**.

• Cream of Broccoli Soup

From Theresa Webb of Kitchen Buddy in England. Theresa (at) KitchenBuddy.eu.

This is a great way to use fresh broccoli and is often liked by those who don't like cooked broccoli.

In a high-speed blender, combine until a milk-like quality:
One handful **hemp seeds**
One cup **water**

Add in, and blend until smooth:
Two cups chopped broccoli
One cup chopped **cucumber**
One cup of chopped **celery** or **fennel**

Add in, and blend until fully combined:
One peeled and pitted **avocado**

Two teaspoons ground **flax seeds** (ground in a coffee grinder)

Optional:

Seaweed powder, such as **dulse**, to taste.
One half a chopped **bell pepper**, or one **tomato**, blended in with other ingredients. The tomato or bell pepper may also be diced, and then sprinkled on top of soup as it is in the bowl, as a garnish.

For a thinner soup, add extra water, or for a thicker soup, add extra avocado.

Optional recipe:

This soup can also be used to make **cabbage** or **spinach** soup, instead of broccoli.
Some cabbage or spinach can also be added to the broccoli soup as it is being belended.

• Carrot Soup

Juice:

Enough **carrots** to make one-and-a-half-cups juice
Keep about one cup of the carrot pulp

Juice:

Enough **celery** to make one-and-aphalf-cups juice

Dice:

A palm full of fesh **dill** (or use one tablespoon dried dill)
Two **Romain tomatoes**, or enough of your favorite tomatoes to make a cup of diced tomatoes
One-fourth of a **red bell pepper**
Three inches of a **cucumber**
The flesh of one ripe **avocado**

In a blender, combine:

The carrot juice, celery juice, dill, and avocado.

Pour:

The blender mixture into a large bowl.

Stir in:

The tomatoes, bell pepper, cucumber, and carrot pulp.
Serve chilled. Garnish with a dash of sesame seeds and/or milliet.

Optional:

One-half teaspoon **dulse powder**. Blend in with the liquids.

• Dehydrated Crackers

If you have been around raw food enough, you have likely seen a variety of dehydrated, non-baked crackers. There are as many recipes for these as there are dehydrators in the kitchens that make them.

Step one:
If you have a Champion Juicer, you can take the pulp left over from making half a gallon of vegetable juice, and, using your hands, combine the veggie pulp two cups of flax seeds, a cup of raw pumpkin seeds, a cup of dill, and then let this sit for an hour. If you have to go out, put this in the fridge for up to a day. Letting this seed and pulp mixture sit for a day in the fridge will help the seeds enliving, producing nutritious enzymes and increasing their content of beneficial omega oils.

Step two:
Take the mixture of pulp/flax seeds/pumpkin seeds/dill, and use your hands to mix in a half a cup of raw olive or hemp oil and two tablespoons of pink or sea salt (or no salt, if you are aoiding salt). You may also add a tablespoon of dulse powder. Or, don't use the oil or salt.

Step three:
Spread the mixture approximately one-fourth-inch thick on the dehydrator sheets. Dehydrate them at about 110 degrees for 8 or more hours. How long they take to dry into crackers will be determined by the humidity in the atmosphere, the temperature of the room, and the moisture in the pulp. It may take 8 hours, or it may take 20 hours. As you get used to making crackers, you will be able to determine how long it will take to dry them.

Simple flax seed crackers:
Another version of raw, dehydrated crackers may also only contain three ingredients: Five cups of flax seeds that have been soaked in water for a few hours and drained, and then mixed with a cup of dill weed, a tablespoon of dulse powder and/or salt (or no salt, if you are avoiding salt), and a dash of cayenne pepper. Spread out thinly (about one-fourth-inch thick) on dehydrator sheets and dehydrate at about 115 degrees for about 7 to 10 hours.

Simple flax seed crackers, 2nd recipe:
Another recipe for crackers involves combining four carrots in a food processor with one teaspoon salt (or no salt, if you are avoiding salt), one-half teaspoon black pepper, and a dash of cayenne. Then putting this mixture in a bowl and stirring in 3 cups of soaked flax seeds. Spread out about one-fourth-inch thick on dehydrator sheets and dehydrate at about 110 to 115 degrees for 8 to 12 hours. An option with this is to add the flax in with the carrots, black pepper, and dash of cayenne, and also blend in one cup of firmly packed spinach. When you dry this on a dehydrator, it will be more like green tortilla chips, especially if you increase the cayenne, and maybe add a tablespoon of cumin.

Look at various raw recipe books and see what they have in their crackers. You will get your own ideas, and develop your own cracker recipes. Or, like me, you may never pay attention to cracker recipes, and make them different almost every time.

• FRESH TOMATO SALSA

From Matt Amsden of RawVolution
Access: RawVolution.com

In a mixing bowl, stir together:
Two cups chopped **tomatoes**
Three-fourth cup chopped **cilantro**
One-half cup chopped **yellow onions or scallions**
Two tablespoons fresh **lemon or lime juice**
One tablespoon **olive oil**
Four cloves **garlic**, minced
One-fourth teaspoon **cayenne powder**
Three-fourths teaspoon (or less) **sea salt**
One and one-half teaspoon ground **cumin**
Three-fourth teaspoon ground **coriander**

• CHILLED TOMATO SOUP WITH AVOCADO SALSA

From Helen Castillo of TheRawPalate.com

With garden-fresh tomatoes in season, this quick and easy-to-make chilled soup with only five main ingredients is as comforting as Mom's, but made robust and lively with its garnish of avocado salsa that packs a punch of flavor in this savory dish.

In food processor, pulse the following until a puree:
Six large, juicy **tomatoes**, stemmed, seeded and cut into large chunks
Three Tablespoons **olive oil**
Two Tablespoons **shallot**, finely diced
Three Tablespoons fresh **lime juice**
Three-fourths teaspoon **Celtic sea salt** (optional)

In a serving bowl, toss until well combined:
One-half ripe, firm Haas avocado, peeled, pitted and diced
Two teaspoons finely diced shallot
Two teaspoons chopped fresh cilantro
Two teaspoons olive oil
Two Tablespoons fresh lime juice
Himalayan salt to taste (optional)

Transfer the soup from the food processor to salad bowls. Top with garnish.

Serves Two.

• Pine Nut Spread

Some people call this "cheese spread."

Soak:
One and a half cups **pine nuts** for one hour, or for up to a day, then drain water.

Combine in Cuisinart:
The soaked **pine nuts**
Juice of one **lemon**
Three tablespoons **nutritional yeast**
Two tablespoons **dill**
4 raw **walnuts**
One-half teaspoon (or less) **salt** (optional)
One teaspoon **pro-biotic powder** (optional)

Optional:
If you want it spicy, add a dash or two of **cayenne powder**, or **chili powder.**

This can be used as a spread on seed or veggie pulp **crackers**, or on sliced **carrots.**

To make a **collard green burrito**: On a collard leaf, spread some of this pine cheese with **avocado**, **sprouts**, **walnuts**, and a dash of **salt** and/or dash of **dulse powder**. You might also add some of the Mexican Paté from the previous recipe.

• Naise Spread

This is one raw vegan version of mayonnaise.

Soak in water for one to three hours, then drain:
One cup raw cashews

In a high-speed blender, combine:
The soaked **cashews**
One or two pitted **dates**
Juice of one **lemon**
A thumb-sized slice of **brown onion**
One peeled clove of **garlic**
Two tablespoons (or less) **hemp oil** (or no oil)
Two tablespoons (or less) **olive or flax oil** (or no oil)
One pinch of **white pepper**
One pinch **dulse powder**
One teaspoon (or less) pink or **sea salt** (optional)
A little **water**, just enough to make the naise the consistency you desire.

Chill.

• Sundried Tomato Butter

From Anand and Runi of Raw Power Australia, LiveFoodEducation.com

In a high speed blender, blend into almost a powder:
Eight **sun-dried tomatoes**
Add the rest of the ingredients, and blend until smooth, using the tamper to fully blend all ingredients.
One large **avocado** (large)
One tablespoon **tamari**
One-half clove of **garlic** (optional)
Two teaspoons **parsley** (optional)

This is a yummy vegan butter alternative and is delicious on flax crackers and raw breads. Alternatively, you can use it any savoury recipe where you'd normally use butter.

• Matboukha

By Maya Melamed of ChangingMaya.com.au, in Sydney, Australia. Moroccan style red capsicum relish.

In a Cuisinart or food processor, combine the following until completely smooth:
One and a half cups **sun dried tomatoes**
One cup seeded chopped **tomatoes**
One-half red hot **chili pepper**
One-eighth teaspoon **cayenne pepper**
One-fourth teaspoon sweet **paprika**
One teaspoon **garlic powder**
One-fourth cup **olive oil**

Dice:
Two **red bell peppers**, chopped
One-half **green bell pepper**, chopped

Place in serving bowl and combine the diced bell peppers with the other ingredients. Chill.

Serve with dehydrated veggie and/or seed **crackers**, coin slices of **cucumber**, and two-inch long slices of **celery** for dipping.

• Simple Nut Milk

Some people spell it *mylk* when they are referring to non-dairy drink.

Some people like to soak the seeds or nuts for several hours in water first.

In a high-speed blender, combine:
Six pitted **dates**
One cup of your choice: **hemp seeds or almonds** (or some of both)
One teaspoon **vanilla** (or seeds from one vanilla bean)
Pinch of **dulse seaweed powder**
Enough **water** to make the milk the consistency you desire.
Chill.

Optional:
Instead of hemp seeds or almonds, you can use raw **hazelnuts**.
Instead of water, use the **water from a coconut** or two.
Add a **banana** or **berries**. Or some **chia** seeds to make it creamy.

• Holiday Nog

Rinse in water, than soak in water for half a day:
Four cups **Brazil nuts**
Then rinse a second time.

Soak in water for half a day:
Twentyfive to thirty pitted **dates**
Four **vanilla beans**, slit open and cut into small pieces

Combine in high-speed blender:
The soaked **Brazil nuts**
The soaked **dates** and **vanilla beans**
One-half of a ripe **banana**
One teaspoon **nutmeg**
One teaspoon ground **cinnamon**
Enough **water** to make it into a creamy liquid consitency – about eight cups of water – and more if you want it to be thinner.

After blending, you can either strain it by placing a nutmilk bag or cheesecloth into a large bowl and pouring the contents of the blender container into the bag or cloth and straining out the pulp, or you can serve it unstrained.

Chill.

This can be made a day ahead of time to allow the nutmeg, cinnamon, and vanilla flavoring take hold.

Optional:
One tablespoon raw **tahini**

• Banana Nut Smoothie

From Julie Tolentino, a private chef in California. Julestolen (at) yahoo.com

For this recipe, you can use the nut milk from the previous recipe.

In a high-speed blender, combine until creamy and smooth:
Two cups of **almond milk** (or any variety of nut milk, hazelnut, cashew, hemp milk works as well too)
Two frozen **bananas**
One-half cup of fresh or frozen **mango**
Two or three large **kale** leaves
Two tablespoons raw **hemp** powder
One tablespoon **almond butter or tahini**
One teaspoon **maple syrup, or raw honey, or half a date**
One-half teaspoon **vanilla**
If you want it to have crunchies, after you are done blending, add one of the following, and blend for a few seconds:
One-fourth cup **cacao nibs**
Or, one-half cup fractured **walnuts**

Pour into tall glasses or wine glasses and garnish with a scattering of: cacao nibs or powder, **hemp seeds**, **coconut shreds**, and a sprinkle of **cinnamon**.

A delicious treat or meal. I make this smoothie very thick and creamy. Feel free to add more or less of any ingredient to suit your palate.

Serves 2-4 depending on serving size

• BRAZIL HEMP MILK

Soak for several hours, then drain:
12 raw **Brazil nuts** - about 12, raw, NOT toasted or roasted - soaked for several hours, and rinsed.
In high-speed blender, combine:
12 soaked **Brazil nuts**
One ripe **banana**
Pinch of **cinnamon**
Two tablespoons **vanilla**
One teaspoon raw **tahini**
Pinch of pink or sea **salt** (optional)
Pinch of **dulse powder**
Four dates
Two tablespoons **hemp seed powder**
Pour in enough **water** to fill container halfway

Blend on high. Chill.

Optional:
Two or three tablespoons **raw carob powder**
One-half teaspoon **nutmeg or cinnamon**
Berries

• Chia Seed Pudding

From Vicki Veranese of Alchemia Luquid Nutrition Restaurant in Byron Bay, Australia. Alchemialiquicnutrition.com.

High in omega 3 and a great source of soluable fibre.

In bowl, gently mix together, and soak for one to three hours:
One cup of chia seeds (black or white)
One quart of fresh **juice of choice**, we use freshly squeezed organic **pineapple** and **apple**
The seeds of two **vanilla pods**
Combine in a blender:
Two **bananas**
One ripe **mango**
Tiny squeeze of **lemon**
Topping
Fresh **passionfruit**
Shredded **coconut**
Goji berries

Take your desired container, if entertaining perhaps a decorative glass, and begin to layer the chia seed mixture and the topping, when full. Sprinkle the topping on.

• Fig Berry Desert

From Julie Tolentino

Take a handful of organic dried **figs** (three or four per serving). Dried figs can be found all year round. Stay away from sulfite dried figs.

Cut off the stems, leaving a small hole around the top. Take one or two halved **pecans** and insert into the hole. Push pecan gently as far as you can inside.

Puree any berry (six berries), preferrably **strawberries or rasberries** with juice from one-half of a squeezed **orange**. Puree in mini food processor or blender.

Spoon and swirl berry puree onto light colored desert plate. Place fig newtons on the swirl of berry, top with **coconut shreds** or **cinnamon**.

• Cantaloupe Mint Sorbet

From Kristina Carillo-Bucaram of RawfullyOrganic.com and FullyRaw.com

Fully ripen:
One or more cantaloupes (if you eat enough, this can be eaten as a full meal). Wait until your cantaloupe properly ripens. If you wait until it is soft at the stem end, and smells potent, it will be significantly sweeter!

Cut:
The skin off the **cantaloupe**, getting close to the edge to prevent waste. Cut the cantaloupe into chunks.

Freeze:
The canteloupe in a bag or sealed container.

Combine in a food processor:
Frozen canteloupe chunks
A few **sprigs of mint**
Blueberries (optional)

Scoop:
The whipped sorbet into serving bowl(s), and top with mint sprigs.

Enjoy this sweet treat! Best if savored in the sun!

• Carob Crumble

From Theresa Webb of Kitchen Buddy in England. Theresa (at) KitchenBuddy.eu.

In food processor, combine until mixture resembles crumbs:
One cup **walnuts**
One cup **dates**
One-forth cup **carob powder**
One teaspoon **Lacuma powder**

Serving suggestions:
For breakfast, combine some carob crumble with nut or seed milk (such as **almond milk**) and fresh **coconut** and chopped **Brazil nuts**.

Use as a crumble topping to a seasonal **fruit pie** or a **pudding**, such as pureed apple or plums.

• Strawberry-banana Dessert

In bowl, stir well with a spoon:
Four tablespoons raw **tahini**
Four tablespoons raw **honey** (or don't use any)
One teaspoon **vanilla**
Two tablespoons raw **sunflower seeds**
One-fourth cup raw **buckwheat**

Cut in small pieces:
Two cups **strawberries**

Put the strawberry pieces in the bowl with the tahini, honey, vanilla, sunflower seed, buckwheat mixture. Stir together until strawberries are mosly coated with the other ingredients.

In a small food processor, blend:
The juice from one-half of a **lemon**

Six or seven pitted **dates**
One or two **strawberries**
Two tablespoons **water**

On four dessert serving saucers:
Slice two **bananas** into coins, placing an equal amount of banana slices on each plate. Top the bananas with spoonfuls of the strawberry mix. Drizzle a little of the date sauce over each platter of the strawberry-topped bananas.

Serve fresh or chilled. Four servings.

• Lemon Pudding

In a blender or food processor, combine:
Two pealed **lemons**
About one-cup pitted **dates**
The meat of one **avocado**

This can be poured into dessert cups and topped with **fresh berries** and a sprinkle of **buckwheat**.

• Apple Cobbler

In a bowl mix:
Two cored **apples** diced or cut into small cubes. (Don't peel them.)
One cup **raw oatmeal** (not heated)
Lemon juice from one-half of a lemon
Full tablespoon of raw **tahini**
Heaping tablespoon **lucuma powder**.
One tablespoon **vanilla** (more if you like)
Big pinch of **nutmeg**
Big pinch of **cinnamon**
One teaspoon **bee pollen** (unless you don't eat bee products)
A tablespoon or more of **water**

Optional (one or more of the following):
A little **maple syrup** or honey (or rely on the sweetness from the apple and lucuma powder).
Two tablespoons **buckwheat**.
One or more of the following: Several sliced **cherries**. A palmfull of **raisins**. Several fractured raw **walnuts** or slivered raw **almonds**. A palmfull of **blueberries**. One tablespoon **sunflower seeds**. One tablespoon or more of **buckwheat seeds**.
Pinch of pink or other natural, unprocessed, unheated **salt** (optional).

Stir well with a spoon until the moister of the water, lemon juice, vanilla, and tahini moistens the lucuma powder.

Put in pie crust, or in four desert cups. Chill.

Also, you can put this in a breakfast bowls and chill overnight to have for breakfast.

• PIE CRUST

Process in a Cuisinart
About one-half cup of raw **coconut meat**
Then add the rest of the ingredients to the Cuisinart:
Four **dates**
Three tablespoons **sunflower seeds**
One-half cup raw, uncooked **oats**
One-half teaspoon **cinnamon**
One-fourth teaspoon **nutmeg**
One-half teaspoon (or less) pink or sea **salt** (optional)
One tablespoon **vanilla**
One teaspoon raw **tahini** and …
Three tablespoons **sesame seeds**
Six raw **walnuts**
Eight raw **macadamia nuts**
Two tablespoons raw **carob powder**
Water (very little - minimal - just enough to make the crust stick)

After processing in the Cuisinart, press into glass pie pan and chill.

Fill with your favorite chocolate/carob pudding/mousse, or use as a crust for cheesecake, or raw fruit pie filling.

• FRUIT PIE CRUST

In a Cuisinart, combine:
One-half cup of your choice, raw **macadamia nuts or pecans**
One-half cup raw **walnuts**
Five large dates, or seven or eight small **dates**, pitted
One-half teaspoon **cinnamon**

Optional:
Pinch of **nutmeg and/or** pinch or **cloves**

Combine until all ingredients are well mixed.
Press into a glass pie pan and chill.

Fill with your choice of thin slices of fruit, such as bananas, peaches, pears, apples, and berries.

You can also make a **berry sauce** to drizzle all over the top by blending:
Half a cup of **berries** (either blueberries, strawberries, raspberries, blackberries)

Flesh of one half of a ripe **mango**
A squeeze of one half of an **orange**
Optional for berry sauce:
One **plum**, pinch of **cinnamon**, tablespoon **Yacon root syrup**, or tablespoon **maple syrup**

• Fruit Pie Filling

Core (apples or pears) or pit (peaches) and then thinly slice:
Three **apples or** ripe **peaches or** ripe **pears**

Stir together in a big bowl:
The sliced fruit
An even teaspoon of **cinnamon** (some people like a little more cinnamon)
A small pinch of **cloves**
A pinch of **nutmeg**
Lemon juice from one-fourth of a lemon
Orange juice from one-fourth of a lemon
One tablespoon mesquite **powder**

Optional:
Tablespoon of **maple syrup**
Sprinkling of **sesame seeds**
Top with thin slices of **banana** or **strawberries**

Pour into raw pie crust (from above recipe). Chill.

• Carob Sauce

In a Cuisinart, combine:
One-half cup (or less) raw organic **coconut oil**
One-half cup raw **carob powder** (or raw cacao powder [I prefer carob])
One-fourth cup **maple syrup, or five soaked dates**
One teaspoon raw **tahini**
One tablespoon **lucuma** powder
One tablespoon **mesquite** powder
One dash of **cinnamon**
One tablespoon **vanilla**
One pinch of **salt** (optional)

• Raw Ice Cream

Peel and freeze ripe **bananas** (bananas with freckles) the day before.

Place empty serving bowls in freezer.

In a high-speed blender, combine:
Frozen, peeled bananas – two per person you are serving

One-fourth teaspoon **vanilla** per banana
Blueberries or strawberries

Optional:
Bananas should provide enough sweetness. But, some people add a little raw **honey or yacon root syrup**. Some people also add nuts into the blender, such as **cashews** or **Brazil** nuts. I don't. Also, some people blend in: half teaspoon of **sesame tahini** per banana. Pinch of **salt** or **kelp**.
Put into ice-cold bowls. Eat the raw ice cream right away. It melts fast.

• Simple Carob Truffles

In Cuisinart, combine:
One cup raw **nuts** (**almonds or pecans** – or a mix of both)
One cup **raisins** or chopped dates (or a mix of both0
One-third cup **shredded coconut**
Three or four tablespoons raw **carob powder** (**or cacao powder** – or a mix of both)
Three tablespoons raw **hemp seeds**
Teaspoon raw **sesame seeds**
One-half teaspoon **vanilla**
Pinch of **cinnamon**

Process together until all is combined very well. Should start to form into a big ball. If needed, add one half-teaspoon of **water** as it is processing to help it stick together. Stop, form into cherry-sized balls.

Chill.

Optional:
If you like the taste of citrus with carob (or chocolate), add one half-teaspoon **orange juice** while the truffle mixture is being processed, instead of water.

If you want to make them fancy, roll the balls in either **shredded coconut**, or fractured **nuts** (such as **macadamia**), or **goji crumbles** (in coffee grinder, blend a heaping tablespoon of dried goji berries until crumbled). You can also roll them in **carob powder**.
Serve as a desert on a small plate with a few truffles, a few berries, and a piece of fruit.

• Liver Cleanse Smoothie

From Victoria Boutenko, author of *The Green Smoothie Revolution*.
Access: RawFamily.com

In a high-speed blender, combine:
Four cups fresh **dandelion greens**

One-half head **endive**
Two cups **cilantro**
Two cups **apple juice**
One **banana**
Two **pears**
One-inch fresh **ginger root**
One cup **cranberries**

Yields 2 quarts.

• STRAWBERRY-PEACH SMOOTHIE

From Cherie Soria, author of *The Raw Food Revolution Diet*
Access: RawFoodChef.com

In high-speed blender, combine:
Two cups coarsely chopped ripe **peaches or nectarines**
Two cups fresh or frozen **strawberries**
Two peeled **oranges** coarsely chopped
One cup coarsely chopped **kale or romaine lettuce**, firmly packed
Enough **water** to give it the consistency you desire

Optional:
Two tablespoons **green powder** supplement (such as Infinity Greens)

• BASIC GREEN SMOOTHIE

For more green smoothie recipes, see Victoria Boutenko's book, *The Green Smoothie Revolution*. RawFamily.com.

In a high-speed blender, combine:
Eight leaves **Romaine lettuce**
Eight leaves **spinach**
Two **bananas**
One pinch of **dulse powder**
Enough **water** to make it the consistency you desire.

Optional:
Use **chard** or **kale** instead of lettuce or spinach. **Mango** instead of banana. One **apple**, or **berries**. One-teaspoon **spirulina powder** or **green supplement powder**. One or two **dates**. One tablespoon **hemp powder**.

• WARMING SAVOURY GREEN SMOOTHIE

From Anand Wells of LiveFoodEducation.com

In a high-speed blender, combine:
Two or three **tomatoes**
One **celery** rib (cut up to make easier to blend)

One-half of a **cucumber**
Several leaves of leafy greens: **kale, spinach, lettuce, or bok choy**
Half a cup of fresh herbs: **parsley, basil, coriander, or dill**
Half of a **lime or lemon**
Palm full of **dulse**
One teaspoon of **kelp** powder
One-forth of an **avocado**
One cup of **water** (or more if you like)
One **chili**
A bit of a **ginger root**, sliced to make it easier to blend
One teaspoon **blue green algae**

Pour into two glasses. Sprinkle with **spirulina.**

• TURQUOISE BARN GREEN SMOOTHIE

From Michelle Premura of upstate New York's Turquoise Barn retreat. TurquoiseBarn.com.

In a high-speed blender, combine:
One bunch of **Italian parsley**
Two cups **lambsquarters or spinach**
Three cups frozen **mango**
One cup fresh **spring water**
Add more water to adjust desired consistency.
Optional:
One teaspoon **bee pollen.**
Pour in glass and sprinkle with **bee pollen.**

• WINTER GREEN SMOOTHIE

From Victoria Boutenko, author of *The Green Smoothie Revolution.*
Access: RawFamily.com

In a high-speed blender, combine:
One cup organic frozen **berries** (any kind)
Two cups fresh **spinach** greens
Two cups **water**
One-fourth-inch fresh **ginger root**, or to taste

Decorate with a **slice of fruit.**

Yields: One quart.

• MANGO ORANGE SPINACH SMOOTHIE

From The Rawfully Organic Co-op, Texas. RawfullyOrganic.com; KristinaBucaram.com; Kristina (at) RawFullyOrganic.com; FullyRaw.com.

In a high-speed blender, combine:
One **mango**
Three to four peeled **oranges**
Large handful of **spinach** or **lettuce**
Optional:
For a kick, add either **strawberries** or **pineapple**.

• SPIRULINA SMOOTHIE

In a high-speed blender, combine:
Two frozen **bananas**
Several frozen **strawberries** (include the leaves)
Coconut water from one coconut
Coconut meat from one coconut
One tablespoon **vanilla**
One tablespoon **tahini**
Three tablespoons raw **carob powder**
Three tablespoons **mesquite powder**
One tablespoon **spirulina powder**

• GREEN POWER MORNING JUICE

By Chef Cristina Gonzalez of La Vie En Raw Café, Coral Gables, Florida; lavieenrawcafe.com.

In a high-speed blender, combine:
One cup chopped **apple**
One handful **sunflower sprouts**
Two tablespoons **coconut oil**
One tablespoon **spirulina**
Two teaspoons freshly minced **ginger root**
Four fresh **mint leaves**
Six **figs**
One-half of a chipped **cucumber**
One-half rib of chopped **celery**
One and one-half cups **water**
One pinch Celtic **sea salt** (optional)

• BLUE GREEN SMOOTHIE

In a high-speed blender, combine:
Two cups **water**
Four **pitted dates**
One **banana**
Several leaves of **kale**
Tablespoon **hemp powder**
Tablespoon freshly ground **flax seeds or chia seeds**

One-forth cup **blueberries**
Half-teaspoon **dulse powder** (or exclude)
One pinch **cinnamon**

• RUNNER'S DRINK

Juice:
Several **oranges**

In a high-speed blender, combine:
The **orange juice**
One chopped **cucumber**

This is a common drink among low-fat raw foodist athletes. You may also like to add one or more of the following:
One **banana**
Several leaves of either **lettuce or spinach**
Berries, such as **blueberries**
A spoonful of freshly ground **hempseed powder** or freshly ground **chia seed powder**
A cup or two of **water**

"Iv'e always felt that animals are the purest spirits in the world. They don't' fake or hide their feelings, and they are the most loyal creatures on Earth. And somehow we humans think we're smarter. What a joke."

– Pink

• ABOUT THE AUTHOR

"Every morning I wake up saying, 'I'm still alive – a miracle.' And so I keep pushing."
– Jacques Cousteau

JOHN MCCABE'S first book was *Surgery Electives: What to Know Before the Doctor Operates.* First published in 1994, and now out of print, it was an exposé of the financial ties of the medical school, hospital, pharmaceutical, and health insurance industries whose unethical business practices result in the deaths of tens of thousands of people in the U.S. every year. The book was endorsed by some congresspersons and by all of the patients' rights groups in North America.

McCabe also wrote a similar book specific for those considering cosmetic surgery. *Plastic Surgery Hopscotch* was published in 1995. With a mix of social criticism, the book detailed many of the serious risks involved with the various surgeries, and in dealing with the vanity surgery industry in general.

Realizing that following a plant-based diet is the way to avoid a wide variety of common health conditions that lead people to take toxic prescription medications, to undergo surgery, and to early death, in 1995 McCabe began writing a book on the vegan diet. That book became *Sunfood Living: Resource Guide to Global Health.* It was published in 2007 as a companion book to David Wolfe's *The Sunfood Diet Success System.*

McCabe did research for, helped compose, and ghost co-authored the first edition of *The Sunfood Diet Success System*, which was published in 2000. McCabe worked to overhaul the manuscript for the succeeding five revised editions. He also did the same, working as a ghost co-author on the first two editions of Wolfe's 2003 book *Eating for Beauty.*

In the 1990s, McCabe overhauled the manuscript of an already published book titled *Nature's First Law: The Raw Food Diet.* Wolfe and two co-authors were presenting this irreverent book written with an absurdist surfer-dude tone as an original work. Wolfe and company used the book to publicize themselves as authorities on the raw food diet, to travel to several countries to give seminars and conduct retreats, and to set up a company selling packaged raw food and kitchen supplies. However, McCabe did not know until 2007 that the material in the *Nature's First Law* book was largely plagiarized from a book titled *Raw Eating*, which was written and published during the middle 1960s by an Armenian man, "Aterhov" Arshavir Ter Hovannissian, living in Iran. Sadly, it was because of Aterhov's rightful criticism of the society in which he lived, including his work advocating clean drinking water and reducing government pollution, that he ended up in prison.

McCabe was the ghost co-author of Frederic Patenaude's 2002 recipe book, *Sunfood Cuisine.* McCabe also overhauled the manuscript for a revised edition. McCabe also helped Patenaude with his quarterly raw food publication, *Just Eat an Apple*, which was sold internationally.

Using his vast knowledge of the raw food industry, McCabe authored the 2010 book *Sunfood Traveler: Global Guide to Raw Food Culture.* It is an international reference covering the raw and organic food lifestyle and industry. In addition to listing raw restaurants, health food stores, organic food co-ops, organic orchards, retreats, and raw chef training schools in many countries, the book contains chapters on everything from yoga to bike culture, organic gardening, seed saving, composting, slow food, permaculture, protecting the environment, and animal welfare. The book also contains a section of recipes from a variety of raw vegan chefs from various countries. The book was revised for newer editions.

McCabe's *Sunfood Diet Infusion: Transforming Health Through Raw Food Veganism* was published in July 2010, and revised in 2011 and 2012. The book works as a companion to his other sunfood books, and gives more details on the benefits of organic foods and plant-based nutrition, including for humanity, wildlife, and the environment.

McCabe also wrote *Marijuana & Hemp: History, Uses, Laws, and Controversy*, which details the world's most useful plant, and how corrupt politicians and corporate leaders worked to outlaw industrial hemp farming.

In 2011, McCabe's book, *Extinction: The Death of Waterlife*, was published. It details what is causing what scientists consider the final extinction of life on Earth.

In addition to the books mentioned above, McCabe has been a content and research editor and a ghost co-author on health, medical industry, and animal welfare books by other authors.

For more information, access:
IgnitingYourLife.com
SunfoodTraveler.com

To contact the author:
John McCabe
C/O: Carmania Books, POB 1272, Santa Monica, CA 90406-1272, USA

McCabe is not associated with the company Sunfood, other than that they may sell his books.

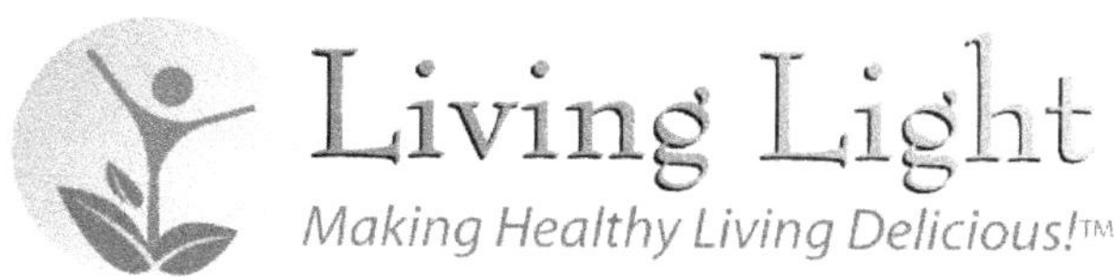

LIVING LIGHT CULINARY INSTITUTE is the world's leading gourmet raw vegan chef school. Located on the beautiful Mendocino coast of northern California, it was founded in 1997 by Cherie Soria, who is known as "The mother of gourmet raw vegan cuisine." Her graduates are a virtual who's who in the world of raw foods.

People from over 50 countries have attended the Institute to study raw vegan culinary arts and the science of raw food nutrition to become certified chefs, nutritional consultants, instructors, and recipe book authors. Many of the raw restaurants around the world are owned by graduates of Living Light.

To subscribe to the Living Light newsletter, access their site, RawFoodChef.com. Scroll down and enter your email address in the "subscribe" box.

Besides Living Light Culinary Arts Institute, Cherie and her husband, Dan Laderman, own and operate several other eco-friendly, raw vegan businesses.

The Living Light Café and Living Light Marketplace share the same building as the Institute. The Marketplace also has an online store providing gifts for chefs and products for healthful living. (Access: RawFoodChef.com/store/marketplace). The historic Living Light Inn is located nearby in a restored mansion.

Cherie and Dan have received numerous awards and occolades for Living Light International, which is recognized as one of the leading raw food businesses in the world.

•••

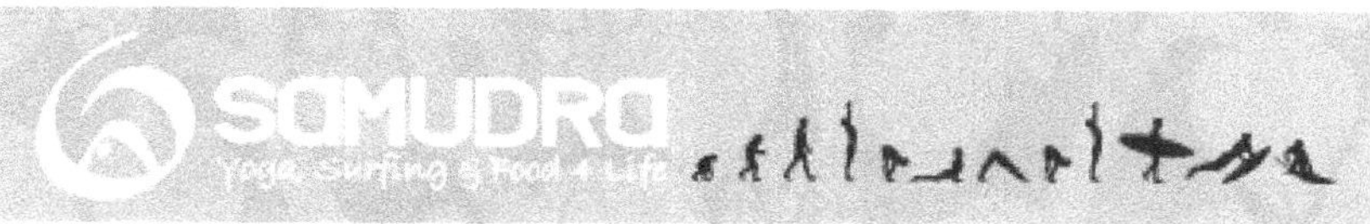

In addition to Living Light as an epicenter of raw food, there is alsa **Samudra**. Located in Dunsborough, Western Australia, the facility runs yoga and surf retreats. Their raw food café and organic store opened in 2008. Chef training courses began in 2010. They have also been adding culinary gardens and fruit orchards to provide the healthiest food possible to their guests and students. (Access: Samudra.com.au)

"The purpose of learning is growth, and our minds, unlike our bodies, can continue growing as we continue to live."
– Mortimer Adler

"I prefer you to make mistakes in kindness than work miracles in unkindness."
– Mother Teresa

"Let us endeavor so to live that when we come to die even the undertaker will be sorry."
– Mark Twain

"How wonderful it is that nobody need wait a single moment before starting to improve the world."
– Anne Frank

Eat
a plant-
based
diet.

Know
that you can
change the world by
changing your diet.

Protect and preserve forests and the habitat of wildlife.
Plant mass quantities of native trees and wildflowers.
Grow organic food. Support organic farmers.
Outlaw the genetic engineering of plants.
Legalize industrial hemp farming.
Compost your kitchen scraps.
Nurture your talents.
Uplift the weary.
Do yoga.
Ride a bike.
Love your way.
Peace your path.
– John McCabe, *Sunfood Traveler*

"Nothing will ever be attempted, if all possible objections must first be overcome."
– Samuel Johnson

AncientTrees.org
NRDC.org
EarthIsland.org
EarthFirst.org
EarthEcho.org
y2g.org
KitchenGardeners.org
MonsantoWatch.org
WilderUtopia.com
SeaShepherd.org
FoodNotLawns.net
OccupyMonsanto360.org
SayNoToGMOs.org
OKRaw.com

"Unless someone like you cares a whole awful lot, nothing is going to get better. It's not."
– Dr. Seuss, *The Lorax*

• **What People are Saying about John McCabe's Book** *Igniting Your Life: Pathways To The Zenith Of Health and Success*

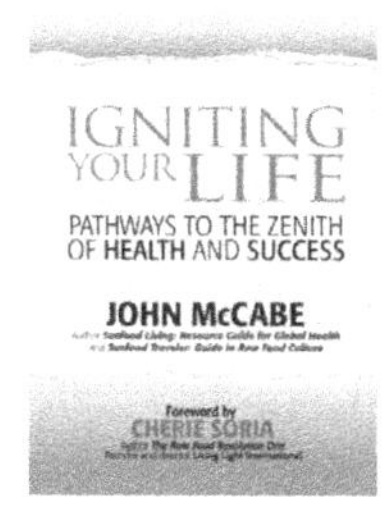

"*Igniting Your Life* will kindle your innermost desires."
– **Cherie Soria**, author *The Raw Food Diet Revolution.* Founder and director Living Light International. RawFoodChef.com

"**An** uplifting and empowering collection of worldly work."
– **Sheridan Hammond**, Australia. Samudra.com.au.

"**We** defy you to not be inspired by this book!"
– **Matt Amsden**, author *RawVolution*, and **Janabai Amsden**, ELR restaurant, Santa Monica, CA. EuphoriaLovesRawvolution.com

"**An** impressive collection of eclectic quotations and thoughtful commentary. Inspiring and motivating."
– **Victoria Moran**, author *Living a Charmed Life: Your Guide to Finding Magic in Every Moment of Every Day.* VictoriaMoran.com

"**In** this book McCabe encourages readers to recognise their true potential and work towards a better way of living."
– **Sienna Blake**, Australia's *Vegan Voice* magazine: Veganic.net

"**A** great compilation that shouts inspiration from every page. The more I read it, the more I can relate to it. Gold stuff!"
– **Harley Durianrider Johnstone**, Australian Division One biking athlete and co-founder of 30BananasADay.com

"**After** only a few hours of reading, I was already writing life plans and lists of things I needed to change in my life."
– **Rob Hull**, publisher, London's *Funky Raw* magazine: FunkyRaw.com

"**Open** any page, anytime, and become inspired to live the life of your dreams."
– **Rhio**, author of *Hooked on Raw*, New York; RawFoodInfo.com

"**A** fantastic book."
– **Penni Shelton**, RawFoodRehab.ning.com

"**An** awesome gift for people in your life."
– **Rhonda DeFelice**, The Good Green Witch; goodgreenwitch.blogspot.com

To suggest additions or changes for the next edition of *Sunfood Traveler* book, send information to:

John McCabe
C/O: Carmania Books
POB 1272
Santa Monica, CA 90406-1272, USA

Office: Information@SunfoodLiving.com

Include information such as:

- Name of raw restaurant, raw café, natural foods store, company, retreat, organic orchard, or organization
- Contact person or persons
- Web site address (if there is one)
- Email address (if there is one)
- Street address, including country and postal code
- Phone number (if there is one)
- Reason the listing should be added, changed (or deleted)

"The true self is always in motion like music, a river of life, changing, moving, failing, suffering, learning, shining."
– Brenda Ueland

"In some sense man is a microcosm of the universe; therefore what man is, is a clue to the universe; we are enfolded in the universe."
– David Bohm

"If there is any kindness I can show, or any good thing I can do to any fellow being, let me do it now, and not deter or neglect it, as I shall not pass this way again."
– William Penn

"Twenty years from now you will be more disappointed by the things that you didn't do than by the ones you did do. So throw off the bowlines. Sail away from the safe harbor. Catch the trade winds in your sails. Explore. Dream. Discover."
– Mark Twain

"If the world seems cold to you, kindle fires to warm it.
– Lucy Larcom

www.ingramcontent.com/pod-product-compliance
Lightning Source LLC
Chambersburg PA
CBHW070758280326
41934CB00012B/2961

* 9 7 8 1 8 8 4 7 0 2 0 9 9 *